Sensory-Enhanced Yoga® for Self-Regulation and Trauma Healing

Sensory-Enhanced Yoga® for Self-Regulation and Trauma Healing

Lynn Stoller
OT, MS, OTR, C-IAYT, RYT 500/E-RYT200

Forewords
Stephen Cope
Joseph Le Page

Contributors
Patricia Lillis MD, MHA, RYT
Amanda J. G. Napior MDiv
Alison Rhodes PhD, LICSW, EdM
Danielle Rousseau PhD, LMHC
Gretchen Ki Steidle MBA, BA

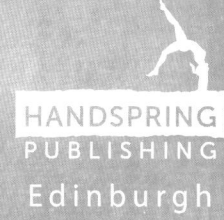

HANDSPRING
PUBLISHING
Edinburgh

HANDSPRING PUBLISHING LIMITED
The Old Manse, Fountainhall,
Pencaitland, East Lothian
EH34 5EY, Scotland
Tel: +44 1875 341 859
Website: www.handspringpublishing.com

First published 2019 in the United Kingdom by Handspring Publishing

Copyright © Sensory-Enhanced Yoga Institute 2019

All rights reserved. No parts of this publication may be reproduced or transmitted in any form or by any means, electronic or mechanical, including photocopying, recording, or any information storage and retrieval system, without either the prior written permission of the publisher or a licence permitting restricted copying in the United Kingdom issued by the Copyright Licensing Agency Ltd, Saffron House, 6–10 Kirby Street, London EC1N 8TS.

The right of Lynn Stoller to be identified as the Author of this text has been asserted in accordance with the Copyright, Designs and Patents Acts 1988.

ISBN 978-1-912085-13-2
ISBN (Kindle e-Book) 978-1-912085-14-9

British Library Cataloguing in Publication Data
A catalogue record for this book is available from the British Library

Library of Congress Cataloguing in Publication Data
A catalog record for this book is available from the Library of Congress

Notice
Neither the Publisher nor the Authors assume any responsibility for any loss or injury and/or damage to persons or property arising out of or relating to any use of the material contained in this book. It is the responsibility of the treating practitioner, relying on independent expertise and knowledge of the patient, to determine the best treatment and method of application for the patient.

All reasonable efforts have been made to obtain copyright clearance for illustrations in the book for which the authors or publishers do not own the rights. If you believe that one of your illustrations has been used without such clearance please contact the publishers and we will ensure that appropriate credit is given in the next reprint.

Commissioning Editor Sarena Wolfaard
Project Manager Morven Dean
Copy Editor Stephanie Pickering
Designer Bruce Hogarth
Indexer Aptara, India
Typesetter DSM Soft, India
Printer Melita, Malta

The
Publisher's
policy is to use
paper manufactured
from sustainable forests

CONTENTS

Acknowledgments ix
Preface xi
Forewords xv
Contributors xix

1. Introduction   1

   PART 1   Stress, trauma, and the neuroplastic brain   7

2. PTSD and sensory processing   9
3. Neurophysiology of PTSD   19
4. Brain changes in PTSD and mind-body practices: the inverse relationship   35

   PART 2   The many faces of trauma   53

5. Combat stress management   55
   Patricia Lillis
   The Iraq Yoga Study   63
   Lynn Stoller
6. Reclaiming body, redefining relationship: yoga with survivors of sexual trauma   67
   Danielle Rousseau and Amanda J G Napior
7. Recovery and empowerment through yoga in prison   77
   Amanda J G Napior and Danielle Rousseau
8. Using mind-body practices among populations of mass disaster and conflict   87
   Gretchen Ki Steidle
9. Yoga for complex trauma survivors   99
   Alison Rhodes

   PART 3   East meets West: the theory and guidelines of Sensory-Enhanced Yoga®   111

10. Sensory-Enhanced Yoga®: healing trauma through the koshas   113
11. **Guideline 1** A sense of safety is essential for healing   125
12. **Guideline 2** The most direct and powerful way to self-regulate is through control of the breath   137

13	**Guideline 3** Yoga can promote effective sensory, motor, and cognitive processing of traumatic experiences and thus aid healing	151
14	**Guideline 4** New beliefs and attitudes more easily take hold when we first prepare the body to receive and accept them	181
15	**Guideline 5** Self-empowerment is born on the wings of the spirit rising from the mind-body connection	193
	PART 4 Putting the practice together	203
16	Structuring the practice	205
17	Description of therapeutic yoga forms	217
18	Sensory-Enhanced Yoga® vinyasas	259
	Appendices	269
	References	277
	Index	307

DEDICATION

This book is dedicated to the combat veterans and the many other traumatized persons who shared their stories with me—you have taught me so much.

PERMISSIONS

Figure 2.1 - Quadrant scores of 12 combat veterans on Adolescent/Adult Sensory Profile (AASP). Quadrant chart copyright © 2002–18 Pearson Education, Inc. Reprinted with permission.

Figure 2.2 - Sensory processing. Used with permission of Sensational Kids Occupational Therapy, Australia.

Figure 3.3 - LeDoux, The Emotional Brain, Simon and Shuster International, 1998,[78] with permission.

Figure 4.3 - A sensory hypothesis of PTSD. Modified from Clancy et al., Restless 'rest': intrinsic sensory hyperactivity and disinhibition in post-traumatic stress disorder. Brain, 2017, Volume 140, p. 2041–2050, by permission of Oxford University Press.

Figure 12.1 - Relationship between respiration and the ANS (Elliot, Coherence,[40] adapted with permission).

Figure 14.1 - The power of language in the context of yoga (adapted with permission from Alan Fogel[7]).

Table 14.1 - Recommended mudras for PTSD and related disorders* *Columns 3 and 4 are from the second edition of Mudras for Healing and Transformation, by Joseph and Lilian Le Page © 2014. Reprinted with permission. The numbers refer to numbers in the book. The affirmations were also inspired by it.

Table 14.2 - A sampling of mudras for self-regulation and trauma healing* *These mudras are from Mudras for Healing and Transformation, by Joseph and Lilian Le Page (2014) which provides two full pages of information for each (including a guided meditation) plus 98 additional mudras. This brief version of the mudras is presented here with the authors' permission, but advanced training is highly recommended.

Table 15.1 - Wellness Survey for Post-Traumatic Growth* by Lynn Stoller, M.S., OTR/L, C-IAYT, RYT 500/E-RYT © Sensory-Enhanced Yoga Institute, 2018. All rights reserved. *Many of the items used in this form were inspired or taken from materials developed by Joseph Le Page and were chosen based on their relevance to trauma healing and reorganized into the kosha model format, with his permission.

ACKNOWLEDGMENTS

I would like to take a moment first to express my deep appreciation to all the organizations and individuals who supported me along this journey. I know I will inevitably forget to mention some but hope you all know who you are and forgive me for the momentary memory lapse.

To Sarena Wolfaard and Andrew Stevenson of Handspring Publishing, who saw the value of my book proposal, and especially to Sarena who provided me with enormous support and excellent guidance along my writing journey.

To Morven Dean, project manager, Stephanie Pickering, copy editor, Bruce Hogarth, art director, Kathryn Mason Pak, proofreader, and the rest of the Handspring Publishing team, whose phenomenal work surpassed all of my expectations and who were so easy to work with.

To the chapter contributors—Dr./Col. (Ret.) Patricia Lillis, Amanda J.G. Napior, Dr. Alison Rhodes, Dr. Danielle Rousseau, and Gretchen Ki Steidle—whose immense expertise and eloquent writings have contributed enormously to the value of this book.

To Dr. Stephen Cope and Joseph Le Page, whose work I so greatly respect, for writing such beautiful forewords to the book—it is such an honor to have their endorsements!

To the late Jane Koomar, PhD, OTR/L, FAOTA, one of the world's most renowned sensory integration experts, who as my Iraq Yoga Study advisor was so generous with her support and guidance.

To Lucy Cimini, one of the first pioneers in using yoga to help heal war trauma, who offered me key opportunities that fueled my deep passion for this work.

To Major (Ret.) Jon Greuel, the PI of the Iraq Yoga Study, who through immense conviction, will, and effort made sure the project was completed while double-tasking as an Air Force instructor pilot in a deployed environment.

To other trauma yoga pioneers and experts who provided me with opportunities and/or offered me help and from whom I learned so much, including Annie Okerlin, Karen Soltes, Robin Carnes, Gail Francisco, Whitney Willman, Susan Pualani Alden, Molly Birkholm, Susan Lynch, and Emily Hain.

To the many organizations and experts whose names fill this book, for the invaluable contributions they made to this field, and especially to those individuals who reviewed portions of the book or provided guidance in other ways for this project, including Dr. Ruth Lanius, Dr. Joseph LeDoux, Babette Rothschild, Dr. David Shannahoff-Khalsa, David Emerson, Dr. Alan Fogel, Stephen Elliott, and Ross Guest.

To all of my teachers and mentors in the Integrative Yoga Therapy Program—Joseph Le Page, Lilian Le Page, Karen Clarke, Ellen Schaeffer, Maria Mendola, Beth Gibbs, Mary Northey, Jennifer Reis, and many others, and for all of my fellow student-friends in the IYT program, who inspired me in their own ways or made me laugh, especially Kate Drake, Jackie Kerstner, and Aggeliki Salamaliki.

ACKNOWLEDGMENTS *continued*

To Lisa Megidesh, Richard Miller, and Gary Kraftsow, who have also greatly influenced my yoga therapy style.

To the Sensory-Enhanced Yoga Institute faculty—Dr./Col. (Ret.) Patricia Lillis, Trisha Barry, Anna Molgard, Marika Paquin, Julie Jack, Jeff Sargent, Dr. Danielle Rousseau, Megan Hennessey, and Erin O'Neill—for sharing their amazing wisdom and supporting and inspiring me along the way.

To my oldest and very dearest friends, Rosanne DeVito, Debbie George, Meredith Brown Fitzherbert, Jerrianne Franklin Anastos, Pat Serrentino, and Eileen Powers-Twichell, for their unconditional love and for being so fun to be around.

To my sister-in-law, Marcelle Ciampa, who is just as dear a friend, for reviewing and advising me on a couple of sections of the book, and to her husband and my brother, Roy Ciampa, for always being there for me with his loving support.

To all past workshop participants, from whom I've learned so much and whose enthusiasm has kept me inspired.

To the combat veterans and many other traumatized persons who shared their stories with me, it is from you I have learned the most and to whom I dedicate this book.

To my two children, Jason and Melissa, who were the models for this book and who bring so much joy to my life.

To my sweet grandson Casey, the apple of my eye and the joy of my heart, for reminding me of what is most important in life.

And especially to my husband Kenny, whom I love very much, for sharing me with my computer, and for the sacrifices he endured for the completion of this book.

Lynn Stoller

PREFACE

I got my first strong whiff of my life's calling on a cold winter morning in 1977 when I was hired as a sensorimotor intern at Belchertown State School (BSS). The large, ominous-looking brick buildings of this notorious institution stood in stark contrast to its bucolic surroundings in the beautiful Pioneer Valley of Western Massachusetts. Inside, some residents sat in their own urine, some banged their heads against the wall, many were fed pureed food to make caring for them easier, and until that winter (just following the resolution of the class action suit against BSS), there was no sensory programming or recreational activities provided to these residents.

It was in this seemingly hellish place that I first discovered the power of sensorimotor therapy, provided within the context of human connection, to promote health and well-being. Working with severely sensory deprived individuals affected me profoundly. Most residents had significant cognitive and/or mental health challenges, and the majority of the ones in the medical unit where I worked had physical challenges as well, most often cerebral palsy and/or legal blindness. One of my most important life lessons was taught to me by Keith, a twenty-one-year-old completely blind, non-verbal, severely sensory deprived young man with quadriplegic cerebral palsy who was kept in a crib all day, as were almost all of the other sixteen men living in his open ward. My treatment sessions with Keith emphasized various sensory experiences, but we especially bonded over the tambourine. He went to town banging that thing with his skinny spastic arm, singing loudly, "Ah, Ah, Ah, Ah, Ah!!!" Keith was *Music Itself* in those moments. It wasn't long before Keith could tell whenever I stepped foot into his ward. He'd start his happy "Ah, Ah, Ah!" calling for me, which filled my heart.

Keith, and so many of the neurologically challenged individuals I have worked with, taught me that quality of life is much less tied to cognitive intelligence or physical ability than it is to the ability to be present in the moment and to have the capability to experience the joy of sensory awareness—whether beholding a beautiful vista, or playing a rhythm instrument, or being aware of the texture of sand against the skin—or the joy of connecting with another person or animal who understands you. It is these abilities that are taken away from many of those who experience severe trauma. Keith was able to relish whatever positive sensory input came his way, despite the severe neglect and sensory deprivation he endured.

At the other end of the spectrum, I have met many combat veterans, most of them very smart and with full use of their limbs and faculties, who were unable to reconcile their war-related traumas and see the world fresh in all of its beauty. One veteran I knew received several war medals for his bravery and military accomplishments, as well as the purple heart, and was incredibly gifted. Yet this same individual found himself in a locked-down ward for a period of time and ended up practically penniless and at high risk for homelessness, due to his PTSD. Until I met him, I had two separate categories for veterans in my head: the extremely accomplished and decorated combat veteran in a soldier's uniform, and the homeless veteran holding a sign on the side of the street. It never occurred to me that these two could be one and the same person.

As different as combat veterans are to the clients I worked with at BSS, the initial foundation of my work with veterans was laid there, where I eventually rose up the ranks to Acting Director of the Sensorimotor

PREFACE *continued*

and Adapted P.E. Department. In the process, I was introduced to Dr. A. Jean Ayres' book, *Sensory Integration and Learning Disorders*. The thought that sensorimotor activity could actually change the human brain was incredibly inspiring to me. Within a couple of years, I had moved to sunny California and was enrolled as an occupational therapy graduate student at San Jose State University, thanks to the passion stirred up in me by Dr. Ayres' book and my experiences working at BSS.

After receiving my graduate degree, I accepted an occupational therapy position at Cotting School, Lexington MA, and soon thereafter, I became certified in Jean Ayres' Sensory Integration and Praxis Tests. However, I found myself stumped as to what to do with my older clients who had outgrown the traditional sensory integration activities designed for young children, so began to integrate yoga into their therapy sessions, with wonderful results. Yet, despite working with many people who had experienced trauma—which included physical and mental injuries caused by parent abuse, fires, accidents, tumors, and many other harrowing events—I was still extraordinarily clueless regarding the effects of trauma on the human brain and spirit. That lesson would ultimately become a very personal one.

Almost three decades ago, way before I learned about PTSD or became aware of the challenges many combat veterans were facing, I experienced an event that made me feel as though I had literally been slammed over the head by a frying pan. The event was always there, reverberating in my head when I brushed my teeth, went to work, cared for my young children, went to sleep at night and awoke in the morning. It was accompanied by strong panic attacks; hyperactive startle reflex; a strong fear of heights and sudden fear of flying; a deep depression; and a deep numbness and sense of disconnection that separated me from the here and now and from the people I loved, and which robbed me of any sense of joy. I had never experienced any of these symptoms before, was terribly frightened my brain would never return to normal again, and in desperation sought the help of several psychiatrists, who were not of much help. Fortunately, I did eventually fully recover, but it took quite a while, and I now recognize my mental health as my greatest blessing in life.

Several years after this was completely resolved and for the benefit of my occupational therapy clients, I was inspired to complete a formal 200-hour yoga teacher training, only to realize during the process that the training was the best thing I could ever do for my own body mind. A few years later, when a good friend of mine shared with me the sensory symptoms of some of the combat veterans who attended her veterans yoga class, I was extremely curious to learn more, which led to a pilot study and later to my role as associate investigator and co-author of the Iraq Yoga Study. Although the sensory processing aspect of PTSD is what drew me into the trauma field to begin with, it is the stories of particular combat veterans and my own history of having dealt with a very distressing trauma-related mental illness myself that has fueled my deep passion for this work. I feel so fortunate that I now have an opportunity to hold up a lantern for those stuck in a quagmire similar to the one in which I found myself all those years ago.

During my journey, I have worked with a number of trauma-informed yoga organizations and have observed some past students start their own organizations to spread this important work. I applaud the amazing work of all of these organizations and suggest we need even more of them. No one trauma yoga

PREFACE *continued*

organization can reach every traumatized individual. There are *millions* of people in need of trauma healing and we need all hands on deck to address the problem. These trainings need to be evidence based, so the more we collaborate and learn from each other, the better the outcome will be for the people we are treating. I am hoping this book will be used in many of these programs, just as I have benefited from the work of so many others. The fact is, there is plenty of work for everyone, and each of us brings an important perspective that we can all learn from. It is only when we work together that we will be able to reach out to every person who needs it in every corner of our own country and across the globe.

Lynn Stoller
April 2019

FOREWORD by Stephen Cope

By now, most mainstream Westerners have become aware of the long-term effects of overwhelming trauma—and of the oft-resulting condition, which we call post-traumatic stress disorder, or PTSD. The stories of those suffering from PTSD fill our nightly newscasts and morning newspapers. As a result of our exposure to this information, many of us have developed, too, at least a vague understanding of the precise causes of PTSD. The most simple, mainstream version of this is, of course: the fight or flight system in the body gets turned on in an extreme situation of danger or perceived danger, and, alarmingly, never really shuts off. The nervous system, then, remains in a state of almost constant hyperarousal—remains on alert, scanning for threat. And we know that an unresolved trauma response can be triggered repeatedly by all sorts of internal and external stimuli.

What most of us do not understand, I think—unless we have been up-close-and-personal to the experience of undigested trauma—is the extreme amount of suffering involved. Indeed, this form of suffering is what the Eastern contemplative traditions, both yoga and Buddhism, have fittingly called a "Hell realm"—a dense, intractable state of mental and physical distress in which we find it impossible to relax, impossible to feel soothed and safe, and unable to enjoy even the simplest pleasures of being human.

Think about this for a moment: what most characterizes the experience of being human is the ability to savor our naturally arising thoughts and feelings, and to experience them as somehow deeply our "self." To get to know them, and to feel friendly with them. Indeed, to make friends with them even when they scare or alarm us. And, of course, to relish moments of authentic happiness. As we grow into adulthood, we learn gradually how to manage our roiling inner life, the arising of thoughts, feelings, and sensations, and we learn how to make sense of them by integrating them into our life story, our identity.

Imagine, however, the experience of our many fellow humans with PTSD. These trauma sufferers cannot do any of this. One sufferer put it this way: "I only barely manage to survive my life, one day at a time. I simply endure." This person is constantly feeling under threat. From where? Well, this is the real nightmare: From within his or her own body. From inside. As a result, no place is safe. Soothing is next to impossible.

Sufferers of post-traumatic stress syndrome, as we know, have an extremely high rate of suicide. We must understand that suicide under these conditions is usually just the wish to rest, to find release, to find an end to the suffering, to lie down even in the arms of great Mother Earth and to at last be safely held and soothed. Can you not feel how this is so? Human suffering takes many forms. But there is perhaps none more insidious than that occasioned by PTSD.

However, for those of us who teach and study the ancient science of yoga, there is some good news. It turns out that the study of human suffering was the prime object of the 2000-year-old yoga tradition. Ancient yogis called this suffering "*duhkha*," which literally means "being ill at ease in the body," or "pervasive unsatisfactoriness." (The Sanskrit word *duhkha* comes from the root that means "awry.") Duhkha is the profound and unsettling experience of being ill at ease in the body and breath, fundamentally not at home in what the Buddha called "this fathom-long body." These great ancient scientists of the mind studied the phenomenon of duhkha for hundreds of years: What is it? How does it arise? What are its precise causes? Can it be attenuated? Can it, even, be ended?

FOREWORD *continued*

Yogis found something fascinating. Suffering arises in the body and is a phenomenon of the body. And therefore it must be addressed directly in the body. And over the course of thousands of years—without scientific instruments, but with the penetrating tool of the human mind and imagination—these yogi scientists discovered a program of healing and regeneration of the self so profound, that it was known to routinely work miracles in the realm of suffering. They discovered that through a series of trainings of mental attention, of breath, and of body movement, this experience of duhkha could be profoundly attenuated, and, finally, ended. The techniques they developed address hyperarousal directly through a series of lifestyle interventions and physical, psychological, and mental trainings.

Over the past 25 years, as yoga has become a mainstream practice in the West, a series of sophisticated research projects have shown precisely how yoga techniques accomplish this attenuation of suffering—and have mapped out the precise mechanisms and effects of these practices.

In recent years, skilled yogis from around the world have discovered that this entire program of recovery—the training to become what yogis called a *jiva mukti*, or a fully alive human being—can be applied to traumatic states with remarkable and reliable success. This program amounts to a kind of Olympic training routine for learning once again to become human—to learn once again how to relax into the ebb and flow of thoughts, feelings, sensations, to savor them, to listen to them, to learn from them. To learn to regulate them when necessary. And to integrate them into the ongoing narrative of our lives.

Now, Lynn Stoller and her co-authors have developed a very sophisticated, highly detailed, and deeply researched program of yoga targeted precisely at the symptoms of PTSD—skillfully adapting the age-old techniques of breathing, yoga postures, meditation, and lifestyle changes, to the particular contemporary problems of trauma.

The program Stoller and her contributors lay out in these pages comes with an extremely sophisticated understanding of the neuroscience of trauma, and it is supported by reams of clinical research. It is user friendly. And it is guaranteed to be effective in repairing the psychological and physiological havoc wrought by trauma. Please recommend this authoritative work to your friends and colleagues, and to all who live with or work with the suffering of unresolved trauma.

Stephen Cope
Scholar Emeritus
Kripalu Center for Yoga and Health
April, 2019

FOREWORD by Joseph Le Page

The healing of trauma is one of the most important areas for the application of yoga therapy. A number of recent books, such as *The Body Keeps the Score*, by Bessel van der Kolk,[1] have pointed out the importance of yoga in the treatment of trauma. This book, *Sensory-Enhanced Yoga® for Self-Regulation and Trauma Healing*, by Lynn Stoller, is an important contribution to this field and is accessible not only to healthcare professionals and yoga therapists but also to individuals in recovery from trauma.

The book begins by outlining the scope of the problem and the important role that yoga can play, especially in light of increased research along with the new certification standards for yoga therapists by the International Association of Yoga Therapists. Lynn carefully describes the foundation of her Sensory-Enhanced Yoga, which must be (1) trauma sensitive; (2) evidence informed; and (3) founded on sound theoretical constructs.

Part 1 of the book is a comprehensive and thorough description of trauma and PTSD from a sensory-processing perspective presented in a way that is accessible to yoga teachers and yoga therapists. It offers a broad range of information about PTSD and also explains in detail the value of yoga in its treatment. Of special interest is the description of the normal stress response and also how that response is modified by those who experience PTSD.

Part 2 comprises accounts from leading therapists in the field, allowing us to see the true face of PTSD in a number of different settings, including combat, sexual trauma, incarceration, mass disasters, and also for complex trauma survivors, those who have suffered repeated or prolonged trauma exposure.

The final sections of *Sensory-Enhanced Yoga for Self-Regulation and Trauma Healing* present a series of yoga practices that are practical, appropriate, and carefully explained in a step-by-step manner that is useful for both teachers and students. There are a number of chapters of special interest to yoga therapists, including the general effects of the different posture families in the context of the treatment of PTSD. Additionally, Lynn's work is very much in line with Integrative Yoga Therapy in the use of affirmations and guided meditations to accompany the yoga postures.

Sensory-Enhanced Yoga for Self-Regulation and Trauma Healing is the only book in the field to include the use of mudras as specific to the treatment of PTSD. It also extensively integrates the model of the five koshas, the dimensions of being, including a wellness survey, which encompasses each of the levels. The final segment of Lynn's book details yoga practices for PTSD and shows how to design yoga programs, including body awareness and relaxation scripts.

Sensory-Enhanced Yoga for Self-Regulation and Trauma Healing is the most comprehensive guide available on the application of yoga therapy for PTSD and is an essential text for every yoga therapist.

Joseph Le Page
Director, Integrative Yoga Therapy
Founder, Enchanted Mountain Center,
Santa Catarina, Brazil
May, 2019

Reference

1. Bessell van der Kolk, The body keeps the score: mind, brain and body in the transformation of trauma, New York: Viking; 2014.

CONTRIBUTORS

Patricia Lillis, MD, MHA, RYT

An experienced clinician physician and decorated former military hospital commander, Col. (Ret.) Patricia Lillis is one of the leading pioneers in drawing awareness and resources to the power of yoga for healing combat stress and war-related PTSD. With more than 30 years of clinical and operational military medical experience, she is the recipient of numerous awards, including the Legion of Merit twice and a Bronze Star. Following her tour of duty in Iraq, she served in the office of the Army Surgeon General and played a key role in establishing the practices of yoga, meditation, and acupuncture as accepted therapies in the Departments of Defense and Veterans Affairs for the treatment of PTSD, traumatic brain injury, and pain. She also co-founded and was the first president of the organization Warriors at Ease and was a contributing editor for the Yoga Service Council's book *Best Practices for Yoga with Veterans*. She currently serves as a senior advisor and faculty member of the Sensory-Enhanced Yoga® Institute.

Amanda J. G. Napior, MDiv

Amanda J. G. Napior is a doctoral student in the Graduate Program in Religion at Boston University, where she studies contemporary US mass incarceration in the context of American religious history. She has taught classes in yoga, creative writing, and history at carceral facilities in the United States. Currently, Amanda is writing her dissertation on how people in prison experience transformation, and on how rehabilitative programming plays a role in shaping such experiences and narratives. She is a contributing editor for the Yoga Service Council's book, *Best Practices for Yoga with Sexual Trauma Survivors*, and has an article forthcoming in the *Journal of Ritual Studies*. Amanda holds an MDiv from Harvard Divinity School, with a focus in Christianity, and a BA in religious studies from the University of California at Santa Barbara, with emphasis in American religious history.

Alison Rhodes, PhD, LICSW, EdM

Dr Alison Rhodes received her Masters and PhD in Social Work from Boston College and is currently a therapist in private practice. She has experience working with adolescents and adults in community mental health, school, and university settings. She is also a certified yoga teacher with 20 years experience in practicing yoga and meditation. Dr Rhodes was part of the research team at the world-renowned Trauma Center at Justice Resource Institute in Brookline, Massachusetts, for the randomized controlled trial and long-term follow-up on yoga for complex trauma survivors, and co-authored the research papers. She has also taught Trauma-Sensitive Yoga classes at the Trauma Center, and now continues her trauma work in private practice.

Danielle Rousseau, PhD, LMHC

Dr Danielle Rousseau is an Assistant Professor at Boston University. She is a social justice researcher and practitioner. Dr Rousseau worked in the field of forensic mental health as a therapist in correctional facilities and served communities doing crisis response and victim advocacy. Dr. Rousseau is a licensed therapist and certified yoga teacher. She serves as the Director of Evaluation 4 Change and has experience collaborating with multiple yoga and mindfulness organizations including Yoga 4 Change, yogaHOPE, the Yoga Service Council, Sensory-Enhanced Yoga, and the Open Spirit Center. Her work is published in the *Prison Journal*; *Criminal Justice Policy Review*; *Gender, Race, and Justice*; *Law and Society Review*; *The Annals of the Academy of Political and Social Sciences*; *Journal of Yoga Service* and other academic journals and books. She is an author on the Yoga Service Council's book *Best Practices for Yoga in the Criminal Justice System* and the editor for *Best Practices for Yoga with Survivors of Sexual Trauma*.

Gretchen Ki Steidle, MBA, BA

Gretchen Ki Steidle is founder and President of Global Grassroots, an international non-profit that catalyzes women change agents in post-conflict Africa through mindful leadership skills and a social entrepreneurship incubator. Gretchen is also a certified Integrative Breathwork and Breath-Body-Mind practitioner. She is the author of *Leading from Within: Conscious Social Change and Mindfulness for Social Innovation* (MIT Press 2017) and a producer of the Emmy-nominated documentary on the Darfur crisis, *The Devil Came on Horseback*. In 2007, Gretchen was honored by World Business Magazine as one of the top International 35 Women Under 35. In 2010 she was chosen as a CNN Hero working in Haiti after the earthquake. In 2011 she was chosen as one of seven Remarkable Women of the World by New Hampshire Magazine. She holds an MBA from the Tuck School of Business at Dartmouth College and a BA in Foreign Affairs from the University of Virginia.

Introduction

Unlike other forms of psychological disorders, the core issue in trauma is reality ... — Bessel A. van der Kolk and Alexander C. McFarlane[1] (p. 6)

The suffering behind the mask

My most compelling observation from conducting private yoga therapy sessions is that, beneath their jovial "hellos" and upbeat personas, many people are in fact deeply suffering. Time and again, my clients have revealed deep emotional wounds, panic attacks or other serious anxiety disorders, deep depression, or even suicidal ideation, which was completely incongruent with my surface impression of them as well grounded human beings moving through life with ease. I quickly learned that first impressions can be deceptive, though it makes sense considering the cultural pressure we are often under to "put our best face forward," both in our relationships and in our work settings.

Statistics bear out the suffering. Almost half of Americans will meet the DSM-IV criteria for a mental health disorder at some point during their lifetime.[2] The lifetime prevalence for anxiety disorders in the general US population is close to 30%. Slightly more than 20% will experience a mood disorder and almost 7% will experience PTSD.[2] Anxiety disorders affect 40 million adults in the US—that is, 18% of the population—within any given 12-month period.[3] They take different forms, with generalized anxiety disorder, panic disorder, and social anxiety disorder listed as the most common. Of the mood disorders, major depressive disorder is the most common and will affect almost 17% of the population at some point during their lifetime and 6.7% within a 12-month period.[2,3] Thus we have a huge need in our society for effective treatments to help individuals self-regulate their emotions and level of stress.

Behavior regulation is another serious issue affecting many people. One quarter of the adult population in the US will experience an impulse-control disorder during their lifetime; this may take the form of an oppositional-defiant disorder, conduct disorder, attention deficit/hyperactivity disorder, and/or intermittent explosive disorder.[2] The statistics provided here actually underrepresent the numbers of people who suffer from these problems, since homeless individuals were not surveyed in the Kessler et al. studies[2,3] and some study respondents may not have acknowledged their mental health issues, due to the fear of stigma. Yet, even these highly conservative numbers make it very clear that many people in the general adult US population have difficulty self-regulating their **emotions**, **levels of stress**, **ability to focus**, and/or **ability to control their impulses**, which can significantly impact their quality of life and ability to fulfill their roles in society.

The incidence of these problems climbs dramatically when you pluck a person out of civilized society and plunk them down in the chaos of a battlefield. In fact, the American Psychiatric Association found it necessary to create a special diagnosis, **post-traumatic stress disorder (PTSD)**, to

Chapter 1

explain the number and magnitude of mental health problems seen in many of the Vietnam era veterans, which have often led to alcoholism, addiction, joblessness, divorce, or even homelessness.[4,5] Even now, some 40 years later, approximately 271,000 Vietnam theater veterans have full or subthreshold PTSD related to combat exposure, and one-third of these veterans have current major depressive disorder.[6] History is unfortunately repeating itself with the next generation of veterans. In a recent meta-analysis involving almost 5 million US military veterans of the wars in Afghanistan and Iraq, 23% were estimated to have PTSD.[7]

The fear of stigma or adverse consequences keeps many veterans from seeking the mental health treatment they need. Of the veterans and military retirees who *do* seek treatment, the vast majority do so outside of the VA system.[5,8] Therefore, the topic of combat stress and war-related PTSD is just as relevant to health providers working in community settings as it is for those working within the military branches or the VA. It is also relevant for health providers working outside the traditional medical establishment, as a strong evidence base is building (and will be presented within these pages) to support the use of yoga as a potentially powerful adjunct treatment for those who suffer from trauma and related conditions. According to the 2016 Yoga in America Study,[9] 34% of Americans say they are somewhat or very likely to practice yoga in the next 12 months, so clearly the potential for stigma is also greatly diminished with regard to this healing modality, and many yoga programs have already become established at many military bases and VA medical centers.

A beacon of hope

Fortunately, treatments for PTSD have become more effective in recent years as awareness has grown regarding the importance of including the body in the treatment process. With this recognition, more opportunities are opening up not only for military personnel and veterans, but also sexual trauma victims and other traumatized populations, including refugees in remote parts of the world, to take yoga classes designed with their unique needs in mind. These opportunities have mushroomed as greater numbers of yoga instructors seek specialized training through one of several trauma-informed yoga programs which have developed across the country (see, for example, Libby et al.[10]), and as *yoga therapy* gains credibility as a bona fide health profession, due to its bourgeoning evidence base and the International Association of Yoga Therapists' new certification standards (www.iayt.org). It is my heartfelt desire that traditional health professionals and yoga therapists will quickly develop an effective and efficient system of collaborative partnerships to help reach veterans and other traumatized individuals who are hesitant to approach the VA or other healthcare system, as well as to provide community-based aftercare.

Sensory-Enhanced Yoga®

It is vitally important that the yoga-based therapy that is provided to those who have been traumatized is: ***(1) trauma sensitive; (2) evidence informed; and (3) founded on sound theoretical constructs***. Sensory-Enhanced Yoga meets these criteria, and is especially designed for combat veterans, active duty military personnel, sexual trauma survivors, and others who suffer from unresolved trauma, anxiety, attention deficit disorders, or mood disorders.

The Sensory-Enhanced Yoga program germinated from the treatment protocol used in the highly successful randomized controlled yoga study conducted with 70 US military personnel deployed to Kirkuk, Iraq, which I co-developed,[11,12] as well as from my experiences teaching yoga to combat veterans in my local community. Over the past several years, my own original ideas and writings have continued to evolve as I acquired more knowledge from trainings and various mentors, made new discoveries in practice, and as new developments in trauma research and theory have emerged. The Sensory-Enhanced Yoga program (including its earlier versions) has been taught to many hundreds of yoga instructors and health professionals who have shared the practice with thousands of military personnel and veterans and with many others outside of the military community. My hope is that by writing this book, the information will reach a far wider audience to support as many people as possible on their healing journeys.

The book approaches the topic of yoga for trauma at a number of levels, in an attempt to weave together bottom-up and top-down healing practices and integrate the primarily reductionist Western science concepts with holistic Eastern yogic philosophy, specifically the kosha model, which is thought to have been created by the ancient yogi sages approximately 3,000 years ago. The aim of this endeavor is a coherently synthesized theory together with practice guidelines that can intelligently inform the healing journey. The model and guidelines provide the context and parameters for the specific practices and techniques that follow, which together are designed to help the trauma survivor reclaim a *sense of safety*, *calm body*, *clear mind*, *uplifted spirit*, and *empowered sense of being*.

The program

The program was especially created to help clients:

- effectively manage stress before it leads to emotional dysregulation and/or inappropriate behaviors
- develop emotional resiliency, that is, the ability to rise to meet a challenge or threat, as well as easily calm once it has passed
- decrease hypervigilance and overreaction to sensory input (e.g. visual, crowds, touch, noise, movement)
- improve quality of sleep and energy level to support wellness and enhance daily productivity
- decrease intrusive thoughts by learning to become present through breath and body awareness
- enhance their sense of self-worth and personal empowerment.

How this book is organized

Part 1, Stress, trauma, and the neuroplastic brain, discusses PTSD from a sensory processing perspective, including symptoms, underlying neurophysiology, and common brain changes that may occur. It also highlights the inverse relationship between brain changes that tend to occur in PTSD and those that tend to occur in response to certain mind-body practices, particularly yoga, thus underscoring yoga's potential value as a healing modality for the condition. **Chapter 2, *PTSD and sensory processing*,** introduces the diagnosis of PTSD and how sensory processing is affected by trauma; **Chapter 3, *Neurophysiology of PTSD*,** describes the normal stress response and what happens on a neurophysiological level when this response does not resolve itself; and **Chapter 4, *Brain changes in PTSD and mind-body practices: the inverse relationship*,** provides a very detailed discussion on how the human brain is affected by an unresolved stress response, down to the level of brain structure and function, and also discusses the potential remediative effects of certain mindfulness-based practices. In the process, **Part 1** presents a clear history of the evolution of theoretical models of PTSD.

Part 2, The many faces of trauma, devotes separate chapters to the discussion of combat-related trauma, sexual trauma, incarceration, global conflict and mass disaster, and complex trauma through the eyes of the expert contributors to this book who are pioneers in using yoga and related mind-body modalities as tools of healing with survivors of these types of trauma. These chapter contributors provide an in-depth overview of their topic area as well as a personal perspective, either by sharing their own professional experiences or sharing the stories of survivors themselves in their own voices.

Chapter 1

Former military hospital commander Col. (Ret.) Patricia Lillis shares her personal experiences and expert perspective on the topic of combat stress in **Chapter 5**, *Combat stress management*. Though the diagnosis of PTSD was originally inspired by the problems seen in combat veterans, many other types of trauma can also cause the condition. Combat exposure and witnessing someone getting severely injured or killed are the most common PTSD-associated traumas for men, while rape and sexual molestation are the most common PTSD-associated traumas for women.[13] Dr Danielle Rousseau and Amanda J. G. Napior are experienced in using yoga as a healing modality for survivors of sexual trauma. They present the topic through an exploration of empirical literature as well as through voices of sexual trauma survivors in **Chapter 6**, *Reclaiming body, redefining relationship: yoga with survivors of sexual trauma*.

In **Chapter 7**, *Recovery and empowerment through yoga in prison*, Napior and Rousseau again join forces to share their expertise in bringing yoga to incarcerated populations. In this chapter, these authors summarize the published research, their own professional insights, as well as the perspectives of a married couple who met in prison and who benefitted enormously from their yoga participation. Their chapter deftly illuminates the public health crisis of mass incarceration that, as they explain, "impacts some people more harshly than others, and which unfolds in a context and history of systemic oppression." Napior and Rousseau also explain how and why embodied mindfulness practices such as yoga can be so powerful in both managing symptoms of trauma as well as the negative impact of the prison environment on personal well-being.

There are many causes of trauma, both man-made and natural in origin. Within the US, we have recently witnessed many natural disasters including the devastating hurricanes Harvey, Irma, and Maria; floods, tornadoes, volcanoes, and fires, as well as man-made causes including gun violence, terror, community violence, and motor vehicle accidents[14,15] In international news, the traumatic ordeals encountered by refugees have made frequent headlines. As we entered the year 2017, a record 65.6 million people worldwide were forcefully displaced, 12 million by the conflict in Syria alone.[16] All of these hard statistics are as difficult to write about as they are to read, and one can hardly be blamed for deciding to avoid the news so as not to become overwhelmed. Yet while some choose to cover their eyes and ears to maintain their own sanity, others, such as Gretchen Ki Steidle, founder of Global Grassroots, heed the call for help and make it their life mission to bring mind-body modalities around the world to those who have suffered from these natural and man-made disasters. You will learn about her important work in Haiti and Africa in **Chapter 8**, *Using mind-body practices among populations of mass disaster and conflict*.

Childhood trauma increases the likelihood of juvenile delinquency and adult criminal behavior, including violent criminal behavior.[17] People who have experienced childhood trauma are also more likely to fit the description of a complex trauma survivor, i.e. one who has suffered repeated or prolonged trauma exposure. The unfortunate truth is that most people have experienced at least one major traumatic event in their lifetime, and likely more than one, and these traumas usually have cumulative effects on the bodymind. The world-renowned Trauma Center at the Justice Resource Institute in Brookline has for many years operated a successful yoga program for complex trauma survivors and has conducted multiple research studies to investigate the effectiveness of yoga as a healing modality for this population. Dr Alison Rhodes graciously shares her insights and expertise on the topic in **Chapter 9**, *Yoga for complex trauma survivors*.

Introduction

One benefit of including the perspectives and stories of field experts in a book that is strongly science-based is the juxtaposition highlights the importance of considering all factors when designing programs for trauma survivors. When we only consider the science, we may end up presenting particular techniques that, though shown to be empirically therapeutic for trauma on a sensorimotor level, may not be appropriate for a specific individual or should be presented with caution, if at all, for a particular trauma population or within a particular culture. On the other hand, programs in the field may miss out on potentially potent therapeutic techniques if they do not take a close look at the science. So how do we reconcile the two? By listening to our students, using nuanced clinical judgment, and offering students a *choice*. This will be discussed in more detail in later chapters.

Part 3, East meets West: the theory and guidelines of Sensory-Enhanced Yoga®, begins by introducing and weaving Eastern yogic philosophy (specifically the kosha model) into the Western perspective that was presented in Part 1, and then presents the model and guidelines of the Sensory-Enhanced Yoga program. **Chapter 10, *Sensory-Enhanced Yoga®: healing trauma through the koshas***, introduces the kosha model and provides an initial "sneak-peek" of the Sensory-Enhanced Yoga guidelines for practice within the context of this model. This leads directly into a description of the *Transdisciplinary Model for Post-Traumatic Growth*, which synthesizes current theoretical concepts from the fields of occupational therapy, neurobiology, and trauma psychology within the framework of the kosha model to create a road map for healing PTSD, anxiety, ADD, and related autonomic nervous system disorders. The *Guiding Principles of Sensory-Enhanced Yoga*, which follow, are aligned with the model and guide clinical decision-making along the healing path.

Many of the practices of the program are presented within chapters in **Part 3** that discuss specific guidelines. These chapters are:

Chapter 11, *Guideline 1: A sense of safety is essential for healing*

Chapter 12, *Guideline 2: The most direct and powerful way to self-regulate is through control of the breath*

Chapter 13, *Guideline 3: Yoga can promote effective sensory, motor, and cognitive processing of traumatic experiences and thus aid healing*

Chapter 14, *Guideline 4: New beliefs and attitudes more easily take hold when we first prepare the body to receive and accept them*

Chapter 15, *Guideline 5: Self-empowerment is born on the wings of the spirit rising from the mind-body connection.*

The final section of the book, **Part 4, Putting the practice together**, presents suggestions regarding how to structure the practice as well as photos and descriptions of the yoga forms and Sensory-Enhanced Yoga flows. **Chapter 16, *Structuring the practice***, includes tips for designing a yoga class; sample scripts such as for initial centering and final relaxation; and a sample yoga class sequence. Both mat and chair versions of the program are presented, as well as strategies for teaching the program to groups of individuals with mixed mobility levels. Tips are also provided regarding class length, sequencing of the yoga forms, the effective use of an assistant, modifications for comfort, and other details as they apply to particular settings and populations. **Chapter 17, *Description of therapeutic forms***, provides photos and step-by-step descriptions of how to assume the specific therapeutic yoga forms. **Chapter 18, *Sensory-Enhanced Yoga® vinyasas***,

Chapter 1

presents the *Sensory-Enhanced Moon Salute* and *Sun Salutation Using a Chair*; as well as a *Choreographed Sun Salutation* designed for a group of individuals with mixed mobility levels—some fully mobile on a mat and others using a chair. Challenging situations such as these require careful planning and use of language to prevent confusion!

Some of the practices presented in this book are ancient, some are more modern or are modified, and all are presented in a fresh new light that ties all of the puzzle pieces together. In a nutshell, this book shows how Western science is validating what the ancient yogis have known for thousands of years: **yoga can be deeply healing at all levels of our being**.

During the course of reading this book, it will become apparent that there are many factors to consider when presenting yoga to trauma survivors—environmental, physical, intrapersonal, interpersonal, the nature of the trauma, cultural, gender, and societal—and that this important work requires a compassionate and highly adept teacher. By choosing this book, you are well on your way to becoming one. I hope you will enjoy and gain much benefit from this learning journey!

PART 1

Stress, trauma, and the neuroplastic brain

PTSD and sensory processing

The sensory system has everything to do with memory. — Babette Rothschild[1(p. 38)]

What is PTSD?

Post-traumatic stress disorder (PTSD) is the only mental health condition listed in the fifth edition of the American Psychiatric Association's *Diagnostic and Statistical Manual of Mental Disorders* (DSM-5) in which specific causal criteria must be met; specifically, this includes directly experiencing or witnessing actual or threatened death or serious injury, learning that a close relative or friend was exposed to such trauma, or being repeatedly and closely exposed to aversive details of the trauma, such as is often the case with emergency medical personnel.[2] However, there is resistance to the idea that only certain types of traumatic events should qualify for the diagnosis of PTSD, as studies have shown that many people who experience a PTSD-type syndrome do not meet the event criteria.[3,4] Furthermore, people exhibit different degrees of sensitivity and vulnerability to stressors, due to genetics and their environmental history.[5] Of those who *do* meet the event criteria in their lifetime, the symptoms and course of the condition cannot be predicted by whether or not the actual *triggering* event fell within these limited parameters.[6]

The reverse situation is also commonly encountered, whereby the symptom criteria fail to fully describe the consequences of a qualifying traumatic event for a particular individual, which leads to additional diagnoses. In fact, many of the conditions in the DSM-5 are often caused by highly stressful or traumatic events. Nevertheless, the four symptom clusters that define PTSD, according to the DSM-5, provide us with a good starting point for our discussion of the condition. These symptom clusters are:

- Persistent ***re-experiencing*** of the event in various sensory forms
  This may include flashbacks (feeling or acting as though the trauma is happening in that moment), distressing dreams (in which the content and/or affect relates to the trauma), and/or intrusive thoughts, memories, images, or perceptions. There may be emotional distress or physical reactions during re-experiencing episodes.

- Persistent ***avoidance of stimuli*** associated with the trauma
  The traumatized person may avoid certain people, places, conversations, activities, objects, memories, thoughts, feelings, bodily sensations (including pain), or stimuli from other senses, i.e. particular sights, sounds, smells, or tastes. Avoidance strategies may be subtle, such as purposeful distraction, or may significantly restrict one's activities and social interactions.

- Persistent ***numbing*** of general responsiveness and ***negative cognitions/mood***
  Numbing is feeling detached from one's own emotions and is associated with restricted affect. It is an involuntary (neurophysiological) form of avoidance, as well as a sign of dissociation, which will be discussed shortly. Unfortunately, in order

Chapter 2

for the mind to suppress painful emotions, it must suppress all emotions, including joy. Examples of negative cognitions include an inability to recall aspects of the trauma, distorted blaming of self or others for the event, and/or distorted negative beliefs about oneself or the world, such as "I am a horrible person" or "the world is a dangerous place."

- Persistent symptoms of **increased arousal** (not present before the trauma)
Symptoms of hyperarousal may include hyperalertness, hypervigilance, having difficulty concentrating, sleep difficulties, rising quickly to anger, and/or exaggerated startle response to sudden unexpected stimuli such as a sound, someone's touch, or a particular sight.

Dissociative subtype

In addition, the DSM-5 identifies a **dissociative subtype of PTSD**.[2] Dissociation is a state in which one loses awareness of the immediate surroundings, and includes even mild forms such as daydreaming or getting lost in a book or a movie. However, during trauma, stronger forms of dissociation may be used as a defense to enable the mind to escape the overwhelming situation, since the body cannot. As the trauma is occurring, the mind blocks off the thoughts, perceptions, feelings, and memories, which makes it difficult to remember the details of the trauma later on. Some forms of dissociation—including numbing and amnesia (a partial or total loss of memory of the traumatic event)—are embedded into the core criteria of PTSD. However, the DSM-5 recognizes that a subgroup of those who have PTSD experience additional dissociative symptoms. They include the following:

- **Depersonalization**—a perception of *one's sense of self* as being unreal. The person feels disconnected from the self, watching the self act while having no control over those actions, and that the world has become less real and more dream-like. Depersonalization is often accompanied by emotional numbing.
- **Derealization**—a perception of the *external world* as being unreal or strange. Familiar places may seem alien or surreal. Derealization often co-occurs with depersonalization.

Alan Schore defines dissociation as "a disruption of primary consciousness."[7(p. 291)] While we often think of consciousness as a reflective thought process controlled by the left hemisphere of the brain, Schore explains primary consciousness as a right brain controlled process which relates our visceral bodily sensations and emotions to the information coming in through the senses from the outside world. It is this process that enables us to feel present inside our skin and in our surroundings. When this process is disrupted, the "here and now" of the present moment loses meaning and can seem distant and beyond reach. Dissociation can be a very debilitating symptom, disrupting how one engages with the world. An intact mind-body connection is essential for finding meaning in one's life, and when one loses that connection, one loses hope. It is therefore not surprising that dissociation is associated with an increased risk of suicidality.[8]

Flashbacks

Flashbacks are vivid and disturbing memories in which the individual feels or acts as though a traumatic event is happening again. They usually lack a space and time perspective and are interpreted by the nervous system as happening in the present moment. Flashbacks are by definition involuntary memories, i.e. they come into awareness without any conscious attempt to retrieve the memory.[9] Flashbacks can be triggered by any stimulus that is similar to one that accompanied the traumatic event (see the section on triggers in Chapter 11) and can be experienced in any of the sensory modalities, e.g. visual, auditory, olfactory, kinesthetic (bodily feelings), as well as in the affective domain.[10] Individuals with PTSD usually avoid triggers that they are aware of, which can significantly affect the individual's functioning in everyday life.[11]

Flashbacks have long been considered to be closely related to dissociative symptoms, as they certainly draw an individual's awareness away from one's surroundings. However, recent neuroimaging research supports the idea that flashbacks are produced by a different neural network in the brain. Whereas flashbacks are associated with increased activity in limbic brain regions (such as the amygdala) and reduced activity in the prefrontal regions (associated with emotional control and regulation), the reverse is true with dissociation, suggesting that dissociation may be an expression of emotional over-modulation (see Chapter 11 for suggestions for handling flashbacks in the context of a yoga therapy session or class).[12,13]

Hyperarousal = core symptom of PTSD

A discussion on flashbacks can't help but lead one back to the symptom of hyperarousal, as the two symptoms are highly correlated. Lanius and colleagues[14] found that 30% of people who meet criteria for PTSD fit into a dissociated subtype while 70% fit into a hyperarousal/re-experiencing subtype. According to several trauma experts, hyperarousal is the key to understanding the whole phenomenon of PTSD, as it underlies the development of the other symptom clusters.[15-17] As trauma expert and social worker Babette Rothschild explained:[18(p. 6)]

> *People who suffer from PTSD are plagued with frightening body symptoms which are characteristic of hyperarousal: accelerated heartbeat, cold sweating, rapid breathing, heart palpitations, hypervigilance, and hyper startle response (jumpiness). These symptoms lead to sleep disturbances, loss of appetite, sexual dysfunction and difficulties in concentrating, which are further*

hallmarks of PTSD. Hyperarousal both instigates flashbacks and is also increased by them, and hyperarousal is the underlying cause of the symptom of avoidance, as traumatic reminders increase ANS arousal. Through understanding hyperarousal, the phenomenon of PTSD becomes comprehendible.

Altered sensory processing is thought to play a major role in the hyperarousal symptoms of PTSD,[19] and vice versa. According to van der Kolk,[20,21] the extreme hyperarousal that is often experienced *during* a traumatic event can disrupt how the event is processed in the brain, resulting in memories that present as vivid yet highly fragmented sensory impressions that often fail to integrate together into a cohesive story that can be verbally conveyed, which explains why talk therapies have had only limited success. *Following* the trauma, those who go on to develop PTSD often show difficulties with sensory filtering, i.e. the ability of the brain to sort relevant from irrelevant information, which reinforces hyperarousal.[22]

While anxiety, stress, and sensory filtering issues have long been known to be associated,[23-25] a study by Stewart and White[22] found evidence that re-experiencing and numbing symptoms are also associated with disruption in sensory filtering. These researchers used self-report measures to compare three groups of undergraduate students: those with PTSD, those with a trauma history but no PTSD, and those with a minimal trauma history. In this study, the sensory filtering issues could not be attributed to the effects of loud combat exposure, as none of their participants had engaged in combat.

The sensory elements of hyperarousal

In 1941, Abram Kardiner described some of the sensory elements of hyperarousal in his landmark book *The Traumatic Neuroses of War*, upon which the current PTSD diagnostic criteria are based:[26,27(p. 320)]

Chapter 2

These patients cannot stand being slapped on the back abruptly; they cannot tolerate a misstep or a stumble. From a physiologic point of view there exists a lowering of the threshold of stimulation; and, from a psychological point of view, a state of readiness for fright reactions.

American combat veterans have reported sensory symptoms since the Civil War. For example, dizziness has been listed as a common combat-related symptom for conflicts from the Civil War, through World War I, the Korean War, World War II, Vietnam, and the Gulf War to Afghanistan and Iraq.[28,29] This makes sense, as there are strong reciprocal neural pathways between the vestibular system, which informs us of our head position relative to space and gravity, and the autonomic nervous system, which is responsible for the stress response.[30] Furthermore, we know that sufficiently loud sounds can stimulate the end organs of the vestibular labyrinth, located in the inner ear,[31] raising the question of whether the explosive sounds of combat contribute to the vestibular symptoms of veterans diagnosed with PTSD. In fact, the auditory system evolved from the vestibular system and the sensory end organs of each of these systems are encased in the same bony capsule where they are well positioned to interact with one another.[31]

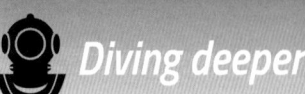

Diving deeper

Interestingly, while the auditory startle reflex has received much attention in PTSD and is listed as one of the diagnostic criteria within the hyperarousal cluster of symptoms, not a single vestibular symptom is mentioned in the DSM-5. We may see vestibular symptoms listed in the next version, thanks to the recent work of Haber and colleagues,[32] who conducted the first known study to identify the nature of vestibular symptoms in veterans both with and without PTSD, using tools specifically designed to measure these symptoms. They used the Post-Traumatic Checklist (PCL) to sort a group of veterans into those who met criteria for PTSD (n=50) and those who did not (n=37) and then used a linear regression to compare their total PCL score with the total score for four symptoms: *feeling dizzy, loss of balance, poor coordination,* and *headaches*. They not only found that veterans with PTSD experienced significantly more vestibular symptoms than those without PTSD (p < .0001), but also that veterans with worse PTSD symptoms experienced a greater number of vestibular-related symptoms within the previous 30 days. Furthermore, statistical analysis showed that their vestibular symptoms could not be attributed to traumatic brain injury or anxiety (though these conditions were common among the study participants). Of most significance, the veterans with PTSD identified these vestibular symptoms as a source of disability.[32]

Researchers are still in the process of identifying sensory symptoms of PTSD and when doing so need to be careful to distinguish between different sources of trauma and the nature of the threats encountered, as sensory symptoms may vary accordingly. For example, Hunt and colleagues[33] observed that combat soldiers serving in Iraq and Afghanistan, where IEDs are commonly encountered, are often triggered by, and hypervigilant toward, external cues such as cars that may possibly be carrying explosives, whereas those who served in the first Gulf War (Operation Desert Storm), where toxic chemical exposure was common, are more often triggered by, and hypervigilant toward, internal or somatosensory cues, for example unusual sensations in the body, limbs, and head (such as dizziness), or related to breathing. They conclude, "It may be that different wars involve different psychological traumas

PTSD and sensory processing

resulting in different manifestations of post-traumatic disturbances in sensory processing, with some syndromes being more internally focused and others more externally focused."[33(p. 709)]

However, van der Kolk and colleagues point out that, in PTSD, heightened physiological arousal does not just occur in response to "triggers," that is, reminders of the trauma, but also in response to intense but neutral stimuli,[34] and this assertion is strongly supported by a recent electroencephalogram (EEG) study.[35] Van der Kolk et al.[34] described this as a "loss of stimulus discrimination." The auditory startle response is the most frequently researched example,[34,36-39] though as far back as 1941, Kardiner observed that this loss of stimulus discrimination can occur in response to temperature, pain, and sudden tactile stimuli as well.[26] The term "stimulus discrimination" in the above context is very closely related to the term "sensory modulation" used in sensory integration theory to describe: (1) the ability to regulate and organize reactions to sensory input in a graded and adaptive manner; and (2) the balancing of excitatory and inhibitory inputs and adapting to environmental changes.[40]

Engel-Yeger and co-workers[41] provide empirical evidence of the association between sensory processing disorder (SPD) and post-traumatic stress (PTS) in their study comparing the sensory profiles of 30 participants with PTS symptoms with those of 30 healthy, matched control subjects. Following consent, all participants completed the Post-Traumatic Stress Disorder Symptom Scale (PSS-SR) and the Adolescent/Adult Sensory Profile (AASP). Those who met criteria for PTS as demonstrated by the PSS-SR scale were significantly more likely to demonstrate sensory sensitivity, sensory avoidance, and low registration, as well as decreased sensory seeking behavior, as compared with the matched control subjects and the population norms (see Table 2.1 for definitions). Significant correlations were found between specific symptom clusters of PTSD and differences in sensory processing in specific sensory modalities. ***Increased arousal*** correlated with a lower tendency to seek touch input and lower registration of auditory input; ***sensory avoidance*** correlated with a reduced tendency to seek visual and touch input; and ***intrusive thoughts*** correlated with higher avoidance to touch, lower registration of auditory input, and a lower tendency to seek vestibular (movement) and touch input. Further studies are needed to confirm these findings.

Pilot study of combat veterans

Several years ago, I became curious about the sensory symptoms of combat veterans and was given the opportunity to conduct a pilot study. Twelve older combat veterans who were all formally diagnosed with PTSD filled out the AASP along with a custom cover sheet, which provided space for optional comments.[42] Figure 2.1 demonstrates the striking similarity of the sensory profiles in this group. The outside edges of the quadrants represent the extreme ranges of that particular characteristic. Table 2.1 defines the terms of the AASP quadrants.

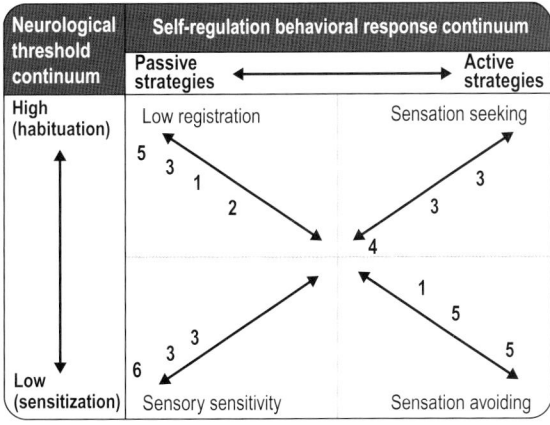

Figure 2.1

Quadrant scores of 12 combat veterans on Adolescent/Adult Sensory Profile (AASP). Quadrant chart copyright © 2002–18 Pearson Education, Inc. Reprinted with permission.

Chapter 2

- **Neurological thresholds** = the way the nervous system responds to sensory input
- **Self-regulation strategies** = the ways that people manage the input that is available to them

As a group, these combat veterans showed significantly higher sensory sensitivity, sensory avoidance, and low registration, and significantly lower sensory seeking behaviors than the normative population, at the .001 level of significance, which is the same pattern revealed in the Engel-Yeger et al. study.

Examples of *sensory sensitivity* that they experienced included becoming dizzy easily, demonstrating a fear of heights and/or fear of movement, showing sensitivity to background noise, and startling easily. Some common forms of *sensory avoidance* were staying away from crowds or noisy settings, only eating familiar foods, and keeping the shades down at home. What interested me most were the *low registration* items, which are less frequently discussed in the literature. They often did not know how they got scrapes or bruises, and a third of them found themselves "frequently" or "almost always" tripping or bumping into things, which is consistent with observations of decreased body sensation that may accompany dissociation. The combat veterans in the pilot study also demonstrated issues related to visual filtering, such as missing road signs or becoming highly frustrated when searching for items in messy rooms or crowded drawers.

They also experienced some difficulties with language processing, revealed by such items as having trouble following what people were saying when they talked fast and asking people to repeat things. According to polyvagal theory, developed by Stephen Porges, auditory sensitivity goes hand in hand with language processing difficulties.[43] Porges explains that we have evolved the capability to contract the middle ear muscles in order to process language. When we do not contract those muscles, we have a better capability of picking up sounds associated with threat, but at the expense of language processing. In a similar vein, the sensory profiles of the 12 combat veterans showed a strong bias toward registering sensory information *external* to the body and which could be potentially threat-laden (captured by the sensory sensitivity items) while also showing reduced registration of sensory information *internal* to the body or which is not typically threat-laden (captured by the low registration items). This is consistent with the fact that most threats encountered by troops of most wars (except the first Gulf War, as discussed earlier) could best be detected by sight and sound. For more information on selected items of this pilot study, please see Appendix A.

In the optional comment section, one of the 12 veterans who scored at the extreme end ranges of the pattern described simply wrote: "I endure most of life." There is a pressing need for society to address

Table 2.1 Term definitions of AASP quadrants*

Sensory sensitivity	"Represents behaviors in accordance with a low neurological threshold. Distractibility, difficulty screening stimuli, and discomfort with sensation characterize this quadrant."
Sensation avoiding	"Counteracting a low neurological threshold, sensation avoiding includes behaviors that limit exposure to stimuli."
Low registration	"Low registration reflects responses in accordance with a high neurological threshold. This quadrant includes a disregard of or slow response to sensation."
Sensation seeking	"Sensation seeking is a counteractive response to high neurological threshold and encompasses pleasure derived from rich sensory environments and behaviors that create sensation."

*Quotations from Brown C, Tollefson N, Dunn W, Cromwell R, Filion D. The adult sensory profile: measuring patterns of sensory processing. American Journal of Occupational Therapy. 2001;55:75–82.

the sensory processing impairments of veterans and others who have experienced trauma as they can have a significant effect on quality of life. These symptoms frequently contribute to the increased irritation, frustration, and anger that many veterans with PTSD experience which can seriously affect personal relationships and work performance. A major premise of this book is that yoga can be very helpful in addressing the core symptoms of PTSD, especially when the practice is explicitly designed to target the aberrant sensory processing that often underlies these symptoms. Toward that end, it is necessary to go into more detail as to what exactly "sensory processing" is.

What is "sensory processing"?

"Sensory processing" refers to how the nerves communicate together to process all of the incoming information from our senses in order to plan our movements, generate ideas, and produce other thoughts and behaviors (Figure 2.2). Single neurons cannot "think," but when groups of neurons all interact together in a focused way for a particular purpose, the result is organized action or thought. The brain sorts through the sensory information, filtering out what is irrelevant, and organizes and integrates the rest, in order to understand the situation and plan an appropriate response. In PTSD, the timing, filtering and processing of sensory information are often impaired.[19,44,45]

Neurons communicate with other neurons by releasing chemicals (i.e. neurotransmitters) within the small gap that exists between them. The "receiving" neurons have specialized receptor sites to allow the neurotransmitters to enter the cell membrane. Some neurotransmitters are "excitatory," that is, they increase the chance that the receiving neuron will fire (i.e. produce an "action potential"), while other neurotransmitters are "inhibitory" and decrease the chances that the receiving neuron will fire. **Glutamate** is the principal excitatory transmitter in the brain whereas **gamma-aminobutyric acid (GABA)** is the principal

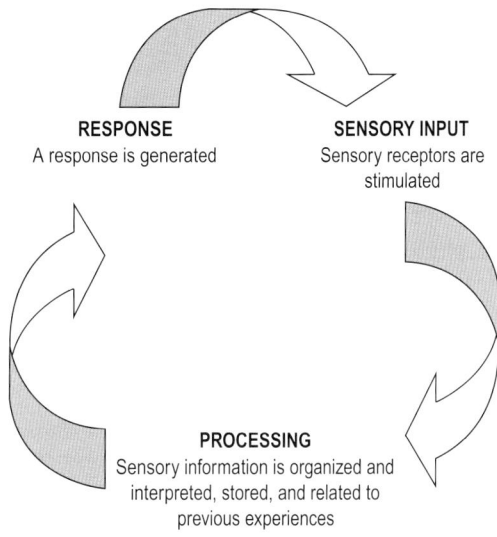

Figure 2.2

Sensory processing. Used with permission of Sensational Kids Occupational Therapy, Australia

inhibitory transmitter.[46] In order for a neuron to fire, the sum of excitatory and inhibitory post-synaptic potentials must be greater than the firing threshold for that particular neuron (Figure 2.3). Though there are more neurons in the brain that release glutamate than there are neurons that release GABA, the ones releasing GABA keep a tight rein on the excitatory neurons and thus regulate activation of the various brain networks.[47]

Inhibitory neural processes have a huge influence on a person's subjective emotional experience. According to Thayer and Lane's[50,51] **neurovisceral integration model**, in order to experience emotion consciously, subcortical emotion-laden information must reach the cerebral cortex, and as this information makes its journey upward, higher-level cortical structures exert their top-down inhibitory influence on this information (such as through the powers of reasoning and memory recall) to shape the nature of the

Chapter 2

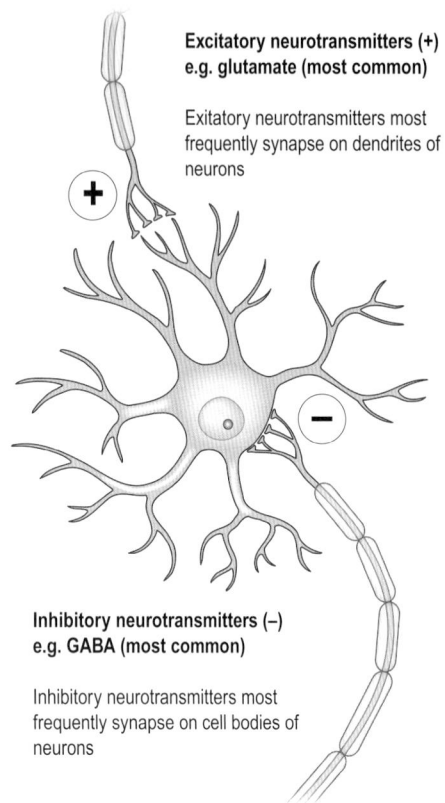

Excitatory neurotransmitters (+)
e.g. glutamate (most common)

Exitatory neurotransmitters most frequently synapse on dendrites of neurons

Inhibitory neurotransmitters (−)
e.g. GABA (most common)

Inhibitory neurotransmitters most frequently synapse on cell bodies of neurons

Figure 2.3

Neuronal impulse transmission. If the excitatory influences exceed the inhibitory influences, an "action potential" (electrical impulse) will be generated within the postsynaptic neuron. The action potential causes a release of transmitters at the end of the axon which are taken up by adjacent neurons. Sensory-based and mindfully-based strategies can be used to enable inhibitory influences to block excitatory influences, i.e. to "close the gate," or to enable excitatory influences to overcome inhibition, i.e. to "open the gate," with the goal to ultimately affect entire brain networks

emotional experience. According to Thayer and Lane, "This is consistent with the more general principle that inhibition serves to 'sculpt' excitatory neural action at all levels of the neuraxis to produce context appropriate responses to environmental demands."[51(p. 83), 52–54]

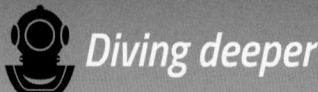 *Diving deeper*

The excitatory transmitters usually synapse on dendrites, whereas the transmitters that block electrical impulses tend to synapse on the cell bodies so they are in position to block the impulses. So, one of two things can happen: either the excitatory transmitters can overtake the inhibitory transmitters to **open the gate** and cause an electric impulse, or the inhibitory transmitters can **close the gate** and block an impulse. Without inhibition, the brain would not be able to filter out irrelevant sensory information. Prager et al.[47] explain that for the brain to function normally, there must be a finely tuned balance of excitatory and inhibitory neuronal activity, which Jean Ayres, the original creator of sensory integration theory and treatment, referred to as "**sensory homeostasis.**"[48(p. 34)] When we use sensory-based and mindfulness-based treatments to affect brain function, we are purposely opening or closing the gates at the neuronal level to help create that balance.[40,48,49] As Streeter and colleagues put it, yoga may "stimulate an under active parasympathetic nervous system and increase the inhibitory action of a hypoactive GABA system in brain pathways and structures that are critical for threat perception, emotion regulation, and stress reactivity."[49(p. 577)] As GABA has been found to be low in the population of people who have PTSD, this is a particularly relevant avenue to explore.[49]

This sculpting of information occurs on a grand scale, as there are approximately 86 billion neurons in the brain[55] and each neuron is connected to tens to hundreds of thousands of other neurons, so numerous summations of potentials are occurring simultaneously. Various sense receptors can initiate the process, as can the brain itself, such as through daydreaming,

PTSD and sensory processing

focused thinking, or meditation. When initiated by sensory stimuli, the input to the brain is usually multi-modal. For example, if we ring a bell, we don't just hear it; we also see it, feel it, sense the movement of our arms when ringing it, and generate an emotional response to it. We also register that information simultaneously, which helps our nervous system to associate these inputs as being caused by the same event. This information is processed in various parts of the brain and is integrated together with much assistance and coordination from the thalamus and other brain structures.

In PTSD, however, the brain may fail to register all of the important sensory stimuli and neglect to filter some of the irrelevant stimuli out—"*relevance*" being dependent upon what is required of the person in order to effectively adapt to the present moment and setting. In fact, the method in which a "post-traumatic stress disordered" brain processes sensory information is actually well adapted for a combat or trauma situation. Thus, the problem isn't one of **dis**organization but rather that the nervous system has **re**organized itself to adapt to the nature of the threat to ensure survival—and then was unable to readapt once the threat had passed. This statement is corroborated by electroencephalograph (EEG) studies showing that, in PTSD, processing of trauma-related stimuli is prioritized over neutral stimuli.[45]

Studies are needed to answer the obvious "chicken or egg" question regarding which came first, the sensory processing issues or PTSD, as a small but unknown percentage of the general population may be more susceptible to PTSD due to pre-existing anomalies in sensory processing. Indeed, Lanius and colleagues[57] hypothesized two pathways of emotional dysregulation and brain dysfunction in PTSD, one due to fear conditioning/stress sensitization following a traumatic event and the other due to inadequate neurodevelopment of the emotional and arousal regulatory systems as a result of adverse events in childhood, which then increases vulnerability to PTSD later in life. The same group of researchers later presented evidence of genetic risk factors for PTSD as well.[58]

Whether predisposed to the condition of PTSD or not, ultimately an event occurred that completely overwhelmed the nervous system, leading to failure of the stress response to resolve itself through the normal negative feedback loop of the hypothalamic–pituitary–adrenal (HPA) axis of the endocrine system. So we will turn our attention now to the hormonal havoc that trauma produces in the brain and pick up the sensory processing pieces of the discussion in Chapter 4.

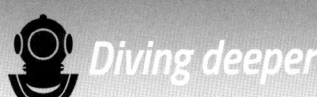

For example, Javanbakht and colleagues' recent meta-analysis of evoked-related potentials in PTSD[56] most consistently found diminished habituation to repetitive stimuli (as evidenced by reduced P50 gating), sensitization of the P300 response to trauma-related stimuli; and diminished P300 response to neutral stimuli.

Neurophysiology of PTSD   3

Until we understand that traumatic symptoms are physiological as well as psychological, we will be woefully inadequate in our attempts to heal them. — Peter A. Levine[1(p. 32)]

Introduction

This chapter is about what actually happens in the brain to cause the symptoms of PTSD. First we need to introduce the key players, which include structures from every tier of the brain, from the primitive brainstem to the cerebral cortex. However, it is the structures in-between, in the nebulously defined **limbic system**, that have traditionally been considered to be the seat of our emotional and survival responses and have been most implicated in PTSD.[2] These structures control the autonomic nervous system (ANS), which is responsible for the fight–flight reaction, and also control the body's hormonal responses to stress. These limbic brain areas interact with higher level cortical structures, which help to shape the responses of these lower centers and give rise to our conscious feelings.[3]

Before describing these structures, I should mention that there is some debate as to whether the term "limbic system" is even valid,[4,5] and consensus has never been reached on the structural and functional criteria that officially define it. As LeDoux[3] cogently pointed out, different emotions are associated with different brain networks that activate multiple levels of the brain, not just structures within the limbic lobe.

Nonetheless, the term is still commonly used among experts to refer to brain areas that play a large role in emotional regulation and homeostatic functions.[2,5] According to Roxo et al., "It is accepted that the prefrontal cortex, amygdala, anterior cingulate cortex, hippocampus, and insula participate in the majority of emotional processes."[5(p. 2429)] We also know that the hypothalamus, pituitary gland, and brainstem nuclei are involved in survival functions such as the fight–flight response, and that the aforementioned emotional areas influence this process.[3,6]

According to Damasio:[7(p. 28)]

It makes good housekeeping sense that [the brain] structures governing attention and structures processing emotion should be in the vicinity of one another. Moreover, it also makes good housekeeping sense that all of these structures should be in the vicinity of those which regulate and signal body state. This is because the consequences of having emotion and attention are entirely related to the fundamental business of managing life within the organism, while, on the other hand, it is not possible to manage life and maintain homeostatic balance without data on the current state of the organism's body proper.

Damasio and his colleagues[8] put this logic to the test by conducting a series of PET (positron emission tomography) experiments with 41 healthy volunteers to examine the neural correlates of emotion and feelings. They targeted four emotions, sadness, happiness, anger, and fear, and found that all of the emotional states activated brain structures related to the regulation or representation of the internal state of the body. The involvement of brainstem nuclei, the insula, secondary somatosensory cortex, cingulate cortex, and hypothalamus in particular highlighted the close physiological connection between emotion and homeostasis. The authors described the neural patterns that emerged as forming "multidimensional maps" of the internal state, which they believe form the basis for feelings. But what happens when a person experiences a highly traumatic event? As discussed in Chapter 2, emotional numbing and dissociation are common symptoms of PTSD, so it can be surmised that these multidimensional maps would be affected.

For many trauma survivors the connection between the body and the mind becomes lost, making it difficult to identify what one is feeling.[2] If not numbed, the feelings may register so strongly as to be overwhelming.[9,10] Since feelings arise in large part through awareness of visceral and other bodily sensations, disturbances in somatosensory processing would by definition affect the neural patterning of emotion in the brain. Neuroimaging studies have found altered activity in many of these brain areas in PTSD, due to the failed resolution of the fight–flight response. Thus, in this book, the term *limbic system* will be used broadly to describe the strong neural network connecting traditional limbic structures associated with survival mechanisms, homeostasis, and lower-level emotional processing with cortical structures involved with conscious emotional feeling, which together shape and influence each other.

The sensory filters of the limbic system

The limbic system has long been considered to be a major center for emotion formation and processing, learning, and memory.[11,12] Importantly, it is influenced by all sensory inputs, and dysfunction in this system may lead to defensiveness in all sensory systems. This is thought to be a problem of sensory filtering,[13] which is a major role of the thalamus. However, we now know that the amygdala—considered to be the "chief executive" of the limbic system[14]—shapes initial sensory input to the brain in concert with the locus ceruleus, located in the brainstem.[15] A significant body of evidence is building showing that initial sensory processing (and neuroplasticity) occurs even in peripheral sensory end organs, so there is still much left for scientists to discover regarding how sensory information is shaped and filtered along its pathways to higher centers the brain (see McGann[16] for a review).

Nonetheless, the thalamus is squarely implicated in the sensory filtering issue of PTSD. According to a research team currently studying thalamic-cortical pathways, "All sensory perceptions converge [in the thalamus] first. As the main relay center, it therefore needs to reconcile the flood of incoming information and the brain's limited computing power."[17(p. 2)] So when reading about the key brain structures involved in PTSD (see Figures 3.1 and 3.2), please keep in mind that the information received by most of these structures (except those in the brainstem) has been filtered through the thalamus and if this filter is not working properly, it will affect the performance of these other structures as well, and thus our perceptions and understanding of the world around us.

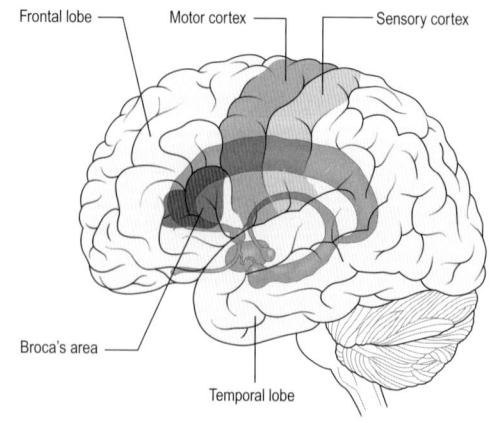

Figure 3.1
Brain structures implicated in PTSD, set A

Neurophysiology of PTSD

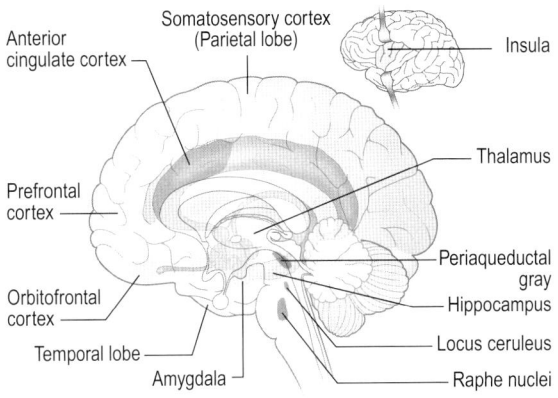

Figure 3.2
Brain structures implicated in PTSD, set B

Key limbic structures and supporting actors

The following brain structures support balanced limbic functioning and thus the ability of a person to regulate emotions, levels of arousal and stress, and attention, as well as control behavioral impulses (see also Figures 3.1 and 3.2). This list goes beyond the classic limbic structures to also include the structures that "anchor" each of the three core brain networks of the triple network model[18] (see Chapter 4). These anchoring structures (marked with this symbol ⚓) typically show altered activity along with the classic limbic structures in individuals who have PTSD.[19,20] The anchor symbols serve as an aid to you when referring back to this mini-encyclopedia of brain structures while reading Chapter 4. The list is intended to lay down the neuroanatomical framework for future discussions.

Before we begin, we should keep in mind LeDoux's warning to "be suspicious of any statement that says a brain area is a center responsible for some function."[3,4(p. 14)] As he points out, nowadays scientists think of brain functions as products of *systems*, not specific brain structures. Thus, when I list roles of specific brain structures, it is intended to mean that the structure serves a key role in a *system of structures* for that particular brain function, as determined by brain research findings. Also, subregions within major brain structures often participate in very different tasks from one another. Some of these subregions are strongly implicated in PTSD and are described in the "diving deeper" (shaded) sections. If you do not have a strong neuroanatomy background, I encourage you to skip these sections for now and refer back to particular structures as you come across them in other sections of the book (i.e. to use this more like a glossary).

Subcortical structures

Locus ceruleus

- The locus ceruleus is located in the pons of the brainstem and consists of a cluster of norepinephrine-containing neurons that project throughout the central nervous system, providing the only source of norepinephrine to the neocortex, hippocampus, cerebellum, and most of the thalamus.[21]

- It is part of the reticular activating system, is activated by stress, and plays a major role in arousal and attention. The locus ceruleus is functionally intertwined with the paraventricular nucleus of the hypothalamus, which controls the hypothalamic–pituitary–adrenal (HPA axis).[22]

Periaqueductal gray (PAG)

- The periaqueductal gray (PAG) is a small midbrain structure that plays an important role in defense responses to threat. There are direct neural projections to autonomic sites in the ventral medulla as well as two-way projections between the amygdala and PAG through which to coordinate defensive responses.

Chapter 3

- The dorsolateral PAG and lateral PAG play a role in active defensive responses associated with **sympathetic nervous system** activation (e.g. fight–flight).[23,24]
- The ventrolateral PAG plays a role in passive defensive responses (e.g. freeze) associated with **parasympathetic nervous system** activation.[23,24]

Amygdala

- Located in the medial temporal lobes, the small almond-sized amygdala is considered a key player of the emotional brain. The amygdala constantly surveys the environment (as filtered through the thalamus and cerebral cortex) and assigns emotional significance to everything coming through the senses, whether positive or negative.[25]
- The amygdala plays a major role in the **detection** of threats and control of the body's **response** to threats.[3,4,26] *It is the trigger that activates the HPA axis of the stress response.*[27]
- However, LeDoux points out that the amygdala likely only contributes to the **feeling** of fear indirectly, and that "the feeling of 'fear' results when the outcome of … various processes (attention, perception, memory, arousal) coalesce in consciousness and compel one to feel 'fear'."[3,4(p. 11)]

Diving deeper

Diving deeper into the amygdala

The *lateral nucleus* is the sensory gateway to the amygdala, as it receives information from the senses (visual, auditory, gustatory, olfactory, and somatosensory, including pain) via the thalamus and cortex. When it detects a threat, it signals other areas of the amygdala to control behavioral and physiological responses.

When alerted by the lateral nucleus that there is a threat, the basal nucleus can disrupt the top-down control of the higher brain centers over whatever the person has been thinking about in order to redirect attention to the threat.

The **central nucleus** controls the expression of the fear reaction, including (but not limited to) the ANS and HPA axis responses. It also activates the arousal systems that release norepinephrine, dopamine, acetylcholine, and serotonin. (Based on J. LeDoux, Anxious[4])

Hypothalamus

- The primary role of the hypothalamus is to maintain the body's homeostasis (state of balance) by regulating temperature, blood pressure, heart rate, the sleep/wake cycle, the fight–flight reaction, feeding, and mating.[28]
- It is responsible for activating the autonomic nervous system and endocrine responses to stress, and has a high level of connectivity with most major brain areas, including the cerebral cortex, hippocampus, amygdala, thalamus, cerebellum, brainstem, and spinal cord.[28]
- When the amygdala detects a threat, it prompts the *paraventricular nucleus* of the hypothalamus to release a hormone called corticotropin-releasing factor to activate the HPA axis.[29] The hypothalamus is intimately connected with the pituitary gland.

Pituitary[30,31]

- The pituitary is a pea-sized gland situated at the base of the skull that controls the function of most of the other glands in the human body; it is thus referred to as the **master gland**.
- The pituitary has two lobes, one anterior and one posterior, which are connected to the hypothalamus by a stalk. The hypothalamus controls the release of hormones from the pituitary through this stalk.

- The anterior lobe secretes at least a half dozen major hormones including adrenocorticotropic hormone (ACTH), which is involved in the HPA axis of the stress response. The smaller posterior lobe secretes only two major hormones, oxytocin and vasopressin.
- Feedback mechanisms allow the hypothalamus or pituitary to determine the levels of hormones in the system and make adjustments.

Thalamus

- The thalamus is the final relay station for sensory information before it is sent to the appropriate areas of the cerebral cortex for further processing.[32,33]
- It distills sensory information into a more interpretable form from which the cortex can then flesh out the details.[34]
- The thalamus also plays a role in regulating sleep.[35]

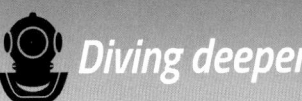

Diving deeper into the thalamus

The **ventral posterolateral nucleus** of the thalamus receives information from nerve pathways that relay sensory information from the body to the brain. It is this nucleus through which the therapeutic modalities of deep touch pressure and enhanced proprioception influence the brain (see Chapter 14). This and other thalamic nuclei also receive vestibular input from the inner ears that register movement of the head through space.[36-38] The integration of vestibular (movement-based) and somatosensory (body-based) input likely occurs in the thalamus.[36]

The **nucleus reuniens** (RE) of the thalamus is a very important link between the medial prefrontal cortex and the hippocampus, both of which are essential for the encoding and retrieval of episodic memories.[39,40] It is believed to gate the flow of information to the hippocampus from the medial prefrontal cortex, likely dependent on states of arousal and attention. Thus, it has been hypothesized that modulating levels of arousal/attention may control the type of information that gains access to the hippocampus for long-term memory storage.[39] This has treatment implications (discussed in Chapter 13).

Cortical structures

Insula ⚓

- The insula has two-way connections to many sensory, motor, limbic, and association areas in the brain and is especially tightly connected with the anterior cingulate cortex (ACC; see below) to enable quick access to the motor system. Working together, these two structures are thought to play a strong integrative role in the brain.[41,42]
- The insula aids in the subjective sense of the inner body and body states; judges the degree of pain; assists in processing of vestibular (movement) sensations; pairs emotion to bodily sensations, giving rise to conscious feelings and the awareness of the "feeling self"; and has an important role in regulating the autonomic nervous system[42-44] and modulating emotions.[19]
- It plays an important role in high-level cognitive and attentional control, especially with regard to detecting salient events, and assists the hippocampus in processing the context of potential threats.[27,42,45,46]
- Furthermore, the insula is believed to mediate between externally oriented attention and self-reflective functioning.[20]

Chapter 3

Diving deeper
Diving deeper into the insula

The **anterior insula** ⚓ is a very important brain structure with regard to the study of PTSD as it is considered the integral hub of the *salience network*. It detects salient events and controls switching between other large-scale networks to attend to the event.

The **dorsal posterior insula** is the location of the primary interoceptive representation (body map) from which emerge basic feelings that include "pain, temperature, itch, sensual touch, muscular and visceral sensations, vasomotor activity, hunger, thirst, and 'air hunger'."[44(p. 500)]

The **right anterior insula** ⚓ is believed to generate a meta-representation of the dorsal posterior insula's body map, which is thought to provide the basis for the experience of emotional awareness.[44] It is involved in the neural representation of somatosensory aspects of emotional states such as sympathetic arousal.[9]

Diving deeper
Diving deeper into the hippocampus

The **anterior hippocampus** has a role in contextual fear conditioning[47] and is also believed to play a key role in regulating activation of the HPA axis through inhibitory mechanisms.[49]

It is also involved in episodic (autobiographical) memory, which provides context for an event.[47,50] For example, it can remind us that most Labrador Retrievers we have encountered in the past have been friendly dogs so the one in front of us likely is, too, which then keeps the HPA axis in check through sensory gating. Neurons in the anterior hippocampus have also been found to code both space and time and can thus remind us where and when we saw that friendly dog.[40]

Hippocampus

- The hippocampus is an essential brain structure for learning, memory, and cognition.[47] It is involved in memory formation and storage and, in particular, assigns emotional meaning, time, and spatial context to our memories.
- It is the most active brain structure for encoding and recalling traumatic memories.[48]

Anterior cingulate cortex (ACC) ⚓

- The **anterior cingulate cortex (ACC)** ⚓ is strongly connected to both the limbic system and the prefrontal cortex and is thus thought to play an important role in emotional regulation[51] and reward-based learning.[52] It is believed to be involved in the experiential and/or expressive aspects of emotion.[53]
- Evidence suggests that the ACC uses contextual information to shape decision-making, socially driven interactions, and empathy-related responses.[54]
- Importantly, the **rostral ACC (rACC)** is believed to have a top-down inhibitory influence on the amygdala; that is, it can help keep the amygdala in check.[55]
- The ACC is considered by many scientists to be part of the medial prefrontal cortex (mPFC) but is usually discussed separately from it, as it is here. Its subregions hold distinct roles.

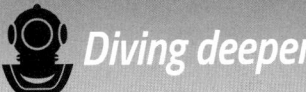

Diving deeper into the anterior cingulate cortex

The *dorsal anterior cingulate cortex (dACC)* ⚓ has a dense two-way connection with the amygdala and is involved with autonomic control of the sympathetic and parasympathetic nervous systems and the evaluation of safety vs danger within the environment.[23,56]

The dACC is a key node along with the insula in the *salience network* of the brain which together guide behavior to the most important actions (see Chapter 4).

The *rostral ACC (rACC)* (which contains both the *subgenual and pregenual ACC)* is associated with resilience; hypofunction in this area is associated with emotional dysregulation such as anxiety or mood disorders.[27]

Posterior cingulate cortex (PCC) ⚓

- The *posterior cingulate cortex (PCC)* ⚓ is a highly complex structure that acts as a connector hub for cortical and subcortical networks.[57] It is famously associated with the *default mode network*[19] as it shows significantly reduced activation during attentionally demanding tasks, although certain subregions do appear to interact with executive, attentional, motor, and language networks.[57]
- The default mode network is described in more detail in Chapter 4, but briefly is thought to be associated with the continuous sense of the self and self-referential processing, autobiographical memory, and social cognition, and is most engaged when a person is resting.[19] The PCC works closely with the precuneus.
- The PCC is also our GPS, providing a physical sense of where we are in space,[2(p. 90)] while the anterior thalamus drives the PCC.[61]

Precuneus (PrCC) ⚓

- The precuneus is adjacent to the posterior cingulate on the medial surface of the hemispheres between the sensory cortex and the cuneus, which contains the visual cortex. It is involved in reflective self-processing, episodic memory, and visuospatial processing.[58,59]
- The PrCC is often lumped together with the posterior cingulate as a single seed region for the study of the *default mode network* of the brain.[60]
- Vogt and Laureys[61] proposed that, together, the precuneus and PCC are considered crucial for conscious information processing and self-reflection. They also reported evidence that the PCC/PrCC has the highest level of glucose metabolism in the human brain.
- In particular, the precuneus is believed to play a large role in integrating current internal experience with past memory and future plans and is also associated with subjective happiness.[62]
- The precuneus is connected to the insula and other sensory areas and the **anterior precuneus** specifically is a sensorimotor area receiving primarily proprioceptive sensory input.[63]

Prefrontal cortex (PFC)

- The *prefrontal cortex* is responsible for planning, reasoning, decision-making, and problem-solving,[64] i.e. processes involved in determining goals and means. It orchestrates our thoughts and can powerfully influence emotions through top-down inhibitory processes. The prefrontal cortex is strongly reciprocally innervated with the thalamus and influences how the thalamus filters incoming sensory information.[65]
- The **orbital and medial PFC (mPFC)** is the portion of the prefrontal cortex most closely tied to

Chapter 3

Diving deeper

Diving deeper into the prefrontal cortex

The **ventromedial PFC (vmPFC)** ⚓, a key node in the default mode network, is concerned with social cognitive processes related to oneself and others.[42,67] It is involved with "on-line decision-making that occurs when one is in the subjective emotional present of **embodied self-awareness** [my emphasis]."[68(p. 321)] It contributes to top-down inhibitory control of the amygdala and is closely connected with structures such as the insula that process interoceptive signals from the body.[69,70] A meta-analysis by Van der Werff et al.[27] found that the structure and volume of the vmPFC is consistently associated with resilience.

The **dorsomedial PFC (dmPFC)** is concerned with **conceptual self-awareness**, i.e. our self-judgments.[68] Hayes et al.[69,70] include the dACC under the umbrella of the dmPFC and state that these areas are associated with appraisal and evaluation. The dmPFC has been shown to be continually active during waking states and is thought to have an important role in the stream of thought that runs through most people's heads most of the time.[68]

The **dorsolateral PFC (dlPFC)** ⚓ is particularly known for its role in **working memory** tasks[64] and is closely connected with the hippocampus.[71] The dlPFC is the primary anchor for the **central executive (CE) network** of the triple network model (presented in Chapter 4), and is active with cognitive tasks requiring focused attention, decision-making, and problem-solving.[18,64]

limbic structures. The mPFC processes internal states relating to affect and motivation and is involved in long-term memory processing. The mPFC can suppress the HPA axis in response to stress by exerting inhibitory control over the emotional limbic system, including the amygdala. That is, it can help to reason away our fears. The mPFC includes the subcallosal cortex, anterior cingulate cortex, and medial frontal gyrus,[66] though the ACC is usually separated out in discussion, as in this book.

Posterior parietal cortex (PPC) ⚓

- The **posterior parietal cortex (PPC)**, located between the primary sensory cortex and visual cortex, is involved in attention and salience, saccadic eye movements and visual working memory, response selection, decisions to act on a sensory stimulus, planned movements, and spatial reasoning.[72,73] It plays an important role in sensorimotor and visual-motor integration[73,74] and works closely with the dlPFC to perform a variety of cognitive tasks requiring attention and working memory.[75]

Somatosensory cortex (aka sensory cortex)

- The sensory cortex is located in the postcentral gyrus of the cerebral cortex and is subdivided into regions that interpret body-based sensory information in greater detail and perform higher-order sensory processing. These regions consist of the **primary somatosensory cortex (S1)**, with subregions 1, 2, 3a, and 3b, and the **secondary somatosensory cortex (S2)**.[76] The sensory cortex is frequently represented by the sensory homunculus, a map that reflects the amount of space allotted to different parts of the body. Actually, a somatopic map exists within each of the subdivisions whereby neurons are lined up in columns that represent specific body areas, though the one in S2 is coarsely grained.[77] The sensory cortex receives its information from the thalamus and S2 also has two-way connections with the posterior insula.

The normal stress response and what goes wrong

Now that we have introduced the entire cast of actors for Chapters 3 and 4, we are ready to tell the story of how PTSD develops and the effects it has on the brain. We need to begin by describing the normal response to threat. As you will recall, all sensory information (except for some olfactory input) gets filtered through the **thalamus** before being sent to the **amygdala** and higher-level brain structures for further processing.[33] Using his famous high road/low road analogy,[4,78] LeDoux explained that thalamic information arrives in the amygdala more quickly than information processed in the cerebral cortex, for survival reasons; however, this information is fuzzy, lacking the detail that only the cerebral cortex can fill in (Figure 3.3). It is thus dubbed the "quick and dirty" low road. More specific information regarding the nature of the object or situation arrives just a bit later on the "slow but accurate" high road from the cerebral cortex, which has the potential to calm you down if the perceived threat turns out to be something innocuous (e.g. your brother, who you forgot had a key to your house, as opposed to a burglar).

Assuming for the purposes of our story that this is a genuine and serious threat, a full-blown stress response results. The amygdala triggers the **hypothalamus**, which responds to threat two ways:

- *Through the nervous system*, via the **locus ceruleus** and **periaqueductal gray** of the brainstem, which control the sympathetic branch of the **autonomic nervous system (ANS)**
- *Through the endocrine (hormonal) system*, by initiating a series of hormonal responses of the **HPA axis**.

Figure 3.4 depicts the series of events that occurs in the stress response, which will be discussed in more detail on the following pages.

The autonomic nervous system

The autonomic nervous system (ANS) is the branch of the peripheral nervous system that transmits signals from the central nervous system to all of the tissues and organs of the body except for the skeletal muscles; hence, it is often referred to as the "involuntary nervous system" as we typically have little control over it unless we are specifically trained in mind-body methods. Historically, the autonomic nervous system has been depicted as having two opposing branches, the **sympathetic nervous system (SNS)** (aka the fight–flight system) and the **parasympathetic nervous system (PNS)** (aka the rest and digest system) that operate similar to a see-saw: when one becomes more active, the other is less activated, and vice versa (Figure 3.5). However, this analogy is a bit misleading as it leaves one with the impression that when the SNS (or PNS) becomes more activated,

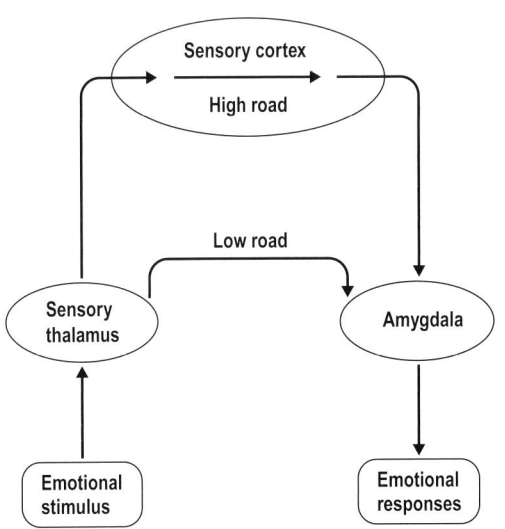

Figure 3.3

The low and high roads to the amygdala. Reproduced from LeDoux, *The Emotional Brain*, Simon and Shuster International, 1998,[78] with permission

Chapter 3

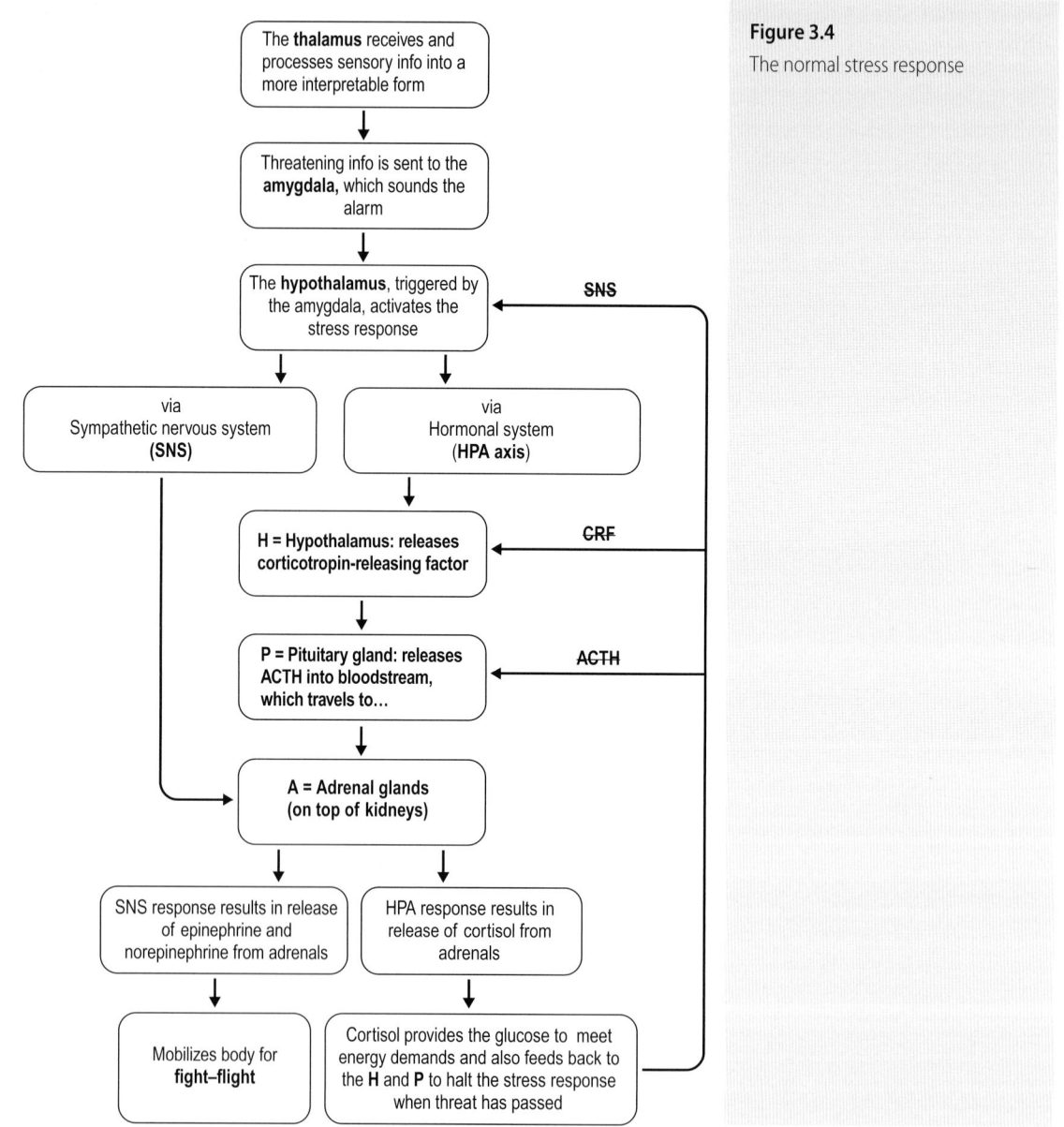

Figure 3.4
The normal stress response

it always does so as a whole body response and not just at a localized level.

In reality, these systems work together in a much more complex fashion, and usually at the same time to varying degrees, depending upon the activity, circumstances, and unique physiology of the individual, utilizing many different functional pathways to target particular organs and tissues.[79] In the face of a serious threat, however, there is typically an all-out,

Neurophysiology of PTSD

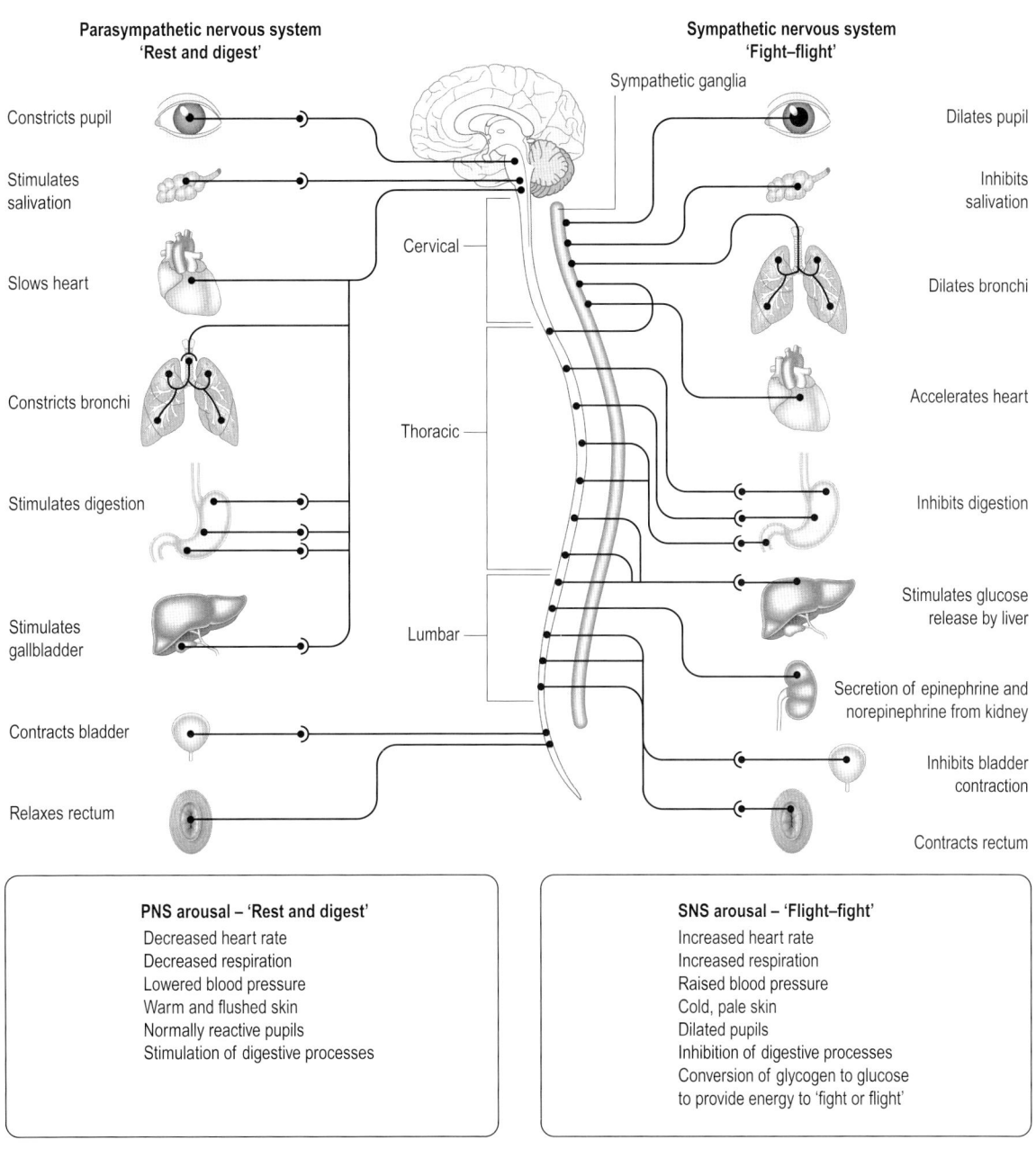

Figure 3.5
The autonomic nervous system

Chapter 3

no holds barred effort on the part of the SNS to deal with it, with an associated nosedive in activation of the PNS at the whole body level, so the simplified explanation is still highly useful as a teaching tool when discussing the stress response specifically. However, we do need to add one important layer of complexity to this schematic representation.

Porges' polyvagal theory

According to Porges' polyvagal theory,[6] there are actually three divisions to the autonomic nervous system (ANS): one sympathetic and *two* parasympathetic (see Figure 3.6). The parasympathetic system is divided into:

- a primitive **unmyelinated vagus**, which is responsible for both the freeze response during life threatening situations as well as homeostatic rest/digest functions during states of perceived safety
- a newer **myelinated vagus** that has evolved in mammals and regulates the organs above the diaphragm (including the heart and lungs). This system is closely neurophysiologically linked to the cranial nerves that are responsible for facial expression and contraction of the middle ear muscles. These cranial nerve functions facilitate language comprehension and have a direct role in modulating hyperarousal.[6]

According to Porges' theory, humans have a hierarchical response system to stress that is based on our evolutionary history. If we sense safety in the environment, we employ our most highly developed system of engagement, which is the **ventral vagal branch of the parasympathetic nervous system** (otherwise known as the *social engagement system*), which keeps us in a state of optimal arousal. This system can modulate the fight–flight system and its associated symptoms of hyperarousal (which has clinical implications in itself, to be discussed later). If we sense danger, the **sympathetic system** kicks in which is responsible for the *fight–flight response*. During the fight–flight reaction, the body releases high levels of adrenaline and cortisol to face the challenge. The heart races, the breath quickens, and blood is shunted to the extremities to aid in fighting or fleeing. Once the threat has passed,

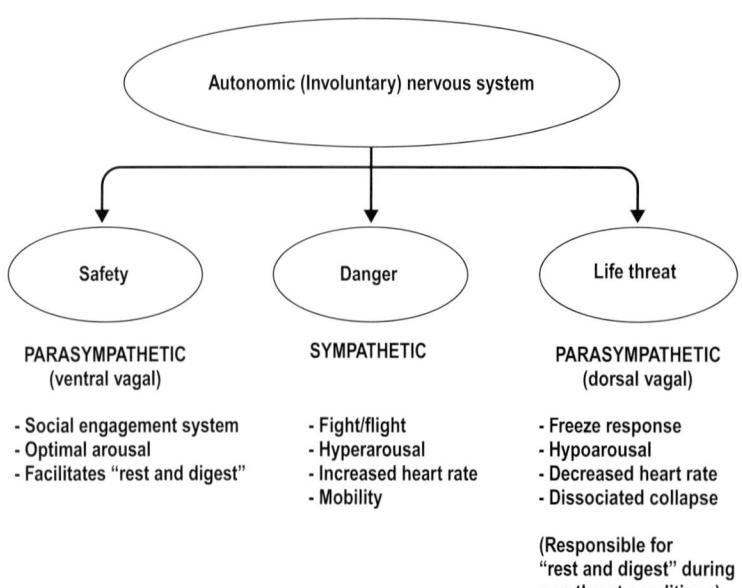

Figure 3.6

Porges' three divisions of the autonomic nervous system. Based on Stephen Porges, *Polyvagal Theory: Neurophysiological Foundations of Emotions, Attachment, Communication and Self-Regulation*[6]

Neurophysiology of PTSD

normally cortisol resolves the fight–flight response through a negative feedback loop to the brain, and then life resumes as usual with no lasting effects.

However, if we are in a situation of threat to life with no perceivable means of escape, we employ the most primitive branch of the parasympathetic nervous system, which is the **dorsal vagal system**, responsible for the **freeze** or immobility response and characterized by extreme hypoarousal. The freeze response is accompanied by an "opioid-mediated analgesia,"[6] presumed to spare animals from agonizing pain when being devoured by a predator.[1] According to Levine,[1] it is the residue of undischarged energy from the freeze response (i.e. **dorsal vagal response**) that is said to be responsible for the symptom of **dissociation**, in which the mind has lost its connection to the body and to the here and now of the present moment. In his highly recommended book, *Waking the Tiger*, he writes:[1]

> *Traumatic symptoms are not caused by the "triggering" event itself. They stem from the frozen residue of energy that has not been resolved and discharged; this residue remains trapped in the nervous system when it can wreak havoc on our bodies and spirits. The long-term, alarming, debilitating, and often bizarre symptoms of PTSD develop when we cannot complete the process of moving in, through, and out of the "immobility" or "freezing" state.*

Window of tolerance

Porges' polyvagal view of the ANS closely parallels the concept of the **window of tolerance**, often discussed in clinical treatment in reference to self-regulation.[80–82]

Normally, in everyday life, people fluctuate between higher and lower states of alertness but usually stay within the normal range, which is represented by the middle bar in Figure 3.7. However, when experiencing an extremely stressful or traumatic event, it is common for people to veer far outside the window of tolerance into hyperarousal, controlled by the sympathetic nervous system, or into hypoarousal, controlled by the dorsal vagal system.

Scaer[83] has observed that many individuals with PTSD cycle in and out of arousal and dissociation immediately following a traumatic event. However, Bremner[84] and Lanius[85] report that, over time, many become stuck in one of two general patterns of PTSD: approximately 70% fall into a flashback/re-living/hyperarousal PTSD group and 30% fall into a hypoaroused, dissociated PTSD group. Yet even in the hypoaroused state, there is an increase in circulating adrenaline, which still needs to be discharged, even though the heart and metabolic rate are slower while in this dissociated, dorsal vagal state.[1]

The HPA axis: the brain's hormonal response to stress

To explain how and why the undischarged energy from an unresolved fight–flight response wreaks havoc in the bodymind, we need to dive deeper into the brain's hormonal response to stress, the **hypothalamic-pituitary-adrenal (HPA) axis**. During the fight–flight response, the hypothalamus not only activates the sympathetic fight–flight branch of the nervous system, it also activates a chain of hormonal responses, which was briefly mentioned earlier. As with the sympathetic

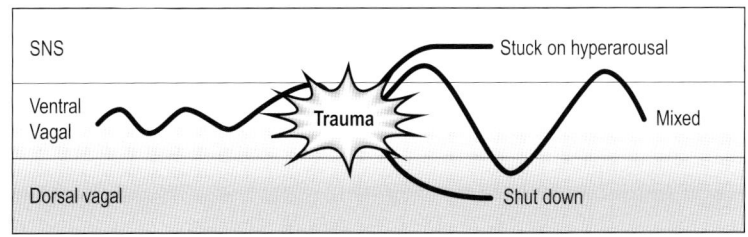

Figure 3.7
Window of tolerance[80–82]

Chapter 3

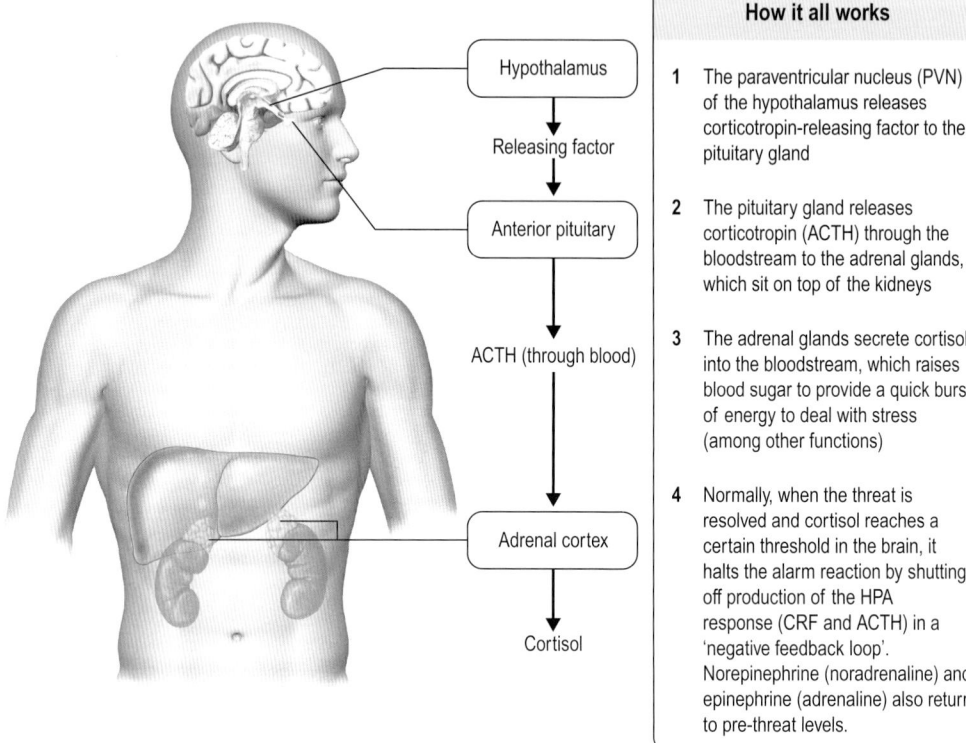

Figure 3.8
The HPA axis

nervous system, the HPA axis is always operating to maintain homeostasis with regard to many bodily functions and particularly with regard to an organism's energy needs. During our everyday lives, the HPA axis is kept in balance by the inhibitory influences of other brain structures on the ***amygdala***, including the ***anterior cingulate cortex***, ***dorsomedial*** and ***ventromedial prefrontal cortices***, and ***hippocampus***.[9,10] In turn, the ***thalamus***—when working well—helps to keep those structures humming sweetly along so they can perform their roles effectively.

The neurotransmitter serotonin (5-HT) also helps to regulate the HPA axis. Serotonin modulates stress and affective responses and is implicated in mood and anxiety disorders. Neurons that secrete serotonin originate in the dorsal and medial nuclei raphe in the brainstem and project to the amygdala, thalamus, hippocampus, prefrontal cortex, as well as many other areas of the brain, and interact with other neurotransmitters to help keep the nervous and hormonal systems regulated.[86,87] So for people who are not under chronic stress, experiencing other mental health issues, or dealing with the sequelae of prior traumas, this is the situation on the ground before the "tiger" shows up, as the person experiences the normal ups and downs of nervous system arousal but generally stays within the window of tolerance.

Neurophysiology of PTSD

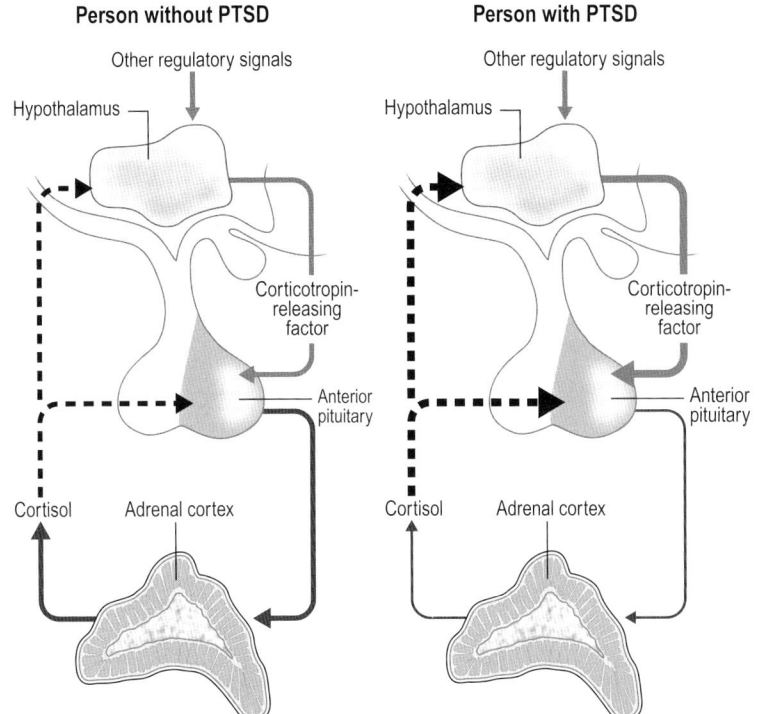

Figure 3.9
Failure of the negative feedback loop in PTSD

However, in response to a highly stressful or traumatic situation (the tiger), the normal HPA drive is greatly boosted to meet the challenge.[88] This HPA chain reaction is depicted in Figure 3.8 (see also Figure 3.4). The hypothalamus significantly increases its release of corticotropin-releasing factor (CRF), which stimulates the anterior pituitary to release more ACTH. The ACTH travels through the bloodstream to the adrenal glands (located on top of the kidneys), causing the adrenals to pump out a rush of cortisol. Cortisol produces various effects to promote short-term survival, one of which is to raise the blood sugar to provide energy to respond to the threat. Normally, once the threat has passed and the cortisol reaches a certain threshold in the brain, it **turns off** the fight–flight response, similar to how a thermostat works. This is called a negative feedback loop. Glucocorticoids (i.e. cortisol) do this by binding to receptors in the hypothalamus and pituitary.[89]

In PTSD, this negative feedback loop fails; this is believed to be due to exaggerated cortisol negative feedback at the level of the pituitary. This in turn causes the pituitary to release an insufficient amount of ACTH (Figure 3.9).[86] Studies have implicated pituitary glucocorticoid receptor binding as the likely mechanism, reflecting increased pituitary sensitivity to glucocorticoids.[89,90] So corticotropin-releasing factor continues to be released from the hypothalamus, reinforcing the hyperarousal and causing damage to brain structures. The failure of the HPA axis to resolve itself typically results in lower cortisol levels and higher norepinephrine and epinephrine levels in the bloodstream, which biases the nervous system toward hyperarousal and hypervigilance.[89] Interestingly, several genes involved in glucocorticoid signaling have been found to express differently in people with current PTSD, suggesting that some people may be genetically predisposed to developing PTSD.[20,90]

Chapter 3

The process described here occurs not only as a result of an acute traumatic event but also in response to chronic stress due to a prolonged HPA axis response.[89] In either case, the resulting chemistry changes in the brain can produce structural changes as well. For example, in animal studies, chronic activation of the amygdala due to prolonged stress leads to increased branching of neuronal dendrites in this brain structure while the same stressor leads to dendritic atrophy and de-branching of neurons in the hippocampus, consistent with the symptoms of PTSD.[91] This is also consistent with findings of increased/decreased activity levels and/or volumes in various brain structures as revealed by human neuroimaging studies, which will be discussed in the next chapter.

The effect of yoga on the ANS and HPA axis

From the foregoing discussion, it is clear that we need effective ways to help people better manage the neuroendocrine response to challenging stressors so they do not lead to such destructive brain changes and symptoms. Among the current treatments for PTSD, yoga is arguably among the best for this purpose and there is recent evidence to back up this assertion.

A systemic review and meta-analysis was conducted of 42 randomized/controlled trials that each included yoga (with or without mindfulness-based stress reduction), an active control group, and physiological measures of comparison. The researchers found that "practices that include yoga asanas [forms] appear to be associated with improved regulation of the sympathetic nervous system and hypothalamic–pituitary–adrenal system in various populations".[92 (abstract)] When compared to active control, yoga asana interventions (which varied between studies) were associated with reduced evening cortisol, waking cortisol, ambulatory systolic blood pressure, resting heart rate, high frequency heart rate variability, fasting blood glucose, cholesterol, and low density lipoprotein—all without any pharmaceutical intervention!

In the next chapter, we will discuss changes that tend to occur in specific brain structures and networks of individuals who have PTSD and compare them with brain changes that have been shown to occur following engagement in mindfulness-based practices, including yoga. The inverse relationship between the two provides yet another level of empirical support for the idea that yoga can be a potentially powerful healing modality for survivors of trauma.

Brain changes in PTSD and mind-body practices: the inverse relationship

[The brain is a] plastic, fluid, and ever-changing electrical/chemical/structural system that generates new synapses and neurons and discards old ones in response to sensory input from changes in the environment.
— Robert C. Scaer[1(p. 16)]

The last chapter ended in the midst of a crisis, with the failure of the stress response to resolve itself causing numerous changes in the chemistry of the brain. When someone is in this state of disrupted homeostasis, the hypothalamus continues to release CRF while cortisol, epinephrine, and norepinephrine continue to feed back to the brain from the bloodstream. These alterations in brain chemistry produce structural and activity changes in the brain that first came to light in the 1990s, following the invention of functional neuroimaging techniques.[2] The imaging processes used to investigate PTSD have included functional MRI (fMRI) and more recently, SPECT, PET, and MEG (see the text box **Brain imaging techniques** for explanations of these terms). In this chapter, we present the neuroimaging findings for PTSD as well as those for mindfulness-based practices to show the inverse relationship between them.

A word of warning: this chapter is quite complicated, to cater to those who wish to understand the brain science underlying PTSD at a deeper level. It is not necessary to fully understand this material to provide yoga therapy for traumatized individuals, so if you are not interested in diving so deep, please feel free to skim the chapter, focusing on the bold text.

Brain imaging techniques: The brain imaging techniques used in the studies presented in this chapter include the following:

Functional MRI (fMRI): Uses *blood oxygenation level dependent* (BOLD) signals to measure blood flow to various regions of the brain, which is a strong though indirect indicator of neuronal brain activity.[3]

Positron emission tomography (PET): Uses radiotracers to analyze regional cerebral blood flow (rCBF) or regional cerebral metabolic rate for glucose (rCMRglu, i.e. sugar metabolic rate) to determine approximate levels of neuronal activity in the brain. A dye containing the radioactive tracers is ingested, inhaled, or injected and is then absorbed by organs and tissues. The radiotracers decay, producing small particles called positrons, which are then detected by the scan.[4–5,7]

SPECT: Is a *single-photon emission computerized tomography* scan which uses a radioactive substance and a special camera to produce 3-D images in order to analyze the function of certain organs.[6,8] A SPECT scan differs from a PET scan mainly with regard

> to the type of radiotracers used.[7] Instead of measuring positrons, a SPECT scan measures gamma rays.
>
> *Magnetoencephalography (MEG)*: Uses magnetic fields outside the skull to record neural activity, which is spatially analyzed to determine the location and then superimposed on anatomical images, such as MRI, to measure both the structure and function of the brain.[9,10]

The neurocircuitry model of PTSD

While participants are in a scanner, they are often asked to look at images or listen to auditory stimuli that are emotionally laden and/or neutral, or are asked to perform specific cognitive tasks. With regard to PTSD, a brain pattern emerged early on from these experiments, referred to as the **neurocircuitry model of PTSD**.[11] The neurocircuitry model is characterized by the following:

> ↑ *Increased activation* of the **amygdala**, the brain's threat detector, which instigates "knee-jerk" emotional reactions in the face of danger or a significant challenge.
>
> ↓ *Decreased activation* of structures within the **medial prefrontal cortex**, which are involved in rational thought processes and allow us to "reason away" our fears.
>
> ↓ *Decreased activation* of the **hippocampus**, which puts situations into context based on personal memories.

According to the neurocircuitry model, there is **inadequate top-down control of the amygdala** by the medial prefrontal cortex and by the hippocampus, causing the amygdala to overreact in the face of threat.[12-14] The neurocircuitry model has been supported by numerous studies, including a large meta-analysis by Hayes et al.[15]

An important conductor behind the scenes

The **thalamus** is also implicated in PTSD, showing **decreased activation**.[16-21] For some puzzling reason it was not included in descriptions of the neurocircuitry model; however, the Sensory-Enhanced Yoga program has always included it in its own model since it pointed toward a bottom-up method for addressing the issue of PTSD. All sensory information (except for smell) is filtered through the thalamus before it reaches the amygdala, hippocampus, or cortical brain structures, including structures of the medial prefrontal cortex, so *if the thalamus is not working properly, the functioning of these other brain structures will likely be impacted*. As mentioned in Chapter 2, Jean Ayres'[22] sensory integration theory is based on the concept that carefully selected sensory input can influence the functioning of subcortical brain structures, including the thalamus, which in turn theoretically affects higher level brain functioning. So when occupational therapists see a sensory processing issue, they also see a potential remedy.

The concept that therapeutic sensory input, provided within the context of a mindful yoga practice, may help heal trauma is very compelling given the sensory processing symptoms of combat veterans. Even before neuroimaging studies were conducted, Krystal et al.[23] hypothesized that high levels of arousal during traumatic experiences may impair thalamic sensory processing, thus impacting transmission of sensory information to the frontal cortex, anterior cingulate gyrus, amygdala, and hippocampus. They further hypothesized that this would affect emotional behavior and possibly underlie dissociation and flashbacks. Bergmann[24] reported that altered thalamic functioning explains the cognitive and memory impairments, hemispheral imbalances, and disturbed somatosensory integration often seen in PTSD, the latter of which may be expressed as fragmented olfactory, auditory, taste, or visual memories or flashbacks, and/or kinesthetic/bodily sensations.

Comparison of the early model with mindfulness-based findings

Interestingly, as fast as neuroimaging studies were revealing brain structures implicated in **PTSD**, other neuroimaging studies were implicating the *same brain structures* with regard to **mindfulness-based practices**—but were showing a reverse pattern. Figure 4.1 depicts these early findings regarding brain changes often seen in PTSD (black arrows) and in mindfulness-based practices (gray arrows), illustrating this inverse relationship. To date, this depiction is still accurate, especially in terms of depicting the brain structures most consistently implicated in PTSD; however, there has subsequently been a proliferation of neuroimaging studies that have uncovered other relevant brain structures, subregions, and networks to add to the picture.

Expansion of the neurocircuitry model

As more research was conducted, the ***dorsal anterior cingulate cortex (dACC)*** and ***insula*** were gaining attention in the trauma field due to findings of altered activity in traumatized individuals.[8] The dACC has a strong bilateral connection with the amygdala and helps control the sympathetic and parasympathetic nervous systems by assessing safety vs danger within the environment, while the insula registers internal visceral sensations and is more involved with the somatosensory aspects of emotional states such as sympathetic arousal. These two brain structures work closely together to determine what is most important to attend to in the moment and to guide behavior to the most important actions.

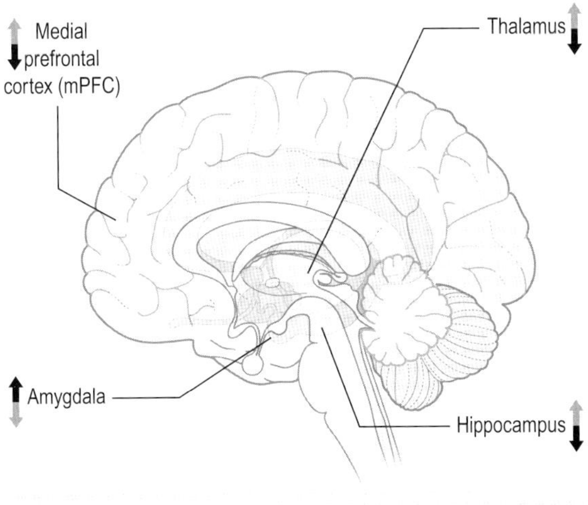

Most (though not all) neuroimaging findings showed hyperactivity of the dorsal anterior cingulate cortex (dACC) in PTSD, which was hypothesized to underlie the exaggerated fear learning seen in the condition.[14] This is in keeping with studies of healthy people which have generally shown activation of the amygdala and dACC during fear conditioning and activation of the vmPFC (in the medial prefrontal cortex) during fear extinction and extinction recall.[15,25] VanElzakker and colleagues characterize the relationship as follows:

> *Essentially, in PTSD the fear '**accelerators**' (amygdala and dACC) fail to turn off while the '**brakes**' (vmPFC and hippocampus) fail to turn on. These are the brain correlates to the increased psychophysiological responses during conditioning and extinction seen in PTSD.*[25(p. 15)]

With regard to the insula, study findings appeared inconsistent until Lanius and colleagues[26-29] discovered that different patterns of brain activation are elicited during the ***dissociative*** vs ***hyperaroused/re-experiencing*** states of PTSD. Hence, they proposed a dissociative subtype, which ultimately became incorporated into the DSM-5. The ***dissociative subtype*** is characterized by ***emotional overmodulation***, in which structures of the medial prefrontal cortex overinhibit the neural substrates of emotions, specifically the amygdala and insula, leading to detachment/numbing and other symptoms of dissociation (Figure 4.2). It is assumed that this is at least

Figure 4.1
Selected brain changes in PTSD and mindfulness-based practices: the early findings
Black arrows = typical direction of activation in PTSD
Gray arrows = typical direction of activation following mindfulness-based practices

Chapter 4

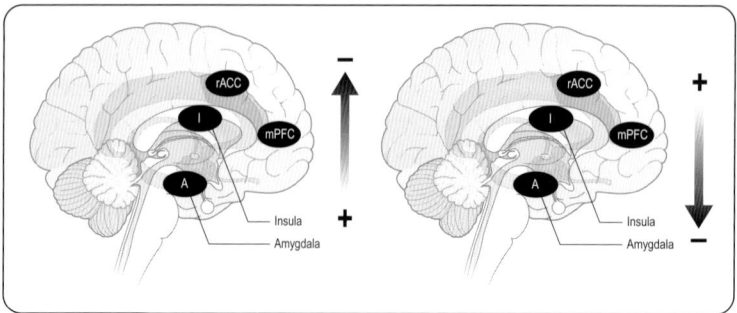

Figure 4.2
The two basic subtypes of PTSD

Hyperaroused/reexperiencing subtype	Dissociative subtype
Decreased activation of structures within the medial prefrontal cortex, especially the ventral-medial PFC (vmPFC) and rostral anterior cingulate cortex (rACC) results in undermodulation (inadequate inhibitory control) of lower brain centers implicated in emotional arousal	**Increased activation** of structures within the medial prefrontal cortex, especially the ventral-medial PFC (vmPFC) and rostral anterior cingulate cortex (rACC) results in overmodualtion (excessive inhibitory control) of lower brain centers implicated in emotional arousal
Increased activation of neural substrates of emotion (amygdala and insula) overtake the regulatory influences of the mPFC	**Decreased activation** of neural substrates of emotion (amygdala and insula) are overpowered by the regulatory influences of the mPFC
Either or both scenarios may result in symptoms of hyperarousal and re-experiencing	Either or both scenarios may result in symptoms of dissociation, including emotional detachment and numbing

Traumatised individuals can also cycle between these two states or fall along a sliding scale from hyperarousal to hypoarousal
(Lanius et al. 2002, 2005, 2010b; Hopper et al. 2007; Stark et al. 2015, p. 217)

partially a conscious process in the beginning, to avoid a state of overwhelm.[26,30] Decreased activation of the insula is also more associated with chronic PTSD.[31,32]

In contrast, the more common **hyperaroused/re-experiencing subtype** is characterized by emotional **undermodulation** due to failure of the medial prefrontal structures to inhibit limbic structures.[26,29] Increased right anterior insula activation is associated with this subtype. It is also recognized that traumatized individuals can cycle between these two states (Figure 4.2)[26,33] or fall anywhere along a continuum from hypoarousal to hyperarousal.[34(p. 217)]

The triple network model of PTSD

As the neurocircuitry model was being refined, a major paradigm shift was occurring in the field of brain imaging. The old adage "neurons that fire together, wire together" evolved into a more complex understanding that the brain is organized into coherent, large-scale functional networks. More advanced statistical techniques have enabled investigators to better understand the dynamics of networks, including the direction in which information is flowing.[35] Soon, three core global brain networks emerged from a field of many networks and were formulated by Menon[36] into the *"triple network model"* that has piqued the interest of trauma researchers and others in the mental health field.

Menon characterized these core networks as consisting of a collection of brain regions, referred to as "nodes," and the connections that link them. He stated that a network may become altered by either faulty node functioning or faulty connections between nodes, which explains why functional impairments may not only relate to the area of an actual brain lesion but also to a totally different part of the brain as a result of impaired connectivity with that lesion. Lanius and colleagues[33] have pointed out that alterations in these networks affect the balance between excitatory and inhibitory neural microcircuitry.

The three core global networks are considered to be the *salience network (SN)*, *central executive network (CEN)*, and *default network (DMN)*.[30,33,35-37] In brief:

- The **central executive network (CEN)** is anchored in the *dlPFC* and the *posterior parietal cortex (PPC)*, and is especially important for attention, working memory, decision-making, problem-solving, as well as other executive functions that enable people to exert cognitive control over their thoughts, emotions, and behavior. The clinical marker of dysfunction is *impaired cognitive function*.[30,33]
- The **salience network (SN)** is anchored in the *insula* and *dACC* and has extensive connectivity with the amygdala, thalamus, other subcortical regions associated with reward and motivation, as well as the hippocampus.[36,37] It registers, filters, and integrates interoceptive (body-based sensory input), autonomic, and emotional information and also assists other brain regions in generating appropriate behavioral responses to salient information through changes in sympathetic tone.[38] Clinical markers of dysfunction are *hyper- or hypoarousal* and *altered interoception*.[30,33]
- The **default mode network (DMN)** is anchored in the *posterior cingulate cortex (PCC)/precuneus* and *medial prefrontal cortex (mPFC)* and also involves the lateral parietal cortices. Van der Kolk has called the midline structures of the default mode network *"the Mohawk of self-awareness"*. [32(p. 90)] This network is active when engaged in task-irrelevant self-reflective thinking,[31,33] such as related to one's own emotions, social situations, personal memories, or thinking about the future.[30] The PCC is considered to play a particularly important role in the default mode network as it links past information with whatever is happening in the current situation and assesses its relevance to the self.[31] A clinical marker of dysfunction is *altered self-referential processing*.[30,33]

Typically, the central executive network (CEN) and default mode network (DMN) function independently from each other: when one is "on", the other is "off." In other words, the brain is either focused on a specific task at hand (CEN) or it is not (DMN). If it is not, it is said to be in default mode, perhaps daydreaming or ruminating over how a recent situation was handled. The salience network (SN) is responsible for switching between these other two networks based on what it considers to be most important (salient) in the moment. However, there are exceptions in which the CEN and DMN do cooperate together, such as when engaged in focused creative thought.[39]

The *right anterior insula*, a key node of the salience network, is thought to control the switching between the on-task/executive and off-task/default networks, while the *posterior parietal cortex* (PPC; a key node of

Chapter 4

the CEN involved in sensorimotor processing and attention) is hypothesized to play a large role in deactivating the default mode network, possibly via a gamma wave control signal from the insula.[33,35] This reflects back to the work of Ayres[22] and her sensory integration theory as we consider that an area of the brain involved in **sensorimotor processes** (PPC) may be the key that activates the **central executive network** involved in focused attention and learning. Yoga, being a rich sensorimotor activity—specifically one that facilitates mindfulness—may thus hold potential to facilitate cognitive development. Table 4.1 is a summary of the triple network model.

Lanius and colleagues[33] reported that individuals who have PTSD often show impaired ability to engage and switch between the central executive network and the default mode network, leading to altered functioning in all three networks, as expressed by the clinical

Table 4.1 The triple network model

Typically ...		
... the salience network (especially the anterior insula) serves as a switch between "on task" (CEN) and "off task" (DMN) behavior		
Central executive network (on task)	**Salience network** 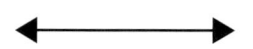 Mediates between externally directed attention and inwardly directed self-reflection based on what is important in the moment	**Default mode network** (off task)
• dlPFC -working memory -executive functions • PPC -sensorimotor processing -attention -may be key in deactivating the default mode network, based on signal from insula	• Anterior insula -interoceptive awareness/"feeling self" -the "switch" • Dorsal anterior cingulate cortex -evaluates safety vs danger and, with the insula, guides behavior to the most important actions	• mPFC -orchestrates thoughts -embodied self-awareness -regulates emotions • PCC and precuneus -self-reflection -integrates current internal experience with past memory and future plans -daydreaming
In PTSD ...		
... the networks are hyperconnected, leading to symptoms of hyperarousal/impaired concentration, re-experiencing, and intrusive thoughts		
Central executive network (on task)	**Saliency network**	**Default mode network** (off task)
Impaired ability to "switch" from the DMN to the CEN may result in **impaired concentration** and **intrusive thoughts** when trying to focus on daily living and work tasks	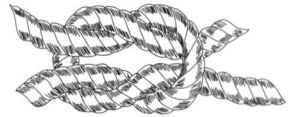 Rather than serve as a "switch," the SN is theorized to become hyperconnected to the other two networks, especially to the default network, effectively tying the networks more closely together	The hyperconnectivity between the SN and DMN may result in **hyperarousal and re-experiencing** during resting periods

Based on references Yehuda et al. 2015; Lanius et al. 2015; Sridharan et al. 2008; Menon 2011; Patel et al. 2012; Akiki et al. 2017; Bluhm et al. 2009; Sripada et al. 2012.

markers listed above.[40] In particular, **the default mode and salience networks show enhanced cross-network connectivity in individuals who have PTSD.**[41] Notably, increased connectivity of the default mode network with the thalamus, amygdala, and insula suggests inappropriate activation of the salience network while the person is resting, thus helping to explain the hyperarousal and hypervigilance seen in PTSD.[41] Then, when the person attempts to concentrate on a given task, intrusive thoughts may hamper the effort due to difficulty switching from the default mode to the central executive network. Lanius et al.[33] also cite over a dozen studies of PTSD demonstrating altered connectivity between brain regions **within** the salience network, including between the amygdala and insula.

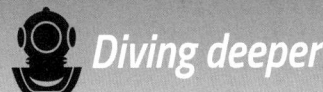
Diving deeper

A study by Nicholson et al.[42] details increased but differentiated connectivity patterns between subregions of the insula and amygdala for the hyper- and hypoaroused subtypes of PTSD. In both subtypes, they found increased connectivity between the left posterior insula and basolateral amygdala, and hypothesized that the basolateral amygdala connection "is altering posterior insula sensory/bodily representation functioning within PTSD patients." [42(p. 70)] In another study, Zhang et al.[43] identified a distinct disruption (weaker connectivity) between the left ventral anterior insula and the ACC in motor vehicle accident-related PTSD. They explained that impaired integration of interoceptive information (i.e. **visceral sensation**, mediated by the insula) with **emotional salience** (mediated by the ACC) would affect the formation of a "subjective bodily representation," leading to emotional dysregulation, circling us back to Damasio et al.'s[44] multidimensional body maps discussed in Chapter 3.

So how does the **triple network model of PTSD** relate to the **neurocircuitry model of PTSD** discussed earlier? In the neurocircuitry model, the medial prefrontal cortex fails to keep the amygdala under control, while in the triple network model, the anterior insula is considered key to switching between on-task and off-task networks and shows altered functioning in PTSD. Based on neuroimaging findings, it has been suggested that **increased activity in the anterior insula may be due to enhanced signaling from the amygdala,**[37] which creates one major link between these models. Both models also implicate the mPFC. Furthermore, in his controlled resting state fMRI study of traumatized adolescent girls, Cisler[45] found a direct correlation between the functional connectivity between the amygdala and mPFC and the functional connectivity between the limbic network and default mode network which, for him, raised the age-old chicken vs the egg question: does an aberrant relationship between the amygdala and mPFC affect the larger networks (salience/limbic and default) or does an aberrant relationship between the larger networks affect the relationship between the two nodes—amygdala and mPFC—that constituted the first consistent findings in PTSD and the basis of the neurocircuitry model?

A sensory hypothesis of PTSD[46]

While we do not yet know the answer to the above question, the following study provides insight into one of the things that may be happening at the neuronal level to cause the brain dysregulation in PTSD. Clancy et al.[46] used Granger causality analysis with EEG to investigate the sensory pathology of PTSD, that is, the neural basis for the threat-neutral sensory hyperactivity often seen in the condition. They evaluated **top-down executive inhibition** (that is, the ability of higher cortical structures to inhibit/modulate the lower brain structures) and **bottom-up sensory inhibition** (that is, the quality of sensory filtering as it moves from the sensory end organs to the higher

Chapter 4

levels of the brain), based on brain wave oscillations in the alpha band, during a resting state and passive picture viewing state.

To provide some background, it is thought that alpha waves may reflect concentrations of GABA, the inhibitory transmitter,[47–49] and also that alpha rhythms may "play a key role in filtering inputs to primary sensory neocortex and organizing the flow of sensory information in the brain."[50(p. 1)] Furthermore, studies have shown that thalamocortical interactions are required to generate alpha rhythms.[9,51–53]

Clancy et al.[46] compared 25 individuals with PTSD, 24 individuals with generalized anxiety, and 20 healthy control subjects. Among the results were the following:

- They found **intrinsic sensory hyperactivity in the PTSD group** as evident from reduced alpha power in the visual cortex (specifically the cuneus and precuneus) and deficient **bottom-up inhibition** (evident from reduced posterior to frontal Granger causality, i.e. reduced influence of the precuneus on the dACC), which correlated with hypervigilance and impulse control deficits. (The generalized anxiety disorder (GAD) control group did not differ from the healthy controls in these indices, ruling out generalized hyperarousal as the cause.)
- The PTSD group also showed **excessive gamma activity** in the frontal lobe, yet this was accompanied by decreased top-town inhibition, suggesting disconnection of frontal activity from top-down inhibition.
- The absence of a correlation between frontal gamma activity and top-down inhibition strongly suggests that the excessive frontal activity was related to passive reaction to sensory overflow as opposed to activating executive control mechanisms.

Based on these results, Clancy and colleagues proposed a "sensory hypothesis of PTSD: constant, spontaneous sensory hyperactivity leads to frontal overload and cognitive depletion, which breaks down executive control, fueling and perpetuating PTSD symptoms" (Figure 4.3).[46(p. 7)] They added that this presents an additional component to the neurocircuitry model of PTSD, forming a **sensory ➔ prefrontal cortex ➔ amygdala circuit** that is present even at rest.

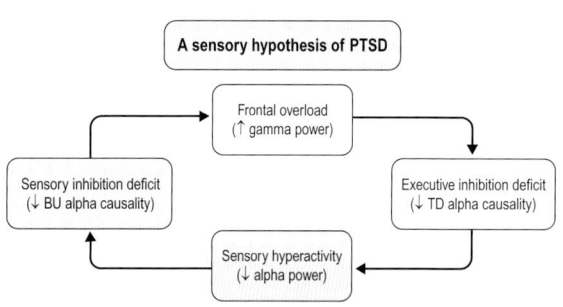

Figure 4.3

A sensory hypothesis of PTSD. Modified from Clancy et al., Restless 'rest': intrinsic sensory hyperactivity and disinhibition in post-traumatic stress disorder. Brain, 2017, Volume 140, p. 2041–2050, by permission of Oxford University Press

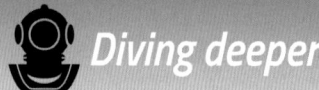

Falconer et al.[54] articulated a similar hypothesis following their fMRI study results, which presented a *go/no-go task* to test the inhibitory mechanisms in PTSD. While in the scanner, participants were asked to press a button when the word PRESS was written in green-colored type (on a black screen) but to refrain from pressing when PRESS was written in red-colored type. The participants with PTSD demonstrated increased inhibitory errors, reduced right cortical activation, and increased activation of striatal and somatosensory areas of the brain. The researchers reported, "Our finding of increased somatosensory cortical (postcentral gyrus), parahippocampal and visual cortical activation in patients with PTSD relative to control participants is consistent with a state of enhanced sensory processing during inhibitory control" (p. 418).

Another study by Huang et al.[9] used resting-state magnetoencephalography (MEG) to compare the brains of 25 active duty service members and veterans with PTSD with healthy volunteers. These researchers found *hypoactivity in the alpha band* from the bilateral precuneus and also identified additional alpha hypoactivity in the right superior frontal gyrus, bilateral dlPFC (R more than L) and bilateral sensorimotor cortices (R more than L) in the group with PTSD. With regard to the high-frequency bands (beta, gamma, and high-gamma), Huang et al. found hyperactivity from amygdala, hippocampus, posteriolateral orbitofrontal cortex, dmPFC, and insular cortex, and hypoactivity from the vmPFC and dlPFC. They reported that the alpha-band hypoactivity likely reflects reduced thalamocortical interactions, possibly leading to reduced functional inhibition in the hyperactive cortical areas.

Tying the Clancy et al. and "Diving deeper" studies in with the triple network model, the more alpha power a brain region has, the less functional connectivity it has with other brain regions,[9,51–53] so we can surmise that the CEN and DMN depend on alpha power to keep them separated from one another, as they should be. If we swing this statement around the other way, the *less* alpha power a brain area has, the more functionally connected it may be with other regions, which explains the excessive cross-network connectivity between the salience and default networks[55] and between the central executive and default networks.[56]

What does this have to do with yoga?

There is direct evidence to support the idea that yoga can help to repair these processes. In Kamei et al.'s[57] EEG study, experienced yoga practitioners exhibited increased alpha power in the frontal areas, suggesting that yoga improved the inhibitory mechanisms in the brain. Other studies have also found an increase in alpha and/or theta band power during meditative states (see reviews cited by Cahn[58]). More recently, Kerr et al.[50] discussed alpha rhythms in the context of a theoretical framework to explain the effectiveness of standardized traditional mindfulness practices, specifically mindfulness-based stress reduction (MBSR) and mindfulness-based cognitive therapy (MBCT). They proposed that the somatic focus of the practices, especially the body scan meditations, helps to modulate the local alpha rhythm in the primary sensory cortex through attention to bodily sensation (subtle changes in tactile and interoceptive feedback) which then "bootstraps to other thalamic-cortical circuits" (p. 3) to enhance filtering and prioritization of information flow throughout the brain. Finally, since alpha power may reflect GABA levels, it is also worth mentioning that Streeter and colleagues' controlled studies found a significant increase in thalamic GABA levels following yoga vs reading[59] or walking.[60]

PTSD and mindfulness: the inverse relationship

Recent years have seen an explosion of neuroimaging and EEG studies investigating PTSD and mindfulness-based therapies implicating more brain structures than depicted in the simple model in Figure 4.1. In creating a new model, there is also the confounding factor of having to account for two subtypes of PTSD, which are hypothesized to have mostly opposing effects on some brain structures. (This was resolved by planting an asterisk next to those brain structures in Figure 4.4 to cue you to swing the black arrow 180 degrees when considering the hypoaroused subtype.)

Chapter 4

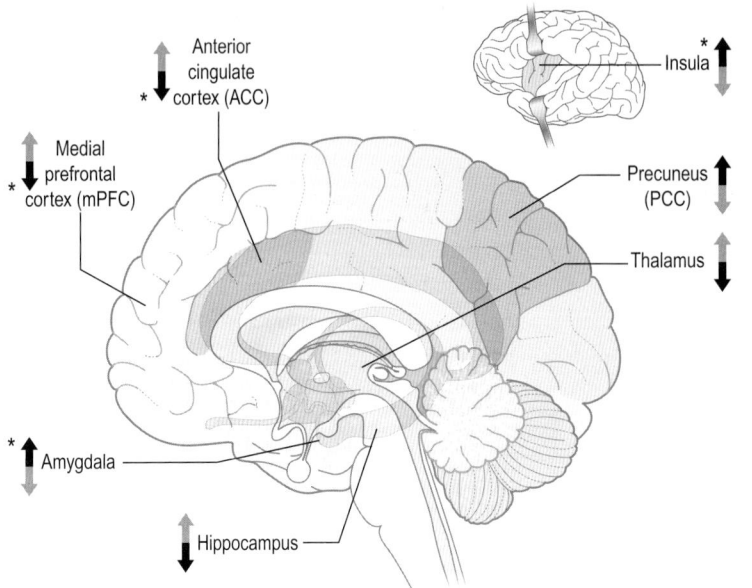

Figure 4.4

PTSD and mindfulness: the inverse relationship.

*Asterisks indicate structures that typically exhibit a reverse pattern of activation to that shown by the black arrows with regard to the dissociated subtype, according to Lanius et al.[26]

Black arrows = typical direction of activation in PTSD

Gray arrows = typical direction of activation following mindfulness-based practices

Furthermore, there are lots of nuances, such as parts of structures that activate while other parts do not; structures that activate more in PTSD than controls with regard to certain tasks but not other tasks; and structures that activate but in an abnormal manner, such as was just described in the sensory hypothesis of PTSD. Thus, it may be impossible to create a 100% accurate model easy enough for the average person (I include myself here) to understand.

What the new model *can* depict is nonetheless remarkable: that even given the expanded cast of characters, *most* of the brain structures currently implicated in *most* studies of PTSD still, on average, show an *opposite activation pattern* in response to mindfulness-based practices (see Figure 4.4 and Table 4.2). The new model incorporates almost all of the key seed nodes from the triple network model but is still not complete; some structures implicated in PTSD are not included here because they are far less discussed in the literature, and the figure does not separate out subregions of the included structures. In fact, from reviewing many studies, it seems like almost every brain area has been implicated in PTSD by one or another. Here, the most consistent findings are presented.

The final caveat is the figure does not depict changes in functional connectivity between brain structures (an attempt to do so produced a "rat's nest"!). Nonetheless, the mere fact of the ***inverse relationship between PTSD and mindfulness states in a multitude of brain structures*** adds strong support to the existing clinical research showing that mindfulness-based practices hold great healing power for PTSD. But not just any mindfulness practice, because the evidence is now pretty clear that, in PTSD, ***the road back to the here and now runs through the body***. As has been stated by van der Kolk[32,61] and by many other trauma experts, trauma is held in all cells of the body and must be released by the body for complete healing to occur. Meditation techniques that emphasize attention focusing through top-down cortical control without addressing the body are usually too difficult for those who have PTSD and can be emotionally overwhelming. Yoga (or another appropriate mind/body modality) is often a necessary stepping stone to draw traumatized individuals away from their intrusive thoughts and back into fully sensing bodies and to the "here and now" of present moment awareness.

Table 4.2 presents many of the neuroimaging findings of PTSD related to specific brain structures, followed by findings from neuroimaging studies of mindfulness practices, most of which incorporated at least some yoga. Many of the mindfulness neuroimaging studies investigated the effectiveness of the eight-week mindfulness-based stress reduction (MBSR) protocol; thus, this program is heavily represented here. However, studies investigating other forms of yoga and meditation, such as kundalini yoga, Iyengar yoga, trauma-sensitive yoga, vipassana meditation, and insight meditation are also included. The MBSR program includes a body scan, hatha yoga, and seated meditation, and thus falls within the definition of a yoga program. In fact, the yoga practice portion of MBSR was significantly associated with several aspects of mindfulness as well as well-being, perceived stress levels, and several psychological symptoms, in a large participant rating study.[62]

Implications of brain studies for yoga practice

Limbic findings

A yoga program carefully designed to reduce hyperarousal may help to repair the destructive neurochemical processes that are responsible for the structural and functional changes in the limbic system. The most powerful means of reducing hyperarousal is through control of the breath, since respiration is typically the only function of the autonomic nervous system that can be controlled by the conscious mind. Yogic breathing practices have been shown to increase parasympathetic activation and heart rate variability, and are theorized to improve GABA levels, which can, in turn, influence brain structures implicated in PTSD to reduce symptoms of the condition.[63] Preliminary evidence also suggests that quiet, natural breathing actively promotes oscillatory synchrony in limbic areas and may thus improve information processing in higher cortical brain areas.[64]

However, voluntarily controlling the breath can sometimes be challenging if one is in an acutely stressed state; combining breath work with sensorimotor input can often be more accessible and particularly powerful—such as by coordinating simple movements with the breath. Carefully chosen sensory input (e.g. deep touch pressure, enhanced proprioceptive input, slow rhythmic movements, and neutral warmth) within the context of yoga is theorized to significantly reduce hyperarousal by enhancing inhibitory mechanisms within the brainstem and thalamus. This, in turn, should help to normalize (reduce) the amount of sensory input reaching the amygdala and higher cortical centers, including the insular, sensory, and visual cortices, thereby reducing hypervigilance and sensory hypersensitivities which drive hyperarousal. Through this process, the salience network becomes disentangled from the default mode (resting state) and central executive (working state) networks, thus helping to draw the mind back to the present moment.

Thalamic findings

The thalamus is the last relay station before sensory input reaches the higher cortical levels and also plays a large role in orchestrating connectivity within and between brain regions.[65,66] Therefore, it needs to function properly for higher brain centers to effectively process information and do their jobs. As discussed in this chapter, alpha waves likely reflect inhibitory neural processes (usually involving GABA as a transmitter) and are generated by corticothalamic interactions, so manipulating thalamic functioning via carefully controlled therapeutic sensory input could conceivably help to correct imbalances between excitatory and inhibitory mechanisms within brain structures and between global brain networks. Furthermore, when therapeutic sensory input is presented within the context of enhanced mindfulness to sensation, such as within Sensory-Enhanced Yoga, the therapeutic effects are accentuated through the combination of both bottom-up and top-down processes of integration. Finally, the thalamic link (i.e. nucleus reuniens) between the mPFC and hippocampus is crucial for the consolidation of memories into long-term storage, so improving function of the thalamus may hypothetically facilitate that process.

Insula findings

Yoga practices that help traumatized individuals befriend their bodies can be expected to be particularly helpful for healing PTSD.[32,61] Lanius et al.[33] hypothesized that body scan meditations in particular, which are designed to increase interoceptive awareness (a primary role of the insula), could be especially beneficial for those who tend toward hypoarousal/dissociation, while they could potentially exacerbate symptoms of hypervigilance and hyperarousal in those demonstrating emotional undermodulation.

On the other hand, Villemure and colleagues[67] found in their study of the effect of yoga on pain that half of the treatment participants thought regular practice would increase *awareness* but also *tolerance* of pain, make the pain more neutral, and/or reduce reactivity to it, thus allowing more control over it. Gard and colleagues apparently agreed, explaining, "Mindfulness practice encourages practitioners to take a meta-cognitive view of their experience, to notice the experience without judging it or modifying it and is thus a form of self-regulation."[68(p. 7)] They explained that yoga allows one to practice mindfulness in this manner, described as "witness consciousness."

In my own professional experience, body scans can help a person shift from an externally to a more internally oriented focus, thereby reducing hypervigilance to external stimuli. As mentioned in Chapter 2, traumatized individuals may be more oriented to external (environmental) or internal (bodily) cues depending upon the nature of the trauma, so their experience of body scans may vary accordingly. It is thus important to be observant and to seek feedback from your clients regarding their own experience.

Cortical findings

Yoga is a powerful mind-body discipline shown to help draw a person back into the **present moment**. This process involves activation of the prefrontal cortex, which is often de-activated by trauma. The prefrontal cortex also plays a large role in **top-down** processing, that is, it can powerfully regulate lower level brain structures including the amygdala. Sensory-Enhanced Yoga promotes bottom-up activation of the prefrontal cortex and simultaneously capitalizes on it through the use of top-down strategies including positive suggestions, guided meditations, and/or inspirational readings, making the practice that much more powerful. The imbalances often seen in the left and right hemispheres of individuals who have PTSD may conceivably correct themselves in the process, since the enhanced inhibitory mechanisms/alpha power generated by a carefully designed yoga program should help to disentangle the central executive, default, and salience networks from each other. Thus, intrusive thoughts and memories (generated by a hyperactive right hemisphere) should interfere less often with working memory processes (in the left hemisphere).

In summary, we now know that the human brain is highly plastic and changes in response to everything we say, do, feel, and experience. As fast as brain researchers are adding to the empirical knowledge base regarding how the brain works, therapists in the helping professions are learning how to manipulate brain processes to promote healing from a variety of conditions. Unfortunately, PTSD is one of the more debilitating of mental health conditions and can affect the brain like a sledgehammer, while certain mindfulness-based practices, including yoga, can exert a highly positive influence on many of the same brain structures affected by PTSD. This points to the huge potential mindfulness-based practices hold for addressing this condition, which will be further described in the chapters ahead.

Part 1 of this book provided an overview of PTSD as well as detailed information on the symptoms,

Brain changes in PTSD and mind-body practices: the inverse relationship

underlying neurophysiology, and brain changes that can occur as a result of this often-debilitating condition. In Part 2, we turn to the nature of the traumas that can cause PTSD and how these specific types of traumatic events can impact individuals, families, communities, institutions, and even entire countries. These chapters are written by contributing authors who are pioneers in using yoga and other mind-body practices as tools for healing certain forms of trauma. They will provide both an academic as well as a personal perspective on their chapter topics, by sharing their own professional experiences or the reflections of some of the trauma survivors they interviewed who have found yoga to be instrumental in their recovery. These experts will also present key factors to consider when developing and implementing yoga programs for survivors of the particular form of trauma. It is a great honor to have these amazing experts share their own insights in this book, and I am confident you will gain a lot from the learning experience.

Table 4.2 Neuroimaging studies of PTSD and mind-body practices

Brain structure	Effect of PTSD on brain activity and structure	Effect of mind-body treatment on brain structure**
Amygdala The **amygdala** constantly surveys the environment (as filtered through the thalamus and cerebral cortex) and assigns emotional significance to everything coming through the senses, whether positive or negative[14] The amygdala plays a major role in the **detection** of threats and control of the body's **response** to threats.[82,83] It is the **trigger** that activates the hypothalamic–pituitary–adrenal (HPA) axis of the stress response[84]	Most studies and meta-analyses show amygdala **hyperactivity*** in PTSD, in both finished and on-going threat[85] * 15,17,37,85,86 However, a hypoactive region lies at the border between the dorsal amygdala and anterior hippocampus that may relate to the emotional numbing and dissociation found in PTSD[17] Most single studies and meta-analyses have shown **reduced amygdala volumes in PTSD***, including a large study comparing OIF/OEF combat veterans with and without PTSD.[88] Smaller amygdala volume has been shown to be a risk factor for PTSD[86] and it is also found in trauma-exposed non-PTSD controls.[175] * 86,87,88,175	Various studies have shown **decreased activity*** in the amygdala following a mindfulness intervention * 107,108,109,110 Of note: Herwig et al.[110] found that directing attention towards the current experience of emotions and bodily sensations without explicit behavioral control reduced activity of the amygdala and increased activation of the dmPFC, vlPFC, ACC, and R insula as compared with controls who engaged in cognitive reflection Reductions in perceived stress following eight weeks of mindfulness-based stress reduction correlated positively with **decreases in right basolateral amygdala gray matter density**[111]
Hippocampus The **hippocampus** is involved in memory storage and formation, and assigns emotional meaning, time, and spatial context to our memories. It is involved in complex cognitive processing; is the most active structure in encoding and recalling traumatic memories; and plays a key role in regulating the HPA axis [92,177]	The majority of studies have produced evidence of **decreased activity levels in the hippocampus*** or diminished neuronal integrity of the hippocampus in PTSD,[90] which is thought to relate to the impaired memory, contextual processing, and regulation of the HPA axis seen in those who have PTSD[14,17] * 17,34,85,91,92,93,94 **Decreased hippocampus volumes*** are commonly seen in PTSD, believed to be both a predisposing and acquired feature[95,96] * 76,87,89,97,98,99,100,101,102,103,104,105,106	Studies have shown **increased hippocampal activation in meditators**[112,113] Studies have also found **increased gray matter density** in the right hippocampus[114] and left hippocampus[115] in MBSR meditators and **increased gray matter volume** in meditators[116] **Increased gray matter volume of the L hippocampus** was found in hatha yoga meditation practitioners vs controls and the effects were dose dependent[117]

continued

Chapter 4

Table 4.2 Continued

Brain structure	Effect of PTSD on brain structure	Effect of mind-body treatment on structure**
Thalamus The thalamus filters and distills sensory information before relaying it to the amygdala and appropriate areas of the cerebral cortex for further processing[66,82,118] A recent theory posits that the thalamus controls functional connectivity within and across cortical regions[65]	Several studies have shown **decreased thalamic activation and/or reduced regional cerebral blood flow (rCBF)*** in PTSD vs controls * 16,17,18,19,20,21 Police officers exposed to traumatic events who had higher re-experiencing scores were found to have **reduced thalamus volumes** (among other findings)[122] **Lower GABA levels have been found in the L thalamus** in veterans with PTSD[123]	*Increased cerebral blood flow in the thalamus* was shown following one hour of meditation by eight Tibetan Buddhist meditators[130] Following 10 weeks of trauma-sensitive yoga, *increased activation of R thalamus* was shown in six PTSD subjects as compared with two matched controls, along with significant PTSD symptom reduction[32] Streeter et al.'s studies found *increased thalamic GABA levels* following yoga vs reading[59] or walking[60]
Insula The **insula** aids in the subjective sense of the inner body and body states; judges the degree of pain; assists in processing vestibular (movement) sensations; pairs emotion to bodily sensations, giving rise to conscious feelings; and has a role in regulating the autonomic nervous system[119,120,121] It is also thought to mediate between externally oriented attention and self-reflective functioning[30]	*Increased activation of anterior insula* is associated with emotional undermodulation (hyperarousal/re-experiencing) while *decreased activation* is associated with emotional overmodulation (emotional detachment) in PTSD*. Many cycle between these extremes. PTSD-related flashbacks** are also associated with *increased activation of the insula* * 29,33,124,125 ** 126,127,128 In general, studies show *increased activation of the anterior insula in acute PTSD* and *decreased activation in severe, chronic PTSD*.[31,32] The latter is attributed to a "shut down" state[32] A study revealed *lower insula GABA* in PTSD than in controls[129] ***Decreased gray matter thickness and volume*** of the insula has also been shown in PTSD* * 102,123,135–144	Nine OIF veterans with PTSD treated with MBSR showed **decreased insula function** in response to traumatic reminders[131] *Greater cortical thickness and gray matter density of R anterior insula* was shown in meditators[114,132] *Increased gray matter of the insula* is also associated with yoga experience consisting of postures, breathing, and meditation* * 117,133 *Increased activation of the R insula* was found in MBSR course completers vs novice meditators[134] and following trauma-sensitive yoga in those with chronic PTSD vs controls[32] Studies have also associated *increased activation of the insula* with meditation-related anxiety relief[145] and meditation-related pain attenuation[109,146,147]

continued

Table 4.2 Continued

Brain structure	Effect of PTSD on brain structure	Effect of mind-body treatment on structure**
Anterior cingulate cortex The **anterior cingulate cortex (ACC)** is strongly connected to both the limbic system and the prefrontal cortex and is thus thought to play an important role in emotional regulation[148] and reward-based learning[149] The **dorsal ACC (dACC)** is involved in evaluating safety vs danger and the expression of fear responses while the **rostral ACC (rACC)** is believed to have a top-down inhibitory influence on the amygdala; that is, it can help keep the amygdala in check[150]	Most studies and meta-analyses have revealed **decreased activation*** of the **ACC** in PTSD, mostly in regions (pgACC and sgACC) that fall within the **rostral ACC** * 17,34,37,90,151–154 Decreased activation of the **rostral ACC** is associated with **emotional undermodulation**, while increased activation of the **rostral** ACC is associated with **overmodulation**[26,29,155] Most studies have found **increased activation*** of the **dorsal** region of the **ACC**, i.e. **dACC**, which, along with the amygdala, has been shown to be a predisposing risk factor for PTSD associated with fear expression. However, decreased activation of the dACC has also been found in PTSD,[17,54] possibly due to testing different sub-regions, which have different roles (see Etkin et al.,[150] for an excellent review) ** 8,14,15,37,86,156,157,158,159,160 Single studies and meta-analyses have found **smaller volumes in the anterior cingulate cortex*** as a whole and in specific sub-regions, including the rACC and pgACC, as compared to non-exposed and trauma exposed healthy individuals. A twin study by Kasai et al.[141] produced evidence that decreased volume of the pgACC in their PTSD group was acquired, not inherited * 84,87,89,102,141,144 Studies have demonstrated **small metabolic ratios** of the cingulate gyrus and **decreased volume of the anterior cingulate gyrus** in PTSD[87,144]	*Increased bilateral activation in the rACC* and dmPFC was found in 15 Vipassana meditators (mean practice 7.9 years, 2 hours daily) vs matched controls[113] A study found *increased pgACC activation in Kundalini meditators*[112] *Increased cerebral blood flow in the cingulate gyrus* was shown following one hour of meditation by eight Tibetan Buddhist meditators[130] OIF veterans with PTSD treated with MBSR improved CAPS and mindfulness scores compared with an active control group. They also showed *increased ACC*, IPL, decreased insula and decreased precuneus function in response to traumatic reminders[131] Meditation-related anxiety relief was found to be associated with *activation of the ACC*, vmPFC, and anterior insula in healthy individuals[145] *Greater cortical thickness of R dorsal ACC* has also been shown in meditators[161]

———— continued ————

Table 4.2 Continued

Brain structure	Effect of PTSD on brain structure	Effect of mind-body treatment on structure**
Prefrontal cortex The **orbital and medial PFC** process internal states relating to affect and motivation and are involved in long-term memory processing. The mPFC is able to inhibit the HPA axis and amygdala in response to stress. The **ventromedial PFC (vmPFC)** is involved with embodied, present-moment decision-making;[72] emotion-labeling based on interoceptive signals (is closely connected with the insula); and exerts top-down inhibitory control over the amygdala[15] The **dorsomedial PFC (dmPFC)** is involved with conceptual self-awareness (including our self-judgments and reflective self-awareness) and has an important role in one's "stream of thought"[72] The **dorsolateral PFC (dlPFC)** is well known for its role in **working memory** tasks[73] and is closely connected with the hippocampus.[74] The dlPFC is active with cognitive tasks requiring focused attention, decision-making, and problem-solving[36,73]	Medial prefrontal cortex dysfunction has frequently been observed in PTSD imaging studies and is associated with deficits in executive functioning[54,71] Studies on PTSD show a reciprocal relationship between medial prefrontal cortex and amygdala function, i.e. increased activation of the amygdala is associated with decreased activation of the medial pre-frontal cortex, and vice versa, especially with respect to the orbito-frontal and ventromedial PFC[13,14,16] Meta-analyses show **hypoactivation of the ventromedial PFC**[15,17] and **dmPFC**[15] in PTSD, while a study of combat veterans found reduced spontaneous neural activity in the **dlPFC**[75] Significantly **decreased cortical thickness of the L and R dlPFC** was found in soldiers with PTSD[76] **A note on hemispheral differences in PTSD** In response to traumatic recall: • Subjects w/ PTSD: show markedly increased activation of **right** hemisphere* • Subjects w/o PTSD: show markedly increased activation in the **left** hemisphere * This may explain why those who have PTSD tend to recall traumas visually (via re-experiencing or flash-backs) while those without PTSD recall traumas through verbal narratives[77] * 77,78,79,80,81	Meditation-related anxiety relief was shown to be associated with activation of the anterior cingulate cortex, **ventromedial prefrontal cortex** and anterior insula[145] **Increased activation of R dmPFC** post-yoga treatment was shown in six chronic PTSD subjects as compared with two matched controls[32] **Increased activation of the dorsal medial frontal lobe** was found in new yoga practitioners following a 12-week Iyengar yoga training[107] Directing attention towards the current experience of emotions and bodily sensations without explicit behavioral control reduced activity of the amygdala and **increased activation of the dmPFC, vlPFC**, ACC, and R insula as compared with controls who engaged in cognitive reflection[110] A study has shown **increased dlPFC activation** in Kundalini meditators[112] **Greater gray matter thickness of prefrontal cortex** was shown in Insight meditators[132] **Greater gray matter volume in orbito-frontal cortex** was shown in meditators[116] **Increased cerebral blood flow in the inferior and orbital frontal cortex and dlPFC** was shown following one hour of meditation by eight Tibetan Buddhist meditators[130]

— continued —

Table 4.2 Continued

Brain structure	Effect of PTSD on brain structure	Effect of mind-body treatment on structure**
Postcentral gyrus (somatosensory cortex) The "**sensory cortex**" (in the **post-central gyrus**) is subdivided into regions that interpret body-based sensory information in greater detail and perform higher-order sensory processing.[162] It is represented by the **sensory homunculus**, a map in each region reflecting the space allotted to different parts of the body[163]	A meta-analysis showed **greater activity in the R post-central gyrus** in the PTSD group vs controls[37] During an inhibitory control task, patients with PTSD demonstrated **increased activity of the post-central gyrus** vs controls[54] An fMRI study of 24 soldiers with PTSD vs 23 control soldiers found **decreased volumes of the L and R post-central gyrus** in the soldiers with PTSD[76]	*Increased postcentral gyrus activation* was found in Kundalini yoga meditators[112] *Increased gray matter of the post-central gyrus (or primary somato-sensory cortex)* has been correlated with current weekly yoga practice[67] and with yoga vs walking or wait-list controls in early psychotic patients.[167] A trend toward significance was also shown in Insight meditators[132]
Posterior cingulate cortex (PCC) and precuneus (PrCC) The **posterior cingulate cortex** and **precuneus** form the caboose of the **midline "Mohawk" structures**[32] that form the default mode network. The PCC and PrCC are important for conscious information processing and self-reflection Vogt and Laurys[164] reported that the PCC/PrCC has the highest level of glucose metabolism in the human brain and that the anterior thalamus drives the PCC/PrCC The precuneus is connected to the insula and other sensory areas; the **anterior precuneus** is a sensorimotor area receiving primarily proprioceptive sensory input[171]	Studies have reliably found **increased activation of the precuneus*** in PTSD. A large resting state fMRI study found that the DMN regions of combat veterans with PTSD were less integrated into the whole brain network except for the **precuneus**, which showed increased integration in the whole brain network.[165] Based on additional evidence, they hypothesized that altered PrCC functioning "may potentially be related to altered memory-and self-referential processes, such as memory deficits, intrusions or flashbacks" (p. 307) * 17,37,159,165,166 *Decreased cortical thickness in the precuneus* was found in veterans returning from Iraq or Afghanistan who were diagnosed with PTSD (n=15) vs those who did not meet the diagnostic criteria (using the CAPS; n=15) and healthy community controls (n=15)[143] *Increased connectivity of the PCC with the R and/or L amygdala*[26,33,172] *or with the anterior insula*[173] have been found to predict who would later develop PTSD or the severity of PTSD symptoms. Hippocampal-PCC connectivity findings have been inconsistent *(e.g. compare Malivoire et al. and Miller et al.)*[174,175]	Studies have shown **decreased activity*** and an **increase in gray matter volume**** of the **precuneus** in response to yoga and/or meditation practices. In the Bremner et al. study, OIF veterans with PTSD were treated with MBSR; they also showed improved CAPS and mindfulness scores compared with an active control group. Simon et al. was a single cohort study of nine participants who undertook a two-week Kundalini yoga/meditation course *168, 131, 169 **170, 133 A recent meta-analysis of[78] PET and fMRI meditation studies revealed **decreased activity of the PCC**[176] *Increased gray matter concentration* has also been found in the PCC following eight weeks of mindfulness meditation practice (MBSR)[115]

PART 2

The many faces of trauma

Combat stress management

Patricia Lillis

Combat comes at a cost—it comes at a moral cost. "The good news is that in the safety of safe, caring relationships, to both human beings and to our God, people can find forgiveness and healing for moral wounds. They don't have to be mortal wounds." — Chaplain (Col.) Thomas Waynick, quoted by Doyle[1(p. 18)]

Introduction

Combat and operational stress reaction (COSR) is a term used by the Department of Defense (DoD) to describe the wide range of mental and behavioral symptoms that can occur in response to combat or heavy operational pace. The effects of battlefield stress on military personnel have been recognized throughout history. Older terms have described the syndrome as "irritable heart," "soldier's heart" (US Civil War), "shell shock" (WWI), "psychoneuroses," "battle fatigue" (WWII and later), among others.[2-3] The term "combat stress reaction" was officially adopted by the DoD in 1999 and just a few years later was revised to "combat and operational stress reaction" or COSR,[4] in order to include symptoms of stress experienced by individuals experiencing a non-combat high operations tempo and those still stateside in high stress jobs, such as Air Force drone operators.

Individuals can be described as experiencing COSR independently of whether or not they meet criteria for a psychiatric disorder. The military does not consider COSR to be a psychiatric or medically diagnosable condition and, unlike PTSD, it is not included in the DSM manual. The Defense Centers for Excellence for Psychological Health and Traumatic Brain Injury[5] differentiates combat stress from PTSD by explaining the former as a normal reaction to combat experiences that can be addressed through some basic self-care strategies (e.g. rest, good diet, connection with others) and the passage of time. In contrast, PTSD is diagnosed when a threshold of symptoms is reached in four cluster areas and persists for at least a month. However, the DCoE cautions that if appropriate steps for self-care are not taken, the symptoms of combat stress could evolve into PTSD, depression, and/or substance abuse.

Prevalence of COSR

There is little information on the prevalence of COSR or the proportion of service members who might experience this in combat, but it is felt to be very high. Costanzo and colleagues[6] studied 78 service members who had recently returned from their deployments to Iraq or Afghanistan, and found that sub-threshold PTSD (which falls under the broader category of COSR) is much more common than full PTSD and presents similar functional impairments across several domains. Only four participants were excluded from the original cohort of 85 service members due to meeting criteria for full PTSD. In contrast, 30 met criteria for increased severity of sub-threshold symptoms and 48 met criteria for decreased severity of sub-threshold symptoms. As one might

Chapter 5

expect, those who presented with increased severity of symptoms experienced greater levels of anxiety and depression and a significantly heightened fear response (e.g. increased startle response and heart rate) to danger cues than those with low severity of symptoms. What is particularly striking about this study is the participants in both groups exhibited physical signs of fear despite the cognitive ability to discriminate between danger and safety. According to the study authors, these findings support the idea that symptoms of hyperarousal precede other PTSD symptoms and may be predictive of future PTSD. The findings also support the notion that the emotional and behavioral symptoms of a COSR-type of response to traumatic stress may be related to the same neurobiological processes that cause acute stress disorder and post-traumatic stress disorder.[7]

Etiology and continuum of COSR

Military personnel may experience combat stress in relation to personal injury, being in combat, witnessing death and injury, or the killing of combatants, while operational stress can be caused by prolonged exposure to extreme environments, the separation from family and normal community, disrupted sleep cycles, long work hours, and austere living conditions.[8] Responses to these events also occur on a continuum and are expected to be transient, with individuals adapting their reactions based on training they have received or interventions by their units. Figure 5.1 depicts a model developed by the military that expresses the continuum of COSR from mild to very extreme, at which point it becomes indistinguishable from PTSD and medical intervention should be sought.[8] At each stage of the continuum adaptive behaviors occur, hopefully positive ones. Some of these are the responsibility of the unit leader, and some are the responsibility of individuals or peers. Each service member in a unit has a designated "battle buddy" or "wing man," the specific

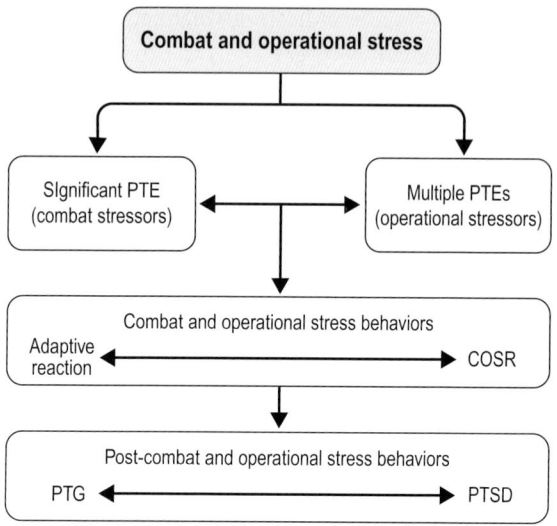

Figure 5.1
Model of stress and its potential soldier and family outcomes (adapted from Brusher[8(Ch. 4)]). PTE, potentially traumatic events; COSR, combat and operational stress reaction; PTG, post-traumatic growth; PTSD, post-traumatic stress disorder

name is service dependent, who is assigned to keep an eye out for you: for example, in a combat zone one would never go anywhere alone without someone else knowing the route, location, and expected return time. Often you might do physical training with this person or go to the dining hall with them. Even though each individual has had many classes on how to identify stress, depression, and healthy behaviors in response to these states, having an extra person watching with you can and has been proven to be life-saving. Prolonged symptoms not responding to conservative measures may warrant medical referral. As a rule of thumb for classic COSR, symptoms are expected to have subsided within 72 hours. However, in a fast operational tempo situation this is unrealistic as the next event often occurs very quickly and thus individuals are constantly in an adaptive state, never having a full 72 hours to recover from any one event. The military has adopted a formal doctrine taught to all service members indicating what actions can be taken to encourage recovery.[9] This also includes guidance on when to refer to the medical community.

Signs and coping strategies

The signs of COSR occur in four specific areas: physical, cognitive, emotional, and behavioral.[10] Physical signs may include both exhaustion and the inability to sleep, as well as palpitations, nausea, sweating, numbness and tingling of the hands or extremities. Cognitively, individuals may have decreased ability to process information, concentrate, or make decisions. They may also have some memory loss as well as nightmares, loss of confidence, and depersonalization. Emotional symptoms may include irritability, anger, sadness, anxiety, fear, or labile emotions. Early on, this may be noticed only by the individual or perhaps close peers. At this stage, useful coping strategies include self-help and advice from friends and close co-workers. When these symptoms become more pronounced, they also become more visible and may come to the attention of leadership, particularly when there is an inability to complete tasks, a decrease in efficiency, evidence of carelessness, and easy distractibility. In close-knit units it is evident quite early if individuals are isolating themselves and if there are inappropriate aggressive outbursts. At the extreme end there may even be outright misconduct.

With effective leadership and strong peer relationships, stressors can also lead to adaptive stress reactions that enhance both individual and unit performance. The *Combat and Operational Stress Control Manual for Leaders and Soldiers: Field manual 6-22.5*[9] provides four examples of adaptive stress reactions: *horizontal bonding* refers to the "strong personal trust, loyalty, and cohesiveness which develops among peers in a small military unit,"[9(p. 12)] whereas *vertical bonding* refers to these factors being present between leaders and their subordinates.

Many are familiar with e*sprit de corps*, a feeling of pride and shared identification with the larger, enduring organization with understanding of its history and mission. The Marines in particular are very well known for this, as are many well-known units such as the First Infantry Division (aka the Big Red One) and the 82nd Airborne. The fourth example, *unit cohesion*, refers to the "binding force that keeps Soldiers together and performing the mission in spite of danger and adversity."[9(p. 12)]

Frontline treatments and combat stress control teams

Since their original inception in WWI, the primary goal of frontline psychiatry doctrines has been to quickly stabilize acutely stressed soldiers and return them to the frontlines as soon as possible to avoid mass evacuations and army attrition.[11] The US Army believes this policy not only serves its own interests but those of the soldier as well. It claims that those soldiers who recover from COSR and return to their original units are welcomed back and are adequately rested, less likely to experience a recurrence of the condition, and "usually become healthy again."[9(p. 3-11)] There is some debate around this issue: for example, Russell and Figley[11] point out that the negative mental health impact of evacuating combat stress casualties is largely based on data relating to conserving the number of fighting troops rather than evidence of superior clinical outcomes in those who return to duty. One must point out, however, that this is in fact just debate, with those who have cared for patients and who have been in the war zones themselves stating there is clearly overwhelming data from years of personal experience in trying to keep the severely "stressed" in theater. The debate may also be largely one of semantics; the interested reader is referred to historical video footage of soldiers with severe combat stress reactions where there would be no question of evacuation to a major medical center.[2]

Chapter 5

Just as an individual may experience COSR, the unit itself can become stressed and, with this in mind, a more recent doctrinal development has been the formation of combat stress control (CSC) teams.[12,13] The mission of the CSC is to ensure "appropriate prevention and management of Combat Stress Reaction (CSR) casualties to preserve mission effectiveness and warfighting, and to minimize the short- and long-term adverse effects of combat on the physical, psychological, intellectual, and social health of Service members."[12(p. 1)] CSCs may be deployed to support various units in response to identified need or as prevention after major operations. If the unit as a whole is under great stress, its needs are assessed in a systematic fashion. Consultation by the CSC may include preventative advice to commanders and staff as well as education in concepts and skills for increasing individual resilience to stress.

The guidelines for treating individuals are based on several principles: brevity, immediacy, centrality/contact, expectancy, proximity, and simplicity, forming the acronym BICEPS.[10,12] Within these principles individuals are treated within their own unit or as close to the unit as possible since their main support system is among their peers (proximity). The initial rest period should last no more than one to three days (brevity) as those who need further treatment are moved to the next level of care. The chain of command stays actively involved (centrality/contact) and great care is taken to reassure the service member that he or she is not a patient but having a normal reaction to very abnormal circumstances and is expected to get well in time (expectancy). Soldiers are encouraged to continue to think of themselves as war fighters. Immediacy refers to the need to intervene as soon as feasibly possible as untreated symptoms may exacerbate and new ones may develop. The CSC can perform a proactive role in further training command and leadership to recognize COSR signs. Simplicity is based on addressing first order needs, such as sleep, rest, food, water, and hygiene. Many of these short-term strategies are often done informally, as there is great reluctance to seek out any avenues that might be construed as mental health care.[8,14,15] Other programs developed were termed "long weekends away" or a workshop on maintaining healthy relationships at home while being separated, titles more acceptable as being non-stigmatizing.

Post-combat operational stress

Stressors of course continue well after combat has finished and occur also among those military members who may have had combat-related missions. This has often been referred to as PCOS (post-combat operational stress). These missions can also impose a combination of heavy physical work, sleep loss, severe noise, vibration, exposure to extreme temperatures, poor hygiene facilities, and exposure to toxic fumes or potentially to infectious diseases. Individuals experience the full range of emotions to these, as well as to any concerns that they may have about problems back home, the ability to manage any perceived or real danger, and perceived skills in accomplishing their mission to their fullest ability. Symptoms may develop after someone has experienced or witnessed an actual or threatened traumatic event. It is also common for stress reactions to persist intermittently or arise long after exposure. If these symptoms interfere with the ability to do jobs and enjoy life, and seem to continually get worse, it could lead to PTSD. Some reactions sharpen abilities to survive while others produce disruptive behaviors. The acronym PTG (post-traumatic growth) refers to the phenomenon in which positive outcomes occur among survivors of traumatic experiences. This may include better relationships, improved appreciation of life, decisions that are now possible with an enhanced sense of personal strength, and even spiritual growth.

Moral injury

Moral injury is defined as an event which shatters an individual's moral or ethical tenets that are deeply rooted in religious, spiritual, or culture-based rules about fairness and the value of life. In the context of armed conflict, moral injury may occur in participating in violence or in the witnessing of the killing or harming of others. For some it may also occur because of not having prevented immoral acts of others that they perceive they could have thwarted. Although killing in war may lead to moral injury, it does not always do so. Military personnel are well versed in the rules of engagement and all societies and religions have accepted concepts of a "just war" which are generally invoked at the time of any conflict. For example, a military member who kills an armed combatant in self defense will likely feel that the death was justified. However, a civilian initially perceived to be armed who is thus killed in self defense may later be a source of moral injury, if subsequently found not to have been armed. Medical personnel who have never injured a single individual are at high risk of coming home with this invisible wound. One must make a clear distinction that moral injury is NOT the same as PTSD although the constructs may overlap. PTSD requires a diagnosis with a DSM code, while moral injury is perceived and judged by the individual and may or may not exist in the context of PTSD. It requires some "transgression" to have transpired while PTSD does not.

The context of this book is the treatment of trauma conditions, including combat-related PTSD, with Sensory-Enhanced Yoga. The focus with body-based techniques is on soothing and supporting the parasympathetic nervous system. The aspect of moral injury is mentioned for the sake of completeness only, and is certainly not to be broached in a regular yoga class, lest the unsuspecting teacher wander into a minefield and inflict more injury to everyone present. The teaching point is that as yoga inspires attention to the present moment, awareness of self, and particularly acceptance of self and gentleness, the seeds of self-nurturing that can start the healing process if moral injury is present are sown.

CASE STUDY A personal perspective

I would now like to share some of my own experiences working in a combat setting. I hope to provide the reader with a "boots on the ground" perspective, following which I will share some key factors to consider when using yoga as a healing modality within military settings.

I came to the army by way of a scholarship for medical school in which the payback was to serve in the military for the number of years of training received. For a variety of reasons, when it was finally possible to leave, I elected to stay as I was engaged in clinical research, assigned two major medical centers, and always involved in training interns, residents, and fellows in my chosen specialty. I was attending and presenting at national and international meetings, not to mention pursuing my favorite activity, which was seeing patients in a relatively unencumbered way in terms of bureaucracy. My patients had no medical bills and got all of their care for free. As one becomes more senior though, more administrative duties are assigned and by the time 9/11 rolled around, I was quite senior and life unexpectedly took a dramatic shift. I became a commander of a CSH (Combat Support Hospital) and was deployed to Iraq early in 2004, within the first year of the initial invasion known as Operation Iraqi Freedom (OIF). My unit was split into three smaller trauma hospitals: one in Tikrit, one in Mosul, and one in a smaller location outside of Baghdad. Later, other units were attached to us: preventative medicine and FSTs (forward surgical teams), among others.

When the outgoing commander hands the unit over to the new commander, a formal Change of Command ceremony takes place.

Chapter 5

This took place in Mosul, on a warm sunny day, during which the flag of the old unit was taken down and a new unit flag was raised in a small but very traditional military ceremony. As the flags were exchanged, a helicopter flew over us and landed at the emergency room entrance. I had a brief internal half smile and thought, *Wow, just like on MASH, would make a great picture*. The ceremony concluded and everyone was told to quickly disburse for safety reasons. Some pleasant chitchat followed, then from the corner of my eye I saw a nurse running up to our chief nurse. A few moments later, both quickly walked up to me, saying, "Ma'am you've got to come right away! The nurses are very upset and crying and it would be very good if you would just come and talk to them." Most were brand new nurses and lieutenants and our CSH was their first military assignment. We had just lost our first soldier, only 18 years old, and the worst part was that he had been talking to the staff on arrival. He had been in the helicopter that had landed during the change of command.

As I turned in that direction, my CSM (command sergeant major) gently touched my left elbow and said, "Ma'am, later—this is more important. I've held this for you for about three hours, until you were in command. You have to address it right now. It is a major problem for us." I walked with him about 50 yards, over to one of our young female medics who was with the first sergeant, and was told that one of the Iraqi soldiers had exposed himself to her while both were on duty in the guard tower. The second young medic came to the group as well and said that the same had happened to her, but she had pushed him away, pointed her M16 at him and left the guard tower. Of course, word of this had spread like wildfire in the unit and others approached the CSM and myself and asked, "What are you going to do?" As a backdrop, the whole issue of our staff pulling guard duty was very unpopular as the prior unit was completely exempt. However, higher headquarters had decided to significantly draw down the number of troops, and we simply had to. By Geneva Convention, medics do carry weapons to protect themselves and their patients; standing guard duty falls into this category. As I stood there, plenty of suggestions came at me: "We should not take any guard duty at all!"; "No more women on guard duty!"; "Hell no, you're not gonna dump this on the men only!" In that moment I was acutely aware of being a female commander; there was an undertone in all of the questions wondering whether I would take care of the women, as another woman, or "betray" them as I much later found out some in fact did think. The next question was how I was going to deal with the Iraqi senior commander who had dug his heels in on the side of his men. I closed my eyes for a brief second and thought, *I've been in command for 20 minutes and I have no idea what to do right now*. My stress level had just risen logarithmically.

Had you asked me then, or even for many years afterwards, I would have said that parts of that year were stressful, but that overall this was outweighed by the times of relaxation and times where we had a lot of fun. All of that would have been true, but in retrospect, I can now see that I never fully relaxed the entire time. Even going to sleep was not always a relief, as I would often lie in bed both wanting to fall asleep, yet fighting it at the same time, thinking, *What if this is my very last memory, lying here closing my eyes, and I just "wake up dead," because a rocket or mortar hit my sleeping quarters and I would never have said anything to my children*. This was not farfetched, as within the first two weeks in Mosul our unit's first Purple Heart was awarded when, without warning, a rocket in fact did hit our sleeping quarters, injuring some not 20 feet from where I was sleeping at the time.

In terms of dealing with stress during the year, I reverted to my tried and true methodology that has always worked throughout my life. I worked hard, I worked late, I worked out virtually every day, and in fact returned home in the best shape I had ever been in. Freed from family responsibilities, I knew I would have more free time and planned to look seriously at my spiritual life; I also took a whole stack of unread books with me. As a higher-level commander, there were very few peers in theater, but when I traveled to other areas, I did try to connect with them.

In dealing with the stress within our unit I was incredibly fortunate to have exceptionally good leaders working for and with me. One of our main thrusts was of course education: teaching about signs and symptoms within the individual, encouraging plenty of sleep, exercise, and a good diet, and learning how to recognize when signs and symptoms crossed the line of being simple things one could cope with by oneself. As medics, we saw and experienced many difficult things and as leaders we encouraged discussion groups to talk things out. We worked not only with US forces but those of many countries, including the Peshmerga from the Kurdish region and Nepalese Gurkha soldiers hired by the British Army. Our own American contract companies subcontracted with firms who hired so-called "third country nationals": individuals from the Philippines, India, and Malaysia, among others. Cultural differences were stressful and often inadvertently led to conflicts.

Larger, more striking activities to relieve stress included our chaplain in Tikrit using his musical background and connections to inspire those with creativity, and the staff working together to build a stand-alone coffeehouse, dedicated to music, improv comedy, games, occasional live music for those who brought an instrument, and creative snacks. The coffeehouse became quite the popular attraction for many who had to visit the hospital. In another location, the senior leaders somehow knew how to provide USDA steaks that, along with our family care packages, formed the basis of quite a few barbecue events with the first sergeant as chef and our onsite commander as his sous chef entertaining and serving all ranks. As our unit had deployed from Germany, somehow Heineken beer surfaced (General Order No. 1 in theater: no alcohol permitted). Intramural sports teams were formed and tournaments were held and the medics always did extremely well. Perhaps it was because we had all the physical therapists—we certainly had the loudest cheering sections and the best time afterwards.

In terms of operational stress control, I cannot go without praising our psychiatrist in Mosul; he, on his own, established for us a mini combat stress unit. With himself in the lead as senior clinician, along with his psych techs and other volunteers from the hospital, he established a separate quiet sleeping area, a separate room for "therapy" away from the hospital, and access to recreational activities, opening the possibility to de-stress to all units in the northern part of Iraq. At that time there was only one unit in Baghdad. This was very early in OIF, just after the initial invasion when only the required combat assets were in place. When we arrived it had been quiet for a few months and other support units were being brought in, but hostility soon picked up again. It was a very intense year with two of my hospitals providing direct casualty care in the battle for Fallujah.

Chapter 5

As this was quite early in the conflict, most of us were not aware of the value of yoga. However, by 2009, the US Army had begun to directly advocate techniques for stress management that, whether they were aware of it or not, are considered integral to many styles of yoga. These include deep breathing (described as inhaling slowly and deeply, expanding both the chest and the abdomen, holding it for two to five seconds, and exhaling slowly through the mouth), diaphragmatic breathing, muscle relaxation (aka tension-release exercises), positive self-talk, imagining "being fully immersed in a deeply relaxing setting," and meditation, i.e. "clearing the mind of all other thoughts by focusing on every breath and silently repeating a single word or phrase."[9(pp. 2-8, 2-9)]

This shift in philosophy toward mind-body modalities evolved as the wars in Iraq and Afghanistan continued and multiple deployments were taking their toll on military personnel. Many of these techniques have been gradually embedded into new Army fitness programs, which may help to promote "buy-in." In 2008, in an effort to strengthen the front end, the Chief of Staff of the US Army, General George Casey, established the Comprehensive Soldier Fitness program, later to be renamed Comprehensive Soldier and Family Fitness (CSF2).[16,17] Each of the services has formed something very similar with their own titles. The purpose of CSF2 is to increase the resilience and enhance performance of soldiers and families. Resilience is defined as "the mental, physical, emotional, and behavioral ability to face and cope with adversity, adapt to change, recover, learn, and grow from setbacks."[17(p. 10)] With this as a backdrop, the Army then developed a program called Total Force Fitness (TFF) as the framework for building and maintaining health, readiness, and performance in the Department of Defense. It views health, wellness, and resilience as a holistic concept. Optimal performance requires a connection between mind, body, spirit, and family/social relationships. The journal *Military Medicine* dedicated its entire August 2010 issue to this new health paradigm that was emerging. TFF had evolved in response to the nature of the Iraq and Afghanistan conflicts and the expectation that the US Armed Forces will be similarly engaged in the years ahead, a type of conflict that we currently see across the globe whether there is formal military engagement or not. It addresses eight domains of human fitness and, in four of those domains, highlights the importance of and supports mind-body practices such as yoga and meditation.[18]

Virtually all of the studies that have investigated the utility of yoga for addressing combat and operational stress have been conducted with service members who have returned from deployments or combat experience. There is in fact only one US study that was actually conducted during OIF in an actual combat zone, showing the excellent benefits of yoga[19] (see the box that concludes this chapter). This study is a landmark investigation as it provides direct support for the idea of using sensory enhanced yoga in a proactive manner for combat stress management. At least one other country is ahead on this topic: I am aware of a study with Indian soldiers in the Kashmir region participating in a prospective study that has demonstrated significant and reproducible results (personal communication from a leading Indian Army senior physician). These results now inform the preparation their soldiers receive prior to going into very high stress areas.

Summary

This chapter has provided a brief glimpse into the most recent war experience of this generation of veterans. The reader should keep in mind that much of this is universal and similar themes can be found as far back as the experiences of Ulysses in the wars in ancient Troy. Also remember that today there are over

18.5 million veterans in the United States.[20] Most did not see direct combat, but they may have deployed or been affected by deployments. Especially important is that US veterans range in age from the late teens into the high nineties, and in experience from individuals who have spent only a few years in the service of their country to those who have spent many decades. Thus they have each been formed and touched by a myriad of experiences. The teacher should, however, keep in mind that at the end of the day they are just people, putting their pants on each day, like everyone else, one leg at a time, wishing to be treated as any other human being: there is no place for pity, or a sense of one being there to help "fix" them. For those who do choose to work with this population though, it is paramount to learn about the culture, the bonds that rinse together over decades and across nations. An in-depth review can be found in the Yoga Service Council's short book *Best Practices for Yoga with Veterans*.[21] While it is focused on US veterans, our colleagues in other countries will be able to extract much helpful information and be able to easily discard recommendations that are not helpful or appropriate for their countries and cultures.

The Iraq Yoga Study

Lynn Stoller

In 2008, while teaching yoga during his off-duty hours as a flight instructor on the Kirkuk Air Force Base in Iraq, Major Jon Greuel came up with the idea of doing a study to gather empirical evidence of its effectiveness in reducing the symptoms of combat stress. Major Greuel ultimately reached out to Lucy Cimini, founder of Yoga Warriors, to ask if she would be interested in collaborating on the study. Lucy in turn delegated responsibility to me (her workshop co-presenter and Occupational Therapy Consultant and Research Coordinator at the time of the study) for forming and managing the stateside team and the writing, and so I was granted the role of associate investigator. Together, Lucy and I developed the treatment protocol, which consisted of treatment principles and a lesson plan. Mary Fowler served as the statistician and the late Jane Koomar served as my professional advisor for the study. Major Greuel served as principal investigator and was also the yoga instructor for the study. The randomized controlled study was managed by the US Army Institute of Surgical Research and was approved by the Brooke Army Medical Center.

The study produced many positive results and was subsequently published in the *American Journal of Occupational Therapy*. The study article ("Effects of sensory-enhanced yoga on symptoms of combat stress in deployed military personnel")[19] is available at: http://ajot.aota.org/article.aspx?articleid=1851541.

Objectives and methods

The ***objectives*** of the study were:

- to examine the effects of sensory-enhanced hatha yoga on symptoms of combat stress in deployed US military personnel
- to compare anxiety and sensory processing in this population with stateside civilians
- to identify any correlations between measures on the State/Trait Anxiety Inventory and the Adolescent/Adult Sensory Profile. (The measures of the Adolescent/Adult Sensory Profile are defined later.)

Of the 70 participants (22 female, 48 male) who participated in the study, 20 were in the Army and 50 were in the Air Force. The average age of the participants was 32. Thirty-five subjects received three weeks (≥ nine sessions) of sensory-enhanced hatha yoga while 35 did not receive any form of yoga. The subjects were required to attend a minimum of two yoga sessions per week. Twenty-five of the 35 subjects met or exceeded the attendance requirements, while 10 did not. The statistical findings were based on the complete treatment group, using "best practices" ITT (intention to treat) analysis, whether or not the subjects actually met the stated minimum treatment criteria.[22]

We used the following three measurement tools. The first two are standardized while the third is a custom designed tool developed by the team.

- Adolescent/Adult Sensory Profile
- State/Trait Anxiety Inventory
- Quality of Life Survey.[23]

The treatment protocol was designed to provide a therapeutic threshold of carefully selected sensory input, breathing techniques that promote calming, and a series of forms to balance the nervous system. The therapeutic sensory input consisted of deep touch pressure, enhanced proprioceptive input, and slow, rhythmical vestibular input (provided by certain rhythmic dynamic flows), which are modalities frequently used in sensory-based occupational therapy interventions for sensory modulation disorders. In addition, each session had to include between two and five positive affirmations per session, and at least 50% of the sessions needed to include an inspirational reading. Thus, the program combined both "bottom-up" and "top-down" interventions in order to maximize the therapeutic effects of the yoga intervention.

Chapter 13 in Part 3 of this book describes ways to incorporate therapeutic sensory input into a yoga session, many of which were used in the Iraq Yoga Study. However, the Sensory-Enhanced Yoga program is not identical to the treatment protocol used in Iraq, but rather evolved from the ideas and writings I contributed to the protocol which remain under my copyright and have been greatly built upon since the time of the study. Among the differences between the programs is the Iraq Yoga Study paired specific positive affirmations with specific yoga forms, whereas the Sensory-Enhanced Yoga program incorporates positive suggestions and may occasionally invite yoga participants to self-generate a positive affirmation that resonates with them while in a yoga form, but does not impose "ready-made" positive affirmations onto participants. An exception is the mudras, in which the positive affirmations are ***process-oriented***. This topic is discussed in detail in Chapter 14. Another difference is we have more props available stateside whereas in Iraq, the military personnel were mostly limited to using rope straps and wooden blocks.

Results

Contrary to our expectations, when comparing the pre-tests between the treatment and control groups, there were no significant differences between the mean values of the deployed military population and the normative civilian population for any of the four quadrants of the A/ASP: low registration, sensory sensitivity, sensory avoidance, and sensory seeking. Nor did the military personnel score higher on state or trait anxiety as measured by the State/Trait Anxiety Inventory. Unfortunately, we did not obtain reliable data with regard to length of deployment or number of deployments, but were told a subgroup of participants had been deployed for less than a month, so it is possible they had not experienced significant combat exposure. Furthermore, all six participants who scored high sensory sensitivity were randomized to the control group, so, as expected, the data also did not yield evidence that the sensory-enhanced yoga treatment would help to increase normalization of sensory processing.

Nonetheless, with regard to the other measures, *the treatment group showed significant improvements in state and trait anxiety, as well as improvements in 16 out of 18 quality of life factors* following completion of the study. These results are particularly striking when aligned with the symptom clusters of PTSD, as shown below.

Hyperarousal

- Decreased state and trait anxiety (≤ .001)
- Improved concentration (≤ .001)
- Reduced irritability (≤ .001)
- Reduced sleep difficulties (≤ .01)
- Reduced outbursts of anger (≤ .01)
- Less "on guard" or "watching my back" (≤ .01)

Avoidance/numbing

- Less avoidance of socializing (≤ .001)
- Feeling more interested in things (≤ .001)
- Fewer feelings of loneliness (< .01)

Re-experiencing

- Fewer intrusive thoughts or images (≤ .01)
- Experiencing distressing 'mini-dreams' (p = 0.023)

Other results from the Quality of Life Survey suggested that the yoga treatment offered some relief for symptoms of depression and also improved daily living performance, as evidenced by a decrease in: "having difficulty performing daily tasks" (p = 0.001), "experiencing feelings of boredom" (p = .001), not attending to my self-care needs (p = 0.002), "feeling 'down in the dumps'" (p = 0.002), and "having bouts of sadness or crying" (p = 0.007). Moral injury relief was suggested by a decrease in "blaming myself for things" (p = 0.011).

The participants were also given the opportunity to write comments following each yoga class: 54% of the subjects reported sleep improvements either during or after class, despite the sounds of gunfire and helicopter sounds; 37% commented that they felt more calm or relaxed; 26% commented on other physical benefits; and 11% reported reduced frustration or anger or better anger management. Reportedly, the sleep comments were of particular interest to the general who visited with the PI while the study was being conducted, since many of the military personnel were reliant on sleep medications due to significant sleep issues.

Correlation Hypothesis

With regard to the correlation hypothesis, a one-tailed Pearson correlation test yielded evidence of a significant positive correlation between the following five measures: *state anxiety, trait anxiety, sensory sensitivity, sensory avoidance* and *low registration. Sensory seeking* was *negatively correlated* with all measures except low registration, which was insignificant. The A/ASP aspect of the correlation pattern matches the sensory profile pattern revealed in the study on post-traumatic stress conducted by Engel-Yeger et al.,[24] as well as the pattern revealed in the pilot study of combat veterans conducted by Stoller and Cimini,[25] both of which were discussed in Chapter 2. Further studies are necessary to determine whether this pattern uniquely characterizes PTSD (and perhaps related ANS disorders) or whether the quadrant measures are essentially measuring the same construct due to a common neurophysiological process, such as might be explained by Porges' polyvagal theory.

Discussion and implications

We attributed the success of the program to the combination of both bottom-up and top-town approaches. It is thought that the sensory-enhanced

Chapter 5

techniques, choice of asanas, and calming breathing practices likely produced autonomic nervous system inhibition, which in turn led to the reduced anxiety scores and to improvements in health and quality of life factors. The pairing of positive affirmations with asanas may have reframed negative thinking patterns, while the readings may have oriented the participants to the present moment vs replaying the past or worrying about the future.

I originally developed the **Transdisciplinary Model for Post-Traumatic Growth** to explain the study implications in preparation for the AOTA Specialty Conference on Warriors in Transition that was held in San Antonio in 2012. This model synthesizes current theoretical and treatment concepts from the fields of occupational therapy, neurobiology, and trauma psychology to create a road map for healing combat stress, PTSD, anxiety, and related autonomic nervous system disorders. Only later did I realize that I had unwittingly reinvented the yogic kosha model using the language of Western medicine. The Transdisciplinary Model for Post-Traumatic Growth is the theoretical model that underlies the current Sensory-Enhanced Yoga program and is introduced in Chapter 10.

Study limitations

There were several limitations of the Iraq Yoga Study, including a lack of clear data on length of deployment and combat exposure, short study duration, reliance on the subjective reports of the participants and, as mentioned earlier, the skewed randomization of all "high sensory sensitivity" subjects to the control group precluded studying the effects of yoga on sensory processing. Furthermore, the study relied solely on the subjective reports of the participants, which would have been bolstered by the addition of objective physiological measures. Finally, the control group did not receive any type of legitimate or sham treatment to match the expectancy of results that may have been experienced by the treatment group. Notwithstanding all of the above, this study is important for the high statistical power of its findings, produced within the context of one of the largest randomized/controlled studies of yoga yet conducted with US military personnel, and the *only* one yet conducted in a deployed environment. The review process was also very stringent as it underwent a total of eight reviews by Department of Defense IRB teams, two in each of four locations. Two locations were in Iraq and two were stateside, with the final review and official oversight conducted by the Brooke Army Medical Center.

Future directions

The results raise the obvious question of whether a carefully designed yoga program might not only reduce the symptoms of combat stress but also possibly preempt the development of PTSD. As we were not able to follow up with the study participants, this question could not be answered in the current study. However, a longitudinal study is certainly warranted to investigate its potential for such purpose, considering the gravity of the problem of PTSD in our society and particularly in the military. Such a study would be most powerful if bolstered by physiological measures and an active control group.

Reclaiming body, redefining relationship: yoga with survivors of sexual trauma

Danielle Rousseau and Amanda J. G. Napior

This stuff is in our bodies, and that's the place of healing. — Keyona (see text)

Introduction

Every year, approximately 321,500 Americans are sexually assaulted or raped. Nine out of 10 of these are women (rainn.org/statistics/scope-problem), and one in six American women has been the victim of an attempted or completed rape in her lifetime. People who are transgender or do not otherwise conform to traditional gender norms are at significantly higher risk for sexual assault than those who do (https://www.rainn.org/statistics/victims-sexual-violence). The risk of sexual assault is also influenced by race and ethnicity, with Native Americans and African Americans at greater risk than Caucasians, Latinos, or Asians.[1,2] Even certain institutional cultures place one at higher risk: each year, 18,900 military personnel report unwanted sexual contact; and 80,600 people in prison report sexual assault or rape (rainn.org/statistics/scope-problem). These numbers are staggering. And yet, because many experiences of sexual trauma are not reported to authorities, we cannot truly know the full scope of sexual violence and trauma.

The impact of sexual violence will be unique for each individual, with social dimensions of violence and trauma bearing on that experience. In the late 20th century, feminist women of color began describing how each person's social position is shaped by an intersection of various aspects of her social identity, such as race, gender, and class. As a result, systemic oppressions hit some harder than others, and advocacy work has often spoken for one group at the expense of the people at its own margins (see writings by, among others, Kimberlé Crenshaw, Gloria Anzaldúa, Cherrie Moraga, and Audre Lorde for how intersecting patterns of racism and sexism impact women of color without being "represented within the discourses of either feminism or antiracism").[3(p. 1243),4] When we look through a wider lens we see how sexual trauma impacts us all: those who have not been personally violated almost always know someone who has. Furthermore, the social norms under which sexual violence occurs are shaped by the culture we create together. And so, as one reads about trauma, it is possible to see hints of their own embodied human experience on the page.

For the purposes of this chapter, we suggest the working definition of sexual trauma proposed by the Yoga Service Council:

Sexual trauma is an experience in which an individual is overpowered, manipulated, violated, betrayed or controlled by another in a position of power. The experience often includes feelings of powerlessness, fear, and a lack of agency or choice. The impact of sexual trauma can result in the person's relationship to their sexual self, sexuality in general and sex in society being influenced by the power differential of the original

Chapter 6

event or events. (Yoga Service Council Symposium, October 2017)

As the definition suggests, a range of experiences or circumstances can lead to sexual violence and trauma. Sexual trauma can result from sexual assault, rape, sexual abuse, incest, intimate partner sexual violence, and abuses in other contexts. The terms *sexual violence and sexual trauma* are non-legal terms we invoke to speak to events and experiences of violence, irrespective of legal action taken against their perpetrators; legal definitions of sex-related crimes vary by state and jurisdiction.

In spite of the saddening scope and impact of sexual violence and trauma, an affirmative central premise the authors of this chapter share is that healing is possible. Humans, both individually and collectively, have a tremendous capacity for resilience, which we have developed across time and place and through modes of self-compassion, connection, ritual, and recovery. This human cultivation of resilience is embodied—which is why the embodied healing modality of yoga can be a powerful tool for survivors of sexual trauma. Yoga can empower practitioners to (re)gain ownership of their own bodies. It can help them tap into and cultivate a sense of inner peace and strength, perhaps even more powerfully than before the traumatic incident(s). Yoga does this, in part, by helping one to recalibrate the physiological stress response that can lead to chronic stress and dis-ease. In short, yoga can be a highly effective tool for promoting self-regulation, resilience, and post-traumatic growth.

The authors come to this subject with personal, experiential, clinical, research and practical connections to the topic of sexual trauma. Both Danielle and Amanda are current collaborators in the Yoga Service Council's best-practices project on sexual trauma. Through Danielle's engagement with yogaHOPE, we were able to connect with the three women—Keyona, Linda, and Jude—who spoke with us about their own healing experiences for this chapter.

Since sexual trauma is so widespread, we recommend that *all* yoga teachers consider themselves to be teachers of survivors, whether they have direct awareness of their students' trauma experiences or not. In the sections that follow, we explicate this topic through a review of literature on yoga studies conducted with sexual trauma survivors, as well as through the voices of sexual trauma survivors themselves. We conclude with recommendations for best practice.

Review of literature

Judith Herman's groundbreaking work *Trauma and Recovery: The Aftermath of Violence, from Domestic Violence to Political Terror*,[5] brought the topic of sexual trauma into clinical conversation and helped to mainstream the feminist discourses of the last two decades. Many practitioners of trauma consider Herman the mother of contemporary trauma studies. She documents how three forms of psychological trauma—"hysteria," combat neurosis, and most recently, sexual and domestic violence—have risen to the forefront of our contemporary consciousness. She suggests that recovery from trauma includes three stages: establishing safety; remembrance and mourning; and reconnecting with others. Herman championed the idea that "establishing safety begins by focusing on control of the body" (p. 160), but only went so far as to make general recommendations, e.g. "relaxation or hard exercise, to manage stress" (p. 160). Nonetheless, her three stages are keenly relevant to understanding the benefits of yoga for healing trauma. Indeed, these can be powerful tools for establishing a sense of safety in the body of the survivor of sexual trauma, making it possible to remember and mourn. As the mind-body connection becomes re-established, reconnecting with others—such as through touch—may become appealing and joyful to the survivor once again.

Reclaiming body, redefining relationship: yoga with survivors of sexual trauma

The first person to advocate yoga as a form of treatment for trauma survivors was Babette Rothschild, in her book *The Body Remembers: The Psychophysiology of Trauma and Trauma Treatment*,[6] which illuminates the psychophysiology of trauma and the phenomenon of somatic memory, drawing attention to the importance of sensation and movement as part of the psychotherapeutic treatment strategy itself. In her follow-up work,[7] Rothschild discusses how she successfully incorporated specific body-based treatment models, including yoga, into her psychotherapy work with clients.

However, it was the scholarly studies and mainstream works of psychiatrist Bessel van der Kolk that brought the body's role in recovery from trauma to the attention of a diverse audience. As a member of the biomedical community, his research on the neurological and physiological effects of trauma and the ameliorating effects of bodymind practices (including yoga) has offered long-awaited scientific legitimacy to healing modalities that have been used for many hundreds of years in various cultural and religious systems. Significantly, his work calls into question the long-held psychoanalytic wisdom that talk therapy, and more specifically exposure therapies, are indispensable to healing. Instead, he advocates therapies that facilitate healing with few words (such as a therapeutic method known as eye movement desensitization reprogramming or EMDR) as well as activities such as collective, rhythmic movement, music-making, and prayer, which he argues ought to be recognized as aids to traumatic recovery. Most significantly for our purposes, he and his colleague, David Emerson, co-developed and have conducted empirical studies on trauma-sensitive yoga (TSY) at the Trauma Center at the Justice Research Institute in Brookline, MA, contributing to the biomedical acceptance of yoga as a therapeutic intervention for persons impacted by trauma.

Studies of TSY conducted by the Trauma Center have primarily focused on complex trauma. Chapter 9 reviews these in-depth, as Alison Rhodes, the author of the chapter, has co-authored some of them and can therefore provide a more intimate perspective on the research. Many of the participants in those studies experienced sexual abuse as part of their trauma history. Indeed, there is a strong association between sexual and complex trauma, as Rhodes explains. In this chapter, we highlight five yoga studies illumining sexual trauma recovery, specifically.

The following three empirical studies were conducted outside of the Trauma Center but have utilized TSY. Each demonstrated improved well-being for survivors. Clark et al.[8] administered a 12-week, 30–40-minute TSY protocol at the end of group psychotherapy sessions, in a study of 17 women with histories of intimate partner violence (IPV). Eight women received this protocol while the other nine received only the typical psychotherapy group sessions. The aim of the study was to test the feasibility of combining TSY and group psychotherapy. Given the high retention of participants, the participants' high level of acceptance of the yoga classes, and their perceived safety and utility of the treatment, this combinatory intervention was considered a success.

Crews et al.[9] assessed how TSY impacted eight women, aged 15 to 60, who had histories of sexual trauma. Noting that the key issue for survivors of sexual violence is not "a mental health diagnosis" but instead about "their relationship with themselves,"[9(p. 142)] these authors conducted interviews with their subjects based on a self-compassion model. Their publication analyzes ways in which the participants' reflections show a shift from "self-judgment to self-kindness" (p. 148), "isolation to common humanity" (p. 149), and "overidentification to mindfulness" (p. 150), over time.

Chapter 6

Third and last, Ong's mixed-methods dissertation examines the use of TSY for five female survivors of IPV. She demonstrates improvements for all of the women across categories of "physiological-," "emotional-," "spiritual-," and "cognitive benefits," as well as through "enhanced perception of self and others," a "shift in perspectives on time," increased "self-care," and "positive coping strategies." These were themes surfaced in interviews with her subjects.[10(p. 185–9)] Ong also administered the CAPS-5 to her subjects, revealing a decrease in PTSD severity and symptomatology for all subjects.[10(p. 143–4)]

Two additional yoga studies beyond the TSY model also address sexual trauma and also demonstrate improved outcomes for survivors. Earley and colleagues[11] conducted a 2.5-year follow-up with 19 adult participants in a study on survivors of childhood sexual abuse (CSA). The original cohort of 26 people had all participated in a mindfulness-based stress reduction (MBSR) intervention, which included "weekly 2.5–3 hour classes [of] sitting meditation, gentle yoga, stretching, and body scanning."[11(p. 934)] At the 2.5-year follow-up, a single clinical visit assessing levels of depression, anxiety, PTSD, and mindfulness demonstrated statistically significant improvements in all measures. The researchers write that "the maintenance of all significant changes observed since the initial baseline demonstrates that, in this sample, an intervention involving meditation, yoga, stretching, and enhanced body awareness was quite effective in reducing emotional distress over the long term."[11(p. 938)]

A study by Hill and colleagues[12] aimed to assess the effectiveness of mindfulness practices in decreasing the rates of re-victimization among survivors of CSA. Twelve female college students participated in the program and 20 women comprised a no-program control group. While the researchers did not use the word *yoga* to describe the practices, they named breathing exercises, a guided meditation, and mindfulness in everyday life among the program's offerings. The authors did not find statistically significant decreases in re-victimization for study participants over the course of the semester-long study; however, a two-month follow-up revealed a "large-magnitude effect," such that survivor-participants were less likely to be sexually assaulted or raped.[12]

Finally, it is worth noting an additional study that did not specifically target sexual trauma recovery yet produced findings that point to benefits of yoga for sexual trauma survivors. Impett and colleagues[13] revealed that the 14 women who completed a two-month yoga immersion program "reported that they cared less about how their bodies appeared to others and more about how their bodies felt to themselves."[15(p. 44)] Being able to relinquish concern for how one's body appears to others can be significant for someone recovering from sexual trauma, insofar as it suggests that one is wrapped up less in the gaze of onlookers and instead experiences greater embodied self-possession. The researchers write, "By reducing the extent to which women objectify their own bodies, yoga may promote improvements in sexual health."[15(p. 45)] This study suggests that yoga can help the individual's locus of bodily validation move inward, as she relinquishes concern over the gazes of onlookers and becomes more viscerally present in her own skin. Such an insight might help us understand one of the mechanisms by which survivors of sexual trauma heal.

While the empirical studies offering yoga modalities specifically to survivors of sexual trauma are few, they demonstrate a growing knowledge base that only adds to what many practitioners of yoga have encountered in practice: that yoga can be a path for healing from sexual trauma. Let us be mindful not to mistake empirical findings as more authoritative knowledge than what practitioners discover on their own. Indeed, we may only be scratching the surface of empirically demonstrating yoga's benefits for survivors. We turn now to the voices of three survivors of sexual trauma, who have experienced the healing benefits of yoga first hand.

CASE STUDY A personal perspective

In order to explore the potential impacts of mindfulness practices for survivors of sexual trauma, we sought out the voices of individual survivors who have participated in mindfulness programs. We conducted a group interview with three women—Keyona, Jude, and Linda—who are past participants and trained facilitators of the Trauma Informed Mind Body program (TIMBo). The five of us met one crisp October evening in a conference room on campus at Boston University. Perhaps due to our participants' shared experiences in TIMBo, an easy conversational intimacy emerged among them. We "facilitators" asked few questions and were instead privy to a conversation in which we participated minimally. Linda, Jude, and Keyona openly shared their experiences with us, riffing off one another's ideas, nodding in agreement, murmuring in recognition. Together, they illuminated the impacts of the TIMBo program on both their daily lived experiences and their attempts to manage the long-term effects of traumatic stress.

TIMBo is the flagship program of yoga HOPE, a Boston-based non-profit organization dedicated to bringing therapeutic mind-body programming to people who identify as women, across the globe. YogaHOPE's aim is "to lead women toward empowerment and recovery by cultivating mindfulness through yoga, meditation, and non-judgmental self-inquiry."[14(p. 1)] The TIMBo program is evidence-based, trauma-informed, and gender-responsive, utilizing the strengths already present in female survivors of trauma. All of the TIMBo curriculum's 16 sessions consist of three central components: (1) group discussion, (2) a focused breath exercise (*pranayama*), and (3) yoga *asana* (physical forms) and meditation.[15] This parallel structure is designed to create safety and predictability for the participants, as is conducive to trauma recovery.

In listening to Linda, Keyona, and Jude's experiences with yoga and trauma-informed mindfulness practices, we noticed their conversation surfaced a variety of themes: the **role of the body** in healing, the experience of **shame and the paradoxical power of vulnerability** in sexual trauma, and a profound sense of **social connection** that can be both one's access to and result of one's own experience of healing. They spoke about how trauma can make one feel strangely *dis*embodied and how TIMBo has been an essential tool, they suggest, for facilitating re-embodiment, for learning about the neurobiology of trauma, and for ameliorating the long term, present day impacts of trauma.

A central theme that shaped our conversation was the **fundamental importance of the body** in healing trauma. For example, all three women discussed being cognitively oriented, by nature, and all noted that they were unable to fully address their trauma without the embodied component of a yoga practice—and the TIMBo program, specifically. Linda said, "I was no longer going to make progress going through the head." As Linda summarized, "When I decided to pursue healing through the body rather than the brain after years of cognitive-based therapy, I turned initially to yoga to begin this process." Keyona agreed: "The whole thing of TIMBo that really was putting everything together for me was that premise that the body is important to

Chapter 6

healing." Jude said, "I need [yoga] for what it's doing up here." She pointed to her head as she spoke. "It's changed my life." The women discussed feeling disembodied because of their trauma—they described themselves as having felt "cut off from the neck down." One woman shared that TIMBo allowed her to "start feeling" for the first time and another suggested that TIMBo provided her with the capacity to work with and through anger and to access vulnerability. Indeed, because trauma is held in the body, addressing cognition alone is not enough. Neurologically speaking, trauma symptoms result from the brain's perception that we are in danger in this present moment; the brain continues to live in and react to the past even when one is no longer at current risk.[16]

Keyona, Jude, and Linda suggested that one cannot simply *explain the impact* of healing trauma through yoga by recourse to scientific or cognitive interpretations. Rather, healing seems to reveal something more basic to our humanity, beyond the reach of scientific explanation. Keyona formed a cup with her hands to say: "The body is holding *this*, and without a lot of words, we can work *this*. It's workable. Everything is workable." She went on to discuss the "simplicity" of the embodied experience, nodding to the wisdom of past generations and cultures in understanding the healing process. "It's like some of the ancient practices. We have been saying this for years. Tribes have been doing this for years. We have literally, for eons, been dancing this out, or breathing this out, or doing this out." Keyona, Jude, and Linda's reflections on body and cognition demonstrate how TIMBo made re-embodiment possible by cultivating and appreciating their bodily capacities to heal.

These three women also reflected on how **shame and vulnerability** play a significant role in trauma and recovery. Shame can be particularly present for those experiencing complex trauma and trauma occurring early in one's development. Because of the fragmented nature of traumatic memory, survivors may not have words for their experience; instead, shame becomes embedded in painful sensation and emotion. A survivor of sexual trauma may believe that something is innately wrong with her. Unlike guilt, which is the sense that "I *did* something wrong," shame suggests "There is something wrong with me. I *am* wrong." Linda echoed this idea when she said,

The message was: I was born with something wrong with me. That something resided in my reproductive organ area. At the age before concrete thinking, this belief turned into I am flawed AND consent is not something that belongs to me. I do not have the right to say no. Other people have the control over consent when it comes to my body, especially my lower body.

Survivors may engage in behaviors to manage this shame. These behaviors may differ from one individual to another and fall along a spectrum from avoidance to hypervigilance and blurring of boundaries. They may not consciously recognize these behaviors as adaptations of survival, nor the physiological impacts that shame and traumatic stress have on their bodies. Linda, Keyona, and Jude suggested that learning to recognize sensation in their bodies and subsequently utilize tools such as breath and movement to regulate sensation has surfaced, in their paths of recovery, a transformative healing power: knowing that they can facilitate their *own* trauma healing has been a source of self-empowerment, which can counter reverberations of shame.

Reclaiming body, redefining relationship: yoga with survivors of sexual trauma

As Keyona, Jude, and Linda discussed their experiences with the TIMBo program, the role of **vulnerability,** accompanied by a sense of safety, arose as a central quality of healing. For example, one of the women discussed being triggered as an opportunity for growth. As they learned embodied practices, they learned how to manage triggers and periods of feeling "down." These experiences became less intense, and in Jude's words, "fewer and far between." Overall, the women described the process of healing as facilitating embodiment and empowerment. They used language of "paradigm shift" to describe what it is like to be one's own healer and to be empowered to administer one's own "treatment" or "intervention." Jude described feeling like she had become a different person, attributing this shift to the TIMBo program. In the women's discussion of participation in the TIMBo program, it became apparent that the practice of embodiment increased their sense of having agency in their own healing.

Given their experiences of self-empowerment, it is no wonder that Jude, Keyona, and Linda identified yoga as a successful complementary and even alternative treatment modality. While all three women had participated in a variety of treatment modalities for managing the impacts of trauma, each indicated that yoga, and specifically TIMBo, was the tool that gave them access to their own healing. One of the participants described the use of yoga, in addition to other approaches like therapy, as "exponential" in the healing process. Another suggested that through a dedicated practice of yoga and participation in the TIMBo program, she was able to reduce and even eliminate psychiatric medications.

As Jude, Keyona, and Linda discussed the history of their yoga practices, the importance of seeking a trauma-informed practice became evident. Not all yoga is the same, and some practices could potentially have a negative impact on survivors. Regarding a more physically vigorous yoga practice she took up earlier in life, Linda noted: "There were things I didn't understand then that didn't work for me. These were felt in my body during the practice as pain and deep psychic discomfort and disappointment in myself." Linda discussed being triggered emotionally, including experiencing anger, during participation in a yoga practice that was not trauma-informed. Outside of a trauma-informed setting, she did not have a way to contextualize what she was experiencing or to use breath or movement to support her in those practices.

Finally, Linda, Keyona, and Jude articulated the **importance of connection to others** in the process of healing. They described the tools offered in embodied practices as being universally applicable, insofar as all populations experience trauma, and all persons have the capacity for healing. It appeared that for these women, this sense of common humanity and connection helped to reveal their own humanity. The women described being able to hold space for others as being healing in their own recovery.

Sexual trauma occurs in relationship; the trauma constitutes a violation of trust and abuse of relational power. As the women indicated, healing results from the transformative power of healthy connection. Linda stated, "connection to others is not only important, I believe it is impossible to heal fully without it." Jude echoed this sentiment in her statement, "Basically for me, I have never truly felt connected to anything or anyone in my life until yoga and TIMBo." The TIMBo program is designed to specifically foster

Chapter 6

such connection. TIMBo facilitators create an environment that is collaborative in support of a healing journey.

Connection is inextricable from our earlier themes of shame and vulnerability. Linda illuminates this point in her discussion of shame in a follow-up communication:

Sexual violence is almost universally met with shame. The deep-rooted feeling of shame. Isolation and silence feeds shame. The one thing that can absolutely reduce the power of shame, the presence of shame, is empathy. Speaking, being heard, being responded to by another or a group of individuals with empathy. Not sympathy, pity, but empathy. The power of a relationship is that it is the basic requirement of empathy. In addition, the connection to others in a TIMBo group allows for an ongoing experience of I'M NOT ALONE, I'm not the only one that this happened to—through empathy, "me too," and the practice of mutuality.

The capacity for connection is also tied to vulnerability; in one's willingness to be vulnerable, connection becomes possible. As Jude shared, "It took me a while to begin to share a little during the groups, but what I noticed was even though it was extremely painful for me to speak up and share, once I did I began to feel a sense of connection."

It became apparent that practicing yoga *with others* was an important component of the healing process for these women. Through practice with others, a survivor may be able to redefine relationship in a way that is safe and healing. As Jude noted:

People still ask me, 'Why do you go to so many yoga classes, can't you just do yoga at home by yourself?' I thought to myself, 'Yes, I could, but for now I personally need that connection with others.' I don't necessarily have to talk with people but just being present with others during a yoga class gives me a deep sense of connection to others in my class. I guess the connection comes from a sense of comfort and safety I feel in my yoga classes. Also a strong sense of feeling safe.

This capacity to experience safety in relationship can be both empowering as well as transformative. In practices that foster healthy connection where both participants and facilitators are on a shared journey, healing becomes mutually supportive. In holding space for another, we empower our own healing and redefine what it means to be in relationship.

To summarize, Linda, Jude, and Keyona stressed the fundamental role of embodied practices in healing the present-day impacts of sexual trauma. They experienced embodied practices positively, as complementary and even alternative approaches to trauma healing. For these three women, vulnerability, accompanied by a sense of safety, was vital to healing. They have experienced this process of healing as empowering, which comes in part from the sense of agency gained in facilitating one's own process. Finally, the participants shared a sense of the universality of the work of healing trauma and acknowledged the mutuality present in the healing relationship. Recognizing the common humanity in the experience of trauma encouraged both compassion and self-compassion. These findings parallel and support the guiding principles of Sensory-Enhanced Yoga.

Summary and considerations for practice

In our review of embodied mindfulness practices that can address the long-term impacts of sexual trauma, we see the promise of these practices for promoting healing, well-being and even resilience in the wake of trauma. Yoga and mindfulness practices offer tools for self-regulation, self-empowerment, and healthy connection. Embodied practices appear to address the impacts of trauma in a way that traditional talk therapy alone cannot. While these tools promise benefit, mindful utilization of techniques is important. Yoga teachers should always seek to employ current best practices and recognize the impact they could have on potentially vulnerable individuals and populations. Here we will note some important recommendations for working with survivor populations. We also honor the reality that sexual trauma is pervasive in our culture and, because of this, we suggest that teachers recognize the significance of these recommendations in each and every class they teach.

Acknowledge diverse cultural perspectives and experiences

Much of the empirical research on trauma actually prioritizes the white experience of trauma[17] and, by extension, of recovery. Teachers must recognize that while anyone can experience sexual trauma, some individuals may be more vulnerable to victimization than others. Teachers must also be careful not to *assume* victimization. The vulnerability and stereotyping of some persons is compounded by a lack of social and institutional structures recognizing their unique precarity. Because yoga and mindfulness practices have the potential to offer refuge for survivors of many backgrounds, we need to ensure that all survivors can access this opportunity in an equivalent way. Teachers can become better advocates and offer classes that are as inclusive as possible by pursuing ongoing education about the potential unique needs and experiences of students of diverse racial, ethnic, and socioeconomic backgrounds as well as students with different gender identities and sexual orientations. Future work in this area may also include the creation programing tailored for sexual trauma survivors whose journeys are inflected by historical trauma.

Maintain awareness of intended and unintended impacts of language and environment

Teachers should use invitational language, rather than commands. When invitations and choice shape instruction, teachers can better create an environment and practice that is as safe as possible, knowing that they can never guarantee safety or define what is safe for any one person. Teachers should be aware of the potential impact of setting up a classroom in a way that reinforces hierarchies or may leave some students feeling vulnerable because of their position in the room. For example, consider arranging mats in a circle or semicircle. Teachers should also maintain awareness of the location of doors and windows within a room, considering how best to position both self and students to minimize vulnerability and avoid triggering a stress response resulting from the perception of threat.

Be mindful in choices of asana, pranayama, and class structure

This work demands that teachers adopt a trauma-informed approach in designing the class structure and selecting *asana* (forms) and *pranayama* (breathing exercises). Consider the value of consistency and repetition in structuring class. Know that some forms, form names, or props can themselves be triggering. For example, it may be best to avoid the use of straps in working with a class designated for sexual trauma survivors and to offer a choice of using one or not in any yoga class. Although no form is specifically off limits, carefully consider the potential impact of each form. Downward Dog or Happy Baby may feel too vulnerable in some settings. Be aware of forms that may evoke sexual connotations and continually monitor the emotional environment created in the classroom.

Root teaching in a foundational understanding of trauma and resilience

Teachers will benefit from active engagement with current literature in the fields of trauma theory and yoga

Chapter 6

service. In October 2017, the Yoga Service Council held a symposium bringing together a diversity of leaders in the use of embodied mindfulness practices with survivors of sexual trauma; the resulting best practices guide can serve as an empowering resource for practitioners (https://yogaservice council.org/best-practices). Teachers should additionally be mindful of the importance of self-inquiry and self-care, and recognizing the negative relational impacts of not addressing their own trauma experiences.

Teachers and embodied mindfulness practitioners have the capacity to share tools that provide the potential for multidimensional healing—healing that is both cognitive and embodied, internal and external, individual and collaborative. By sharing these practices in a trauma-informed way, we can offer individuals who have experienced sexual violence and trauma new avenues into their own healing, resilience, and well-being. Ultimately, we will foster the potential for healing of systems as well.

Recovery and empowerment through yoga in prison

Amanda J. G. Napior and Danielle Rousseau

I can do anything for two more breaths. — Alan (see text)

Introduction

The United States is facing an epidemic of mass incarceration, with roughly 2.2 million people behind bars. As the "world's leader in incarceration," overall incarceration rates in the US have risen over 500% in the last 40 years (www.sentencingproject.org). Disparities of gender and race abound: between the years 1980 and 2014, women's incarceration increased at a rate over 700% (www.sentencingproject.org),[1] and people of color make up 60% of the people in prison.

Mass incarceration constitutes a public health crisis: incarcerated people have a higher rate of mental health concerns and serious psychological distress as compared to others, with women experiencing higher rates than men.[2] Many incarcerated people have histories of multiple and complex trauma and incarceration itself can be both traumatizing and re-traumatizing. The experience of incarceration results in undeniable physical and psychological impacts on people in prison—impacts that are often not only inadequately addressed, but rather exacerbated, in correctional institutions.

Sociologists and legal scholars have linked these carceral increases since the 1970s to the increased criminalization of certain drug-related offenses and systemic racial injustices. These forces have exacerbated poverty and disproportionality disenfranchised African American communities.[3,4] Religious historians and theologians have shown how the criminal justice system's emphasis on personal (rather than communal) responsibility, and its commitment to punishment over rehabilitation, reflects an ideologically disciplinarian and, at times, punitive tradition that runs through American groundwater.[5,6] It has been suggested that the US prison boom has less to do with an increase in crime and more to do with systemic and policy issues (www.sentencingproject.org).[7] Efforts to reverse this increase have ranged from calls for prison abolition to movements which seek to implement more rehabilitative programming, as well as those which embrace both. While prison policy trends continue to sway from goals of incapacitation to rehabilitation, there is no denying the need for holistic, strength-based responses to the multiple impacts of incarceration on the people who endure it. The emergence of programs for embodied mindfulness practices behind bars, including yoga, reflects one such response. To date, there is evidence of the positive—and in some cases, profound—impact of these programs.

Both authors of this chapter have experience working with incarcerated people and know that the facts and figures with which we opened our chapter can be impersonal and dizzying in their magnitude. In an effort to put faces, stories, and lives to these numbers, we interviewed two formerly incarcerated people, Alan and Megan, who are married to one another, and whom we know through an organization we have collaborated with. They met and

Chapter 7

started practicing yoga while incarcerated. Over two individual Skype interviews that bridged the distance between Massachusetts and Florida, Alan and Megan told us about how they each first encountered yoga through the organization Yoga 4 Change, and attribute their sobriety and current life successes to its practice.

We suggest that Alan's and Megan's stories offer a window into a larger reality of incarceration and recovery shared by many, but emphasize that these two stories are unique and in some ways, anomalous. First, most prisons are gender-segregated according to state designations of biological sex. That Megan and Alan met in a rehabilitation group while incarcerated is unusual but provides sweet synchronicity to their love story. Second, Alan and Megan have experienced many successes, both big and small, since leaving jail. Although they both started out living in a halfway house, they now live together in their own home. Alan has been able to find work, first as a tattoo artist, and then a carpenter, with some supplemental income from working for Yoga 4 Change. Megan has been able to stay home with their children. We celebrate these successes and honor the struggles involved in achieving and maintaining them. We also note that this material success contrasts in many ways with the often chronic unemployment, likelihood of recidivating, and greater discrimination against previously incarcerated people of color (Megan and Alan are both white). We hope to tell Alan's and Megan's stories in a way that leaves room for many other, different stories.

After a review of relevant literature, this chapter explores Megan's and Alan's narratives of recovery and empowerment through yoga, which demonstrate how yoga can be a resource for people in prison. We conclude by pointing to the directions toward which we hope prison yoga service and research will go.

Literature review

Embodied mindfulness practices for people who have experienced trauma

Ongoing empirical research is beginning to demonstrate what many yoga practitioners have experienced through practice: that embodied mindfulness practices can facilitate improved physical, mental, and emotional health, and overall well-being. While research exploring the impacts of embodied mindfulness practices on mental health and well-being is relatively new, evidence suggests that these practices can be beneficial and complementary to traditional treatment approaches, ameliorating a variety of mental health symptoms. Research demonstrates improved health outcomes among those participating in such practices, including decreases in the experience of anxiety,[8,9] depression,[10,11] post-traumatic stress disorder,[12] and improvements in self-esteem.[13–15] Research also confirms that embodied mindfulness practices can benefit people who have experienced trauma, and may even provide benefit where other, more traditional treatment modalities fall short.[12,16–18]

Embodied mindfulness practices in the criminal justice system

That embodied mindfulness practices can be a resource and salve for people in prison may be no surprise. As mentioned, incarcerated people demonstrate higher rates of mental health diagnoses and trauma; and the prison system itself constitutes a traumatizing environment. While anyone can stand to benefit from an increased capacity for self-regulation and self-care, people in jails and prisons may especially benefit from increased access to activities that can decrease trauma symptomology and improve well-being. Evidence suggests that embodied mindfulness practices can represent a complementary or alternative approach to mental health treatment within correctional settings.[19–21]

Some studies focus on the effect of embodied mindfulness programs on measures like recidivism or other post-release outcomes. Landau and Gross[22] found that incarcerated participants in a yoga program were less likely to recidivate as compared to those who did not participate. Other studies focus on how yoga can decrease behaviors associated with reoffending. Such studies are often written for policy makers and correctional administrations. These studies can be helpful for bringing new programs to prisons, but often fail to critique the systemic causes of criminality or acknowledge that much behavior associated with it—such as lying or manipulation—emerge as creative adaptations to the coercions of incarceration itself.[23] Auty et al.'s[24] meta-analysis of yoga and mindfulness programs in prisons demonstrates that incarcerated people who participated in yoga or meditation programs experienced an increase in psychological well-being and improvement in "behavioral functioning," a composite measure that grouped behaviors associated with reoffending. Programs that were of longer duration and lower intensity evidenced greater improvement to psychological well-being than those that were shorter and more intense. Muirhead and Fortune[25] likewise found that yoga had a positive impact on impulsivity and aggression, decreasing depression, and improving attention and emotional regulation—variables associated with offending or the ability to participate in rehabilitation activities. Similarly, Barrett[26] demonstrated stress reduction, improvement in emotional regulation, and improved anger management and impulse control among incarcerated men who participated in yoga and mindfulness programs at their facilities.

Other studies focus on measures of well-being from the perspective of prisoner experience. In one of the most rigorous studies, Bilderbeck et al.[27] explored the effects of yoga on incarcerated women and men at seven prisons in Britain, through self-reported measures of mood, stress, and psychological distress. Participants indicated increased positive affect and reduced stress and psychological distress, and demonstrated improved performance in cognitive behavioral tasks, compared to a control group. In another, Ducombe et al.[28] found positive post-release outcomes resulting from participation in yoga programming. Participants exhibited an increase in awareness, self-esteem, hope, and compassion as well as a decrease in depression. Results of a study by Harner et al.[29] revealed decreased depression and anxiety among incarcerated women who participated in yoga. In a study specifically exploring impacts for incarcerated women, Danielly and Silverthorne[30] found a significant decrease in depression and stress and increase in self-awareness for participants in a 10-week trauma-focused yoga program as compared to a control group.

Finally, a recent report from Georgetown University[21] demonstrates the benefit of embodied mindfulness practices for justice-system-involved juveniles and suggests that future programming should be gender-responsive, culturally competent, and trauma-informed. This report suggests myriad positive outcomes for girls participating in programs from the Art of Yoga Project or the Trauma Center at the Justice Resource Institute, to name only two. Benefits include improved emotional development (such as higher self-respect, self-esteem, and self-awareness), an improved sense of agency and self-control, and improved neurological and physical health. In addition, girls engaging in embodied mindfulness programming noted improvements in interpersonal relationships and parenting practices.

Overall, both the empirical data and people's experiences point to the benefit of embodied mindfulness practices for managing trauma and improving well-being for people involved in the criminal justice system. These practices can empower and help people negotiate environments, such as prisons, that can negatively impact well-being. Current research outcomes support bringing embodied mindfulness practices to jails, prisons, and other criminal justice facilities.

Chapter 7

CASE STUDY Megan and Alan

Megan's and Alan's stories are illuminative of how yoga can be a resource for incarcerated people impacted by trauma. Some readers may be surprised to learn that Alan and Megan's struggles during incarceration—such as with drug addiction, poor self-image, and grief—did not center on hardships unique to people in prison, but are those shared in common with many people in diverse circumstances. The yoga they encountered *while* incarcerated, however, helped them manage these human struggles while living in the context of the banality and occasional violence of the prison setting itself. Indeed, yoga meets us where we are, and Alan and Megan happened to meet yoga in jail. Additionally, while only Megan used the word "trauma" to describe her experience, both discussed suffering that led to drug addiction, and which yoga helped them work through and reframe. In this way, their stories can offer insight into yoga's efficacy for working with experiences of profound struggle, whether these are self-identified, formally diagnosed as "trauma," or left unnamed. In the final section, we will offer some recommendations for people offering yoga in prisons. Here, we examine similarities and differences in two stories of recovery and empowerment through yoga.

Megan first started attending Yoga 4 Change classes because they were her "little escape" from the drudgery of prison. She eventually discovered, however, that "once I actually started to get and stay sober, yoga is a tool that I can use because it helps me be OK with being uncomfortable. And no matter what's going on, and what kind of bodily sensation I am going through, I can say: 'I can stay here for two more breaths.'" Alan can also do anything for two more breaths. For him this capacity to weather difficulty amounts to impulse-control: "You might be in a really deep warrior form," he suggested. "Your legs are killing you. Your whole body's screaming to come out of it. But when you're reminded that you can sit for two more breaths in some discomfort, and the world's not gonna end, so much becomes possible." Over "a consistent practice," he told us, these experiences "add up. You learn that you don't have to act on your first impulse."

That Alan and Megan can do anything for two more breaths is an awareness and mantra they share that has made it possible to live differently, in relation to themselves and others. The phrase emerged in both of their stories as a verbal touchstone. Since Megan and Alan are spouses, it is no wonder this phrase has become a shared idea by which they each come back to the breath and to themselves. The phrase expresses a way in which yoga has opened up life's dimension of possibility for Megan and Alan, together and separately.

Besides this pithy embodied wisdom, how do Megan and Alan understand the ways in which yoga has made sobriety and staying out of prison possible? Alan suggests that yoga has been powerful, in part, because of its combination with his previous exposure to 12-Step community and practice, seated meditation, and reading spiritually nourishing books. The following story is powerful and thus worth reproducing in full. Here, Alan speaks to the efficacy of combination and accumulation of his healing practices:

I had the most profound experience, two weeks before I got out of jail. My daughter's mom had just disappeared with my daughter. I was devastated. I laid in my bunk for two days. It was pretty much a breakdown. I had been practicing sitting meditation and yoga and 12-Step for about 10 months and it was the first big deal that I faced clean. So, I shut down for two days. On the third day, I woke up, and I had an overwhelming sense of serenity. I wasn't happy about the situation ... but I didn't have to keep telling stories about it, and torturing myself over it. It was really surreal—the sense of acceptance I felt. I carried around a notebook, and when I found something I could actually do, even if it was a question to ask an attorney ... I did it. And when I couldn't, I accepted it.

The cumulative effects of yoga, 12-Step, and seated meditation are evident by Alan's word choice: the peace he experienced on that third day was "serenity," reminding us of the "Serenity Prayer" practiced in the 12-Step Fellowship. Upon asking him how he understands this "surreal" experience to have been possible, Alan answered by reiterating much of the above: "Everything I had been doing led to that third day. I had been diligently meditating, practicing yoga, taking a moral inventory. It was a really powerful thing. Especially over a 10 month period." Alan suggests that the efficacy of his practices accumulated in this effect. This understanding of the power of combination and accumulation is embedded in the narrative he offers in the quotation above.

However powerful this combination has been, Alan also notes that it was not until yoga entered that sobriety became a reality. He had been in the "Fellowship for seven years before I was able to put together one year [of sobriety]. Yoga is a whole part of that. The awareness, staying in the present." Sobriety may be the effect of this practice—and a powerful one, at that. But, it is only *part* of the main event, which for Alan is actually about this new "awareness" and "staying in the present." During his surreal day of serenity, Alan recalls a kind of self-possession that paradoxically came along with recognizing the limits of his own control.

Megan's story also speaks of the benefit of combining what she has learned in yoga with other practices—namely, seated meditation. She suggests that what made yoga such a helpful tool for use toward sobriety was its ability to make possible a different self-relationship. She describes the asset yoga offered to her seated meditation practice:

There for a while, every single day, I would sit for at least 10 minutes. I would literally sit down and my brain would start screaming at me. But I would say, "OK, take another breath, see how it feels then." That was important to my recovery life ... that what I'd learned in yoga made it possible to pause and take a second. When I get reactive and I'm able to take a step back? That's all from yoga.

In the last sentence of Megan's remarks, she switches from discussing how she uses skills from yoga in her sitting practice to noting how she can use yoga in everyday life. This easy shift in her speech suggests that the habits of yoga have made her life a practice in itself.

Yoga not only planted the idea that sobriety was possible, but over time, shifted Megan's view regarding how she could relate to herself and others. On the one hand, Megan found yoga "definitely helps with stopping using drugs." She remembers a yoga instructor first inviting her class to "[let] go of the things that no longer serve you." At first, she thought, "'Maybe I can let go of a couple pounds! [*Laughter*] But the things of my using and manipulating people, and my lying, they don't serve me anymore and they're not who I am.' I'm not sure I would have learned that without yoga." Megan credits major changes in her behavior to trying on this idea, through yoga. We wanted to know: if yoga could change Megan's behavior, how did it change her

Chapter 7

view of herself? After a beat: "It *gave* me a view of myself!" Her striking answer suggests there had been no prior self-view to change. She continued, "... prior ... It didn't feel like a priority to me to figure out why I did the things I did. It didn't feel important. Yoga made it to where I could look within rather than outside myself for judgment and validation." In granting her access to a self-view, yoga also simultaneously increased her self-regard. Yoga helped her to venture both the challenge of sobriety and new answers to the question of "who I am."

Yoga is not only a tool for sobriety or managing the stresses of incarceration—although those are powerful benefits. Rather, these reflections show that the self which yoga cultivates is a relational one. Alan's and Megan's abilities to notice and sometimes relinquish judgment of their own emotions and bodies and of other people, through a process of self-witnessing, suggests that yoga is a tool for acceptance of self and other. Alan notes how yoga helps him experience greater acceptance around both negative emotions like fear, as well as around physical pain. "I used to relate to my emotions with action and ownership," he said. "I would become the emotion that I felt and let it control me." Due to what he's cultivated over time, he says he can "acknowledge [his fears] and let them go" in a way that he previously could not do. For example, he half-jokingly chided himself for having stepped away from his mat in the past, because the "pain in my wrists didn't allow me to do as many forms that I enjoy, or the rigorous practice I like, and so, like an angry kid, I stopped practicing." More recently, however, Alan can practice yoga even when he is having wrist pain, because he just modifies forms as needed or goes to gentler classes. He finds himself "overwhelmed with gratitude" because he sees "where I was when I stopped practicing because of my wrists, and where I am now. And I can honor my body now." He can witness and have compassion toward the part of himself that desires perfect physical mastery, and instead, accept when his body needs something else.

Alan also recalls how encountering yoga helped him become newly able to relinquish judgments of other people. His jail was a drug rehabilitation facility that some convicted people would be rewarded with sentence reduction for choosing. Alan at first found himself judging people he knew had no real intention of ceasing drug use. Learning yoga, however, repeatedly exposed him to the lesson of "accepting ourselves where we're at and not judging ourselves and others, either." He recognized that he "absolutely would have done the same thing. So who am I to judge these people who were there at [the facility], on their journey?" Learning greater self-acceptance made other-acceptance possible, as well.

Megan has also found greater acceptance of her body and thoughts and feelings about it. A meaningful seed Megan's yoga instructors in prison planted for her was to "experience this class in this body and on this day." At first, yoga made her notice how much her body had changed (seemingly for the worse), since her days as a child gymnast, and "after the years of abuse I'd put [my body] through." Even today, she admits that she sometimes feels discouraged for not "seeing more results than I am," after years of yoga practice. But she also leaves room for the possibility that her body and its progress (whatever those "results" might entail) is not a problem, but rather that her experience of frustration might arise from not practicing as often as she would like. In this vein, Megan notes, "One of the aspects of yoga that I've been able to take into everyday life is to not judge myself for the thoughts that go through my head." Megan's narrative demonstrates that she *is* judging herself. However, yoga has also given her a framework for considering that greater self-compassion and less self-judgment is a worthy aim and more accurate self-perception.

Megan's and Alan's yoga stories also mark a changing relationship to power. This process began for Alan when he found "courage to be vulnerable," countering the competitive masculinity he had been accustomed to and conditioned by:

Some of the forms, even Child's pose, are not a position any male inmate would put themselves in, in a room of other male inmates. Even the willingness to try and fall down on the balance forms, maybe, is huge. Just this experiential understanding of things happening over time ... starts to teach you that it's OK to be vulnerable.

The context of Alan's experience of vulnerability is key. It overcame him, one day, when he found himself weeping on his yoga mat, in this "room of other male inmates." He had lost his sister to suicide earlier that year. "That was hard," he told us. "[Her suicide] started a year of really heavy drug use. The first time I cried for my sister was on my mat in jail in front of a bunch of inmates. And I didn't give it a second thought. At that point I had no need to be tough or hold back." Alan's vulnerability—whether by courage, or a missing inclination to be "tough," or a mysterious combination of both—opened new possibilities for healing his grief. Importantly, he suggests yoga made presence with the loss of his sister possible.

Megan also began a grieving process while incarcerated: her grandfather died while she was in jail. She mentions him by way of discussing how well yoga is suited to healing trauma:

I do associate myself with that word [trauma], because I've been the victim of physical, sexual, and mental abuse, and I lost my grandpa when I was in jail and I didn't have any way to address any of these things, and later on ... I think yoga gives—it gave me a sense of pride, and a sense of goals that I could set for myself. I'm not letting anyone down if I don't achieve it. And it gave me a sense of power. It made me feel like I had some power and some say in what my life was—what I was—to become.

Megan had not yet begun practicing yoga when she lost her grandfather, yet she situates the prospect of healing from her grief within her engagement with yoga.

While Alan's power paradoxically manifests in his newfound ability to show vulnerability, power manifests in Megan's story in the moments in which pride and a sense of possibility emerge. Megan recalls a time in which she assisted other women in the prison to get into handstands. She recalls their self-doubt, her gentle prodding ("All the women were like, 'I can't!' And I'm like, 'I got you.'"), and her exhilaration in witnessing their success, as they hoisted them*selves* into the air. "It did something so good for my heart," she said. Megan described this scene as one of "taking power back." We asked her to say more: "A lot of the women that we ended up doing headstands and stuff with, I know they had the issues of trauma and abuse that I had gone through ... Watching women who don't believe in themselves give themselves a chance to see if they can accomplish something ... it was an amazing experience! And especially for someone who has had someone say 'you're not good enough.' To kick that sentiment's ass ... is just amazing." Through the prism

Chapter 7

of her own experience, Megan witnessed power in others, and by extension, experienced empowerment herself.

Summary and considerations for practice

This chapter began by stating that the present era of mass incarceration in the US is a public health crisis that impacts some people more harshly than others, and which unfolds in a context and history of systemic oppression. We note that most people who are incarcerated have a history of complex trauma, and suggest, further, that correctional environments can be both newly traumatizing as well as *re*-traumatizing. Megan's and Alan's stories give life to but two journeys in an ocean of 2.2 million incarcerated people. Although Alan's and Megan's stories are particular and characterized by unique traumas, hardships, privileges and joys, we hope their narratives of recovery and empowerment through yoga can offer hope about yoga's potential as a life-giving offering for incarcerated people. Furthermore, their reflections surface insights demonstrating the applicability of Sensory-Enhanced Yoga's guiding principles to the journey of healing through yoga.

Research outcomes to date demonstrate that embodied mindfulness approaches may have significant value as alternative and complementary programming options within correctional settings. Several organizations specifically offer Trauma-Informed Yoga (TIY) programming in prisons, including the Art of Yoga Project, Liberation Prison Yoga, the Prison Yoga Project, the Transformation Yoga Project, Yoga Behind Bars, and Yoga 4 Change. These organizations represent positive models for doing embodied mindfulness work within carceral settings. In light of these outcomes, possibilities, and our own observations, we close with some recommendations for people offering yoga to people in prison. For further reading, we recommend consulting The Yoga Service Council's *Best Practices for Yoga in the Criminal Justice System*,[31] co-authored by a diverse group of professionals in the fields of criminal justice and yoga service. It presents a variety of best practices for implementing yoga and other mindfulness practices within a criminal justice setting. Also see the recommendations in Chapters 6 and 9 on yoga for sexual trauma and complex trauma.

Pursue trauma-informed yoga training

Pursuing training in trauma-informed yoga is an important first step for those who wish to teach yoga in prisons. Several modalities of TIY yoga now exist; Sensory-Enhanced Yoga is one. Although TIY modalities vary, most tend to share similar emphases. New teachers might expect to encounter all of the following areas in a training: awareness of language, yoga practices, and forms that are likely to be triggering for people impacted by specific kinds of trauma; the prioritization of breath as a powerful mechanism for self-regulation; conservative use of touch; and the cultivation of practitioner awareness of how personal and systemic power dynamics can shape the student–teacher relationship.

Be aware of intended and unintended impacts of the prison setting

Yoga teachers should know that the prison environment itself creates a unique and potentially precarious setting for yoga practice. Teachers should therefore strive to create an environment and practice that is as safe as possible, knowing that they can never guarantee safety or define what is safe for any one person. Creating a "safe-as-possible" space involves knowing the layout of the room, where security cameras are located, and whether there will be a correctional officer (CO) stationed in the yoga space. The prison setting is thoroughly characterized by surveillance, so teachers must find strategies—like placing mats in particular orientations—to minimize the sense of voyeurism the setting can create. Teachers will also do well to cultivate a working relationship with the CO, which may soften the power dynamic the CO's presence entails (Kimberleigh Weiss-Lewit, conversation with Amanda Napior, YSC Symposium October 2017).

Be mindful of choices in asana, class structure, and language

Choices in asana, class structure, and language are also of great importance in a prison. Familiarize yourself with how some bodily forms may make some people feel more exposed, or how some shapes can replicate positions of submission associated with arrest or abuse. Hands clasped behind one's back, for example, can simulate arrest.[32] Having this awareness does not mean that certain forms will be triggering for everyone; rather, teachers should familiarize themselves with forms or sequences that may be triggering, and then be deliberate about choices they ultimately make. Because the prison setting means student–teacher contact is limited to class-time, teachers should build opportunities for discussion and debriefing into the class structure. Finally, use language that is non-coercive but instead invitational. Commands should be absent or used minimally.

Cultivate self-awareness and understand systemic oppression

The yoga teacher's work in a prison is bigger than relationships with students, administrators, and a host organization. Individuals and organizations must forefront issues of trauma, systemic oppression, and lack of individual and collective agency at every level of their work. Teachers must ask whether they are the most appropriate person to do this work, and to keep self-inquiry and honesty ongoing. They also need to be aware that good intentions are not enough by themselves. However, if practitioners and organizations take care to hold high standards of training, practice, and growing awareness, yoga programming has the potential to be an empowering and healing offering in prisons.

Develop curricula collaboratively, with theory and practice in mind

Organizations offering yoga in prisons should develop instruction and curricula collaboratively, with theory and practice in mind. Developing programming with others allows practitioners to move toward standardized curricula, to make broader and deeper impacts, and to free up energy for meeting individual needs. For some instructors, "standardization" may evoke images of red tape. Consider, however, that working with others to offer consistent programing is well suited to creating *systemic* change.

Employ critical theories and methods in new research

More research on the benefits of yoga for people in prison is needed. Prioritizing strengths-based measures that foreground subjective well-being (such as changes in levels of self-compassion or anxiety) over normative ideas of good behavior (such as compliance with COs) is crucial. Yoga research in prisons should further highlight the experiences of systemically underrepresented people, including queer and transgender people, women, people of color, and people with historically stigmatized and even criminalized religious belonging. Because empirical research generally requires a critical mass of subjects for statistically significant results, marginalized people are systematically underrepresented in research efforts, including studies about trauma.[32] (In this regard, this chapter duplicates research patterns that over-represent those whose voices we can already hear more than others.) Researchers should pursue rigorous methods that employ a randomized control design, when possible, and combine qualitative with quantitative methods that can reach

Chapter 7

multiple audiences and capture multiple dimensions of the program and subjects under study. Research must pursue and abide by Institutional Review Board protocols.

Towards the future

We bring our chapter to a close with future plans and last words from Alan and Megan. After their positive experiences with yoga, Megan and Alan have both made plans to become yoga instructors themselves. This is one way in which their yoga practices have extended beyond their own recovery from addiction and incarceration. Since the time of our interview, Alan has completed a yoga teacher training and will be returning to the prison as an instructor with Yoga 4 Change. He has also been an Alumni Resource Provider for the organization, visiting previously incarcerated people whose sentences have just ended, to share the components of his recovery with them. Megan has wanted to become a yoga teacher for a few years. Since our interview, she has enrolled in Yoga 4 Change's teacher training. Alan and Megan both hope to support their family by helping other people, so Alan's growing employment in yoga service and Megan's pursuit of a teacher training comprise major steps in the right direction. Like Alan, Megan also hopes to return to the jail as a yoga instructor. Megan told us how much she appreciated her yoga teachers while she was incarcerated; however, she imagined what it might be like for incarcerated women if "someone who was a drug addict was able to bring something back to them." She might have a special kind of impact. "At that point," Megan told us, "it's not hope anymore. Look: it's proof."

Using mind-body practices among populations of mass disaster and conflict

Gretchen Ki Steidle

A healing centered approach to addressing trauma requires a different question that moves beyond 'what happened to you' to 'what's right with you' and views those exposed to trauma as agents in the creation of their own well-being rather than victims of traumatic events. — Shawn Ginwright[1(p. 12)]

Introduction

Both conflict and natural disasters have steadily increased in impact on global populations in the last two decades. According to the United Nations Refugee Agency, there are currently 65.5 million people worldwide who have been forcibly displaced from their homes due to persecution, conflict, violence, or human rights violations (double the numbers two decades ago).[2] Of these, over 40 million are internally displaced within the borders of their home country, 22.5 million are refugees, and nearly 3 million are asylum seekers. Although the number of active conflicts has been declining globally, the number of fatalities has steadily increased, with Syria, Mexico, Iraq, Central America, and Afghanistan accounting for the most deadly regions.[3] At the continental level, Africa is disproportionally affected by conflict and mass disaster. War is the primary cause for 70% of displaced populations in Africa; however, severe floods, storms, earthquakes, and droughts also contribute significantly.[4]

In addition to those affected by war, each year since 2008 about 26 million people worldwide have been displaced from their homes by natural disasters.[4] In the 20 years between 1994 and 2013 there were 6,873 natural disasters, affecting 218 million people on average per year, nearly half of whom were in Asia.[5] Climate-related disasters reached a peak in 2005, yet are still more than double their level in the 1980s.[5]

In this chapter, we explore the mental health implications of war and natural disaster on populations—including those displaced from their homes and those who remain to rebuild their communities after crisis. We consider the challenges in treating the traumatized under such circumstances, and the potential for mind-body modalities to address the limitations of conventional Western therapies. And we review the interventions of several non-governmental organizations (NGOs) using yoga-based, mind-body treatment methodologies in sub-Saharan Africa and discuss the best practices and key considerations for working in post-conflict and natural disaster scenarios.

Review of the literature

Common mental health issues of populations surviving conflict and disaster

The impact of war and natural disaster on displaced populations is multifaceted. Individuals may experience a range of traumatic events, such as violence, injury, exposure to combat, terror, torture, rape, witnessing the death or injury of another (including a loved one), life-threatening illness, accident, loss

Chapter 8

and separation from family members and pets, and destruction of property, among others. Guilt among survivors who have witnessed the death or suffering of others compounds their likelihood of developing post-traumatic stress.[6] As a result of the crisis, those displaced are often required to travel and endure extreme circumstances in pursuit of safety. In addition to war and natural disaster, displacement can also be caused by segregation, imprisonment, or forced-relocation, all of which bring a loss of a sense of place.[7] In fact, displacement itself can be a source of trauma. Fullilove describes this loss of place as *root shock*, "the traumatic stress reaction to the loss of some or all of one's emotional ecosystem."[8]

Whether they cross country borders or not, displaced populations experience an elevated risk of anxiety, depression, and PTSD, and frequently these conditions co-occur. Rate estimates for each condition vary widely for war refugees, though are typically 20% or above, and are influenced by the economic, social, and cultural conditions of the countries from which the refugees fled as well as those in which they re-settle.[9,10] Surprisingly, studies have found that post-migration factors are associated with even higher adverse mental health outcomes than the impact of the pre-migration trauma.[11] These factors include socioeconomic stressors (e.g. financial and housing security), social and interpersonal stressors (e.g. separation from family, perceived discrimination in the settlement environment, and change in social roles, such as loss of the role of breadwinner), and the impact of the asylum process and immigration policies on mental health (e.g. length of detention, extended processing times, and insecure visa status).

Furthermore, PTSD experienced as a result of war or natural disaster can inhibit an individual from fully functioning in managing basic tasks, working, and attempting to reintegrate or settle somewhere new. For those living in internally displaced persons (IDP) camps, the primary stressors include lack of employment, dissatisfactory food, and lack of security.[12] Extended detentions are associated with increased rates of anxiety, depression, and PTSD, and these effects can persist long after release.[13,14]

Most mental health studies of internally displaced and disaster-affected populations are country- or crisis-specific. In Rwanda, where I founded my non-profit Global Grassroots, the 1994 genocide resulted in the deaths of nearly 1 million Tutsi and moderate Hutus in just 100 days of horrifying and well-orchestrated violence. Two million refugees—including perpetrators of the genocide—fled the country by the end of the conflict, while 300,000 were left internally displaced. Within two years, Rwanda, a country with a population of only 8 million, had welcomed back nearly 1 million returnees, predominately refugees who had fled previous conflicts dating back to the late 1950s.[15] A study of over 2,000 internally displaced adult Rwandese found that over 75% had been forced to flee their homes due to the genocide, while nearly 25% of the sample met criteria for PTSD.[16] The effects of the genocide on children were especially heartbreaking: over half of the more than 1,500 youth ages 8 to 19 interviewed in the 1995 National Trauma Survey exhibited probable PTSD and over 90% of the entire sample had witnessed killings and had their lives threatened.[17]

Following conflict and disaster, access to mental health services is often limited, and in some cases the mental health infrastructure has been completely destroyed. A study of more than 2,200 people among the 1.6 million internally displaced in the Ukraine determined that 74% of respondents who needed mental health treatment in the previous 12 months did not receive it.[18] The most frequently reported reasons for lack of treatment included not being aware of the need for care, self-medication, lack of affordability, poor quality services, and stigma. In Rwanda, lack of family support, stigma, poor community awareness of mental disorders, societal beliefs in traditional healers and prayers, scarce resources, and gender differences in the willingness to seek help (with women seeking help more than men) are also frequently reported barriers.[19] Other limiting factors include difficulty reaching remote services, lack of childcare, and lack of time.

Trauma from disaster and conflict is not exclusive to survivors. The Antares Foundation[20] and Centers for Disease Control and Prevention (CDC) collaborated on a series of studies looking at PTSD among various groups working in high-stress environments, and found that 30% of humanitarian aid workers, 25% of search and rescue personnel, and 28% of war journalists experienced significant symptoms of PTSD from their exposure in these crises.

Potential of mind-body modalities for populations surviving conflict and disaster

The Western model of individual counseling, while it may have emerged as the predominant treatment methodology in places like Rwanda, has limitations in circumstances of war and disaster. Formal treatment methods are less effective in disaster scenarios when highly trained specialists may be in short supply, inaccessible, or too expensive; where efforts led by foreign practitioners may be seen as lacking cultural relevance; and/or when locally based therapists may have experienced similar trauma. Interventions that rely on some form of talk therapy or sharing of personal narratives can also leave participants vulnerable in their healing process, especially when comprehensive or ongoing follow-up support is subject to the accessibility obstacles mentioned above.

In contrast, mind-body modalities that address the physiological impact of trauma on the nervous system and can be taught safely with basic training, and without triggering the traumatic experiences of those facilitating, can address many of the gaps that exist with more conventional services post-disaster. Sustainability and impact may improve when programs can be offered on-site, in groups, at minimal expense, and can be shared easily with others. Studies have shown that highly resilient people are often characterized by having an active personal coping capacity and the perception that they have control over their destiny.[6] Certain personal qualities, including self-efficacy and emotional regulation, are associated with lower psychological distress in refugees, suggesting that strengthening these skills may reduce the psychological impact of forced displacement and lengthy detentions.[11] Simple but effective mind-body techniques that can be taught easily and then practiced by the traumatized may also be effective because they transfer control over the healing process from the therapist to the survivors themselves. Finally, when trauma is caused by man-made disaster, such as war, sexual violence, torture, or genocide, healing is most effective when it includes not only an individual process of restoration but also a process for one to reconnect with community and find "meaning by joining with others in social action."[6(p. 73)] Those mind-body practices that can be conducted in groups, may provide a sense of connection and community that acts as a support mechanism.

Here, I will feature three NGOs in Africa that have successfully used mind-body approaches to promote healing and self-empowerment in displaced populations.

Africa Healing Exchange's (AHE) Restoring Resiliency Model (healingexchange.org). This model for vulnerable women in rural Rwanda has been designed in partnership with the clients they serve in Rwanda, and helps people to identify and use tools they were born with to move through trauma and manage stress with greater ease and peace. The Restoring Resiliency mindfulness toolkit includes: sensing in, resourcing, grounding, cross-body

breathing, compassion meditation, and full body integration through yoga. *Sensing in* involves noticing the internal and external sensations from one's physical experience, which acts to turn off the stress response system. *Resourcing* involves calling to mind a moment, memory, image or quality that stimulates positive or neutral sensations to help one feel better and then tracking the shift. AHE reports that noticing pleasant and/or neutral sensations connected to personal resources rapidly builds confidence in a person's capacity to soothe his or her nervous system. *Grounding* involves noticing sensations and safety in the present moment. AHE's Restoring Resiliency Model teaches easy-to-learn skills that anyone can use and then teach to their family members. AHE's goal is "to help people rediscover the inherent resiliency of the human nervous system through culturally-aware community interaction, increased ability to practice and enhance the effects of self-regulation skills, and increased awareness of how the body heals from traumatic or stressful experiences" (Africa Healing Exchange website, healingexchange.org).[22] AHE has been offering culturally contextualized trainings for trainers in Rwanda since 2014, and a group of trainers have even gone on to form their own local NGO that has served over 1,000 people throughout the country.

Global Gratitude Alliance (GGA) (gratitudealliance.org) transforms intergenerational trauma into intergenerational healing and resilience through training, mentoring, and leadership programs in the Democratic Republic of Congo, Rwanda, Nepal, and the US. Their trauma-healing model is designed specifically for grassroots communities lacking access to mental health support. Using a train-the-trainer model with teachers, caregivers, and community workers, they build individual agency for self-healing within the communities who need it most. The curriculum takes place in a group and relationship-based environment and leverages evidence-based, culturally adaptable mind-body healing modalities, including: (1) somatic awareness skills that honor the mind-body connection and help regulate the nervous system; (2) mindfulness training in being present with feelings and emotions, informed by the Hakomi method and breath work practices; (3) a social rehabilitation process of healing through relationship and connection to community; and (4) creative arts therapy in drama, music, dance, play, and indigenous/cultural healing rituals. Results have been strong. A key component of trauma is the loss of one's sense of self and identity. GGA works to build a foundation of self-empowerment as a basis for individual healing and for the ability of participants to promote healing within their communities. In fact, in a recent workshop with female microfinance leaders in Nepal, 85% of participants reported experiencing an increase in sense of identity, "faith in own self," and/or empowerment at the conclusion of the training (Amy Paulson, Co-founder, personal correspondence). Furthermore, 93% of participating women reported having developed concrete relaxation strategies while 96% stated that they had developed tools and strategies for self-care as a result of the training. GGA believes building a toolbox of ways to regulate the nervous system when triggered is a key component of the healing process, so that survivors become less prone to over-reactivity. Furthermore, a self-care practice like GGA protects against vicarious trauma and ensures resiliency for participants to act as local healers.

Capacitar International (capacitar.org) uses a similar self-healing and grassroots training approach, teaching and facilitating group practices in breath and body-based relaxation techniques in over 40 countries globally. Groups meet regularly to practice skills designed to support individual personal transformation, such as tai chi, acupressure, visualization and breathing exercises. Dissemination of these wellness skills occurs through a multiplier effect in which newly trained individuals are directly responsible for sharing the practices with others in already-established grassroots groups with whom they work in their home communities. Often, facilitators are professionals who work with community health workers or who facilitate support groups for target populations such as widows or youth. Wellness skills are most often used to complement other approaches, such as the medical support they may already be providing to patients. Capitalizing on this ripple effect allows the knowledge and practice of these wellness skills to penetrate ever-broadening circles.

In all three organizations, building local capacity for healing and resilience, as well as training trainers in skills that are easy to share, extend the impact of mind-body trauma-healing programs. Mind-body methods allow for a direct physiological benefit that can be felt immediately when practiced by the survivor. When utilized over time, these practices have the potential to reset and support autonomic nervous system self-regulation, which is one of the core physiological functions disrupted by trauma. Using group-based methods, mind-body techniques: are easy to learn and teach to laypeople across religious, cultural, and language barriers; do not require a long-term therapeutic relationship as talk-based psychotherapy does; are accessible to communities with little cost; can be made available immediately post-disaster; and can be continued by individuals, families, and grassroots community groups.

In the sections that follow, I describe how this philosophy has been put into action in the context of my own work with survivors of war and mass disaster and discuss some of the key considerations for the design and implementation of such mind-body trauma-healing programs.

CASE STUDY A personal perspective

When the 7.0 earthquake struck Haiti in January 2010, I jumped at the opportunity to volunteer. As the founder and president of an international non-profit organization called Global Grassroots, I had been working for six years in Rwanda to teach extended courses on personal transformation and social entrepreneurship for women war survivors. In Haiti, I would bring my skills as a breath work practitioner to provide trauma healing to earthquake survivors, first responders, and those grieving losses.

With a small group of volunteers, I arrived in Port-au-Prince eight days after the quake. The hour-long journey across the city from the UN logistical base and airport was shocking. UN soldiers stood guard before a sprawling tent camp forged from clusters of bed sheets and an occasional tarp. Buildings were flattened, one after the other. Power lines were dragging and tangled in rebar. People chipped away at concrete. Doctors treated survivors in parking lots. UN trucks and SUVs filled with aid workers and search teams vied for space on the highway with US soldiers in Humvees. Signs hastily painted on cardboard, bed sheets, or standing walls read: *SOS, Urgent – need help, food, water.*

One such sign at the edge of a river valley declared, "Forgotten Village." With another American volunteer, I walked down through the crumbling hillside to see what I could find. As I do in Africa, I began by seeking out representatives among the women to ask about their priorities. A young man we came across led us through the ruins to a house to speak with a local woman. I anticipated their most urgent needs would include water, infant formula, cooking

Chapter 8

fuel or food. Instead, the woman stated simply, "psychological healing."

Earlier that winter, I had attended a lecture at a medical school in Boston given by Richard P. Brown and Patricia Gerbarg, professors of clinical psychiatry at Colombia University and New York Medical College, respectively. They were presenting on a breath-based, mind-body technique they had been refining, called Breath~Body~Mind™ (BBM; breath-body-mind.com). It had been shown to have a measurable impact in reducing the symptoms of post-traumatic stress among a range of populations including 9/11 survivors and first responders, sexual violence survivors, and others. After undergoing their training, I was equipped to bring it to survivors and first-responders in the wake of Haiti's earthquake.

Collaborating with a local orphanage, I convened a group of about 50 Haitian women to offer BBM. Meeting the women assembled on the veranda, safe from the threat of collapsing buildings, I began simply by asking them to share about themselves and how they were feeling. One described feeling shaky. I saw several women nod. Another had pain in her stomach and lower back. Another responded that she had headaches and was feeling distress. One by one they mentioned their symptoms, almost all indicators of post-traumatic stress, and as others listened a sense of common experience grew. A few indicated they had thought themselves crazy, that they didn't know what was wrong, and were afraid to tell others.

Realizing there was little understanding of trauma and significant stigma around mental health issues, I responded by sharing that all of these experiences were a normal response of the body, which had helped them survive a terrible experience. But, I added, when these same responses continue, it is as if our systems are stuck in that emergency mode. Luckily, there are simple exercises we can do that can help "reset" the nervous system. I asked if they were interested in learning these techniques to secure their consent, and they eagerly responded "Yes!"

As I explained the technique, I was careful not to use terms such as "meditation" or any spiritual reference to ensure that I did not engender any skepticism normally associated with such mind-body practices among the largely Christian and partially Haitian Vodou culture. I then led them in the practice of Breath~Body~Mind (see Box).

The response among the Haitian women was palpable as they let themselves relax for the first time since the earthquake. I went on to share this same practice over the course of two weeks with over 150 women and children in regular sessions at the local orphanage and in the surrounding tent cities, attempting to teach any local participant who might be inclined to share this simple, effective practice with others. Later, back in the US, I conducted breath work with first-responders and aid workers who had also served during Haiti's earthquake.

Breath~Body~Mind™

BBM incorporates four main parts: (1) movement; (2) Coherent Breathing; (3) breath-moving visualization and Open Focus meditation by Les Fehmi; and (4) bonding. For movement, we use a series of qigong practices, which help release the outer layers of tension stored in the body, and help individuals who have dissociated from their bodies due to their traumatic experience begin to ground their attention safely in their bodies again. The practices also help synchronize the pace of breathing with slow movements of the body, supporting autonomic balance.

Using mind-body practices among populations of mass disaster and conflict

Second, we use a particular pace of conscious breathing, called Coherent Breathing, at five breaths per minute. Coherent Breathing helps to soothe the stress response system and bring the autonomic nervous system into balance, resulting in cardiopulmonary resonance and optimal heart rate variability, both markers of cardiovascular health.[23,24] At this pace, the electric rhythms of the heart, lungs, and brain are synchronized.[25] Coherent Breathing has also been shown to increase alpha brain waves, which are associated with wakeful relaxation.[23] To practice Coherent Breathing, participants lie down or sit upright, preferably with eyes closed and breathe gently in and out of the nose for between five and 20 minutes. To keep the pace at five breaths per minute, participants can count a six-second inhale and six-second exhale, or the pace can be kept by playing the sound of a bell using a CD (such as Stephen Elliot's *Respire 1* CD, track "2 Bells"), a smart-phone app, or having a designated person keep time and produce a sound for those breathing, such as clicking two sticks together. It is also valuable to combine Coherent Breathing with resistance breathing, also known as Ujjayi breath or ocean breath, where a slight contraction of the throat muscles during both the inhale and exhale, while the mouth remains closed, produces an audible, "white noise" type of sound.[25,26] This further stimulates the vagus nerve and parasympathetic nervous system. The parasympathetic pathways also connect to the cerebral cortex, where they can help calm the thinking, worrying parts of the brain, and to the prefrontal cortex and limbic system, which can calm emotional distress.[27]

Third, participants are guided in a process of breath moving, imagining their breath moving to different parts of their body with their inhale and exhale, which supports self-awareness as well as respiratory and circulatory resonance. Open-Focus attention training uses awareness of space inside and outside of the body to relieve physical and psychological pain and suffering.[28] The final phase is to integrate and ground the experience through singing, journaling, group processes, or open dialogue to discuss participant experiences.

BBM rapidly relieves stress, anxiety, sleep problems and other symptoms of post-traumatic stress, helping to optimize the stress response system.[24,27,29] It can restore the sense of connectedness, the loss of which is a symptom of PTSD. Evidence also suggests it can reduce our defensive over-reactivity and turn on our social engagement system.[24,30] By practicing Coherent Breathing, the body is able to convince the mind that it is safe to turn down the stress response system and turn on the healing, soothing, recharging systems. Over time, the practice helps reset the autonomic nervous system so that it can self-regulate with greater flexibility and stress resiliency.

Soon after completing the program with humanitarian aid workers back home, I returned to Africa to resume Global Grassroots' work with women from conflict-torn countries (globalgrassroots.org). Our Academy for Conscious Change for women and girls from Rwanda, Uganda, South Sudan, and Kenya explicitly incorporates an avenue for personal as well as societal repair. First, the Global Grassroots' program provides training in BBM and a range of other mind-body techniques that help restore balance to the nervous system. Among our trainees, symptoms of PTSD were reduced by 33% following a two-week training that included daily BBM practice sessions.[31] Second, in addition to offering specific mind-body trauma healing skills, Global Grassroots provides opportunities for women to form teams to establish local non-profits. These venture teams serve as support groups for survivors, but without the stigma associated with isolated mental health services. Additionally, the process of working as teams to initiate social change enables survivors to reclaim their sense of agency and self-worth. Finally, Global Grassroots trains participants in mindful leadership. This multi-pronged approach offers a holistic solution to individual and community healing that works in the context of both post-conflict and post-disaster reconstruction.

Summary and considerations for practice

Since my time in Haiti, Global Grassroots has helped bring BBM, breath, meditation, and mindfulness practices to thousands of change agents from Rwanda, Uganda, Kenya, DR Congo, and South Sudan, many of whom are survivors of genocide, gender-based violence, and the chronic stress of life in a post-conflict zone. I have learned several very valuable lessons from these experiences, which are summarized below.

Observe do no harm policies and support local agency

This helps establish ethical standards for delivering psychosocial programming.[32] Under the do no harm principles, local empowerment, capacity-building, and participatory engagement are crucial. "Participation itself is psychologically beneficial since it helps to restore people's dignity and sense of control following overwhelming experiences."[33(p. 2)] Such efforts serve to counterbalance the dependency often created by outsider programs and aid. They also foster a spirit of self-reliance and provide opportunities for healing through participation in rebuilding efforts.[33] When introducing an unfamiliar healing modality into a new context it is important to allow local participants to assess the effectiveness and relevance of the practice for themselves. This can be done most responsibly by partnering with local psychosocial professionals or partner organizations who can help test techniques in a controlled way.

Foster solidarity and community

It is vital to engage communities and groups in trauma healing efforts, capitalizing on community engagement as well as the multiplier effect. It is especially valuable to use existing social networks to leverage resources, disseminate information, and share skills. It must be noted, however, that support groups for ongoing violence faced by women such as domestic violence, sexual violence, or sexual exploitation are more challenging to establish without a significant level of safety and trust. Women report that cultural stigma, propensity toward gossip, and lack of confidentiality have resulted in the disintegration of well-intentioned efforts, and in some cases, have done more harm than good. It is critical that any community engagement process involving trauma healing must first ensure safety, security, and confidentiality.

Honor privacy and consent

Honoring a participant's consent and protecting privacy are imperative for participants to be able to fully relax, which is necessary for balancing the stress response system. It is important to ask the participants themselves, not just representative leadership, what they want, what they need, and what is necessary for them to feel comfortable to participate. This may require identifying an indoor space with window coverings or choosing a more remote location and the most advantageous timing where and when passersby are less likely to come upon and watch participants.

Maximize safety

Ensuring a sense of personal safety is essential when working with traumatized populations. This necessitates an intentional methodology to ensure they feel a form of choice or control. Programs can begin sessions with grounding exercises that allow participants to fully arrive and feel comfortable with their surroundings. This can include taking time to feel the room, touch the ground with hands, sitting bones or feet, identify the exits, and notice other participants gradually. Using prompts that offer choice is also supportive, such as inviting attendees to take action *when they are ready*, or to close their eyes *if it feels comfortable to do so*, or to give them an alternative: keep their eyes open yet gazing softly at the floor in front of them.

Respect religious and cultural differences

Respect for religious and cultural differences requires explanations to focus on the physiological benefits rather than spiritual explanations that derive from differing faiths or wisdom traditions. Limiting explanations to the biological experience of trauma and the physiological treatments for trauma also helps avoid mental health stigma. Furthermore, training local facilitators can go a long way toward mitigating cultural differences, as they can readily adapt or explain the rationale behind unfamiliar practices.

Consider language barriers

Language differences must also be considered. Facilitators should be skilled in recognizing when concepts are lost in translation or when participants are not connecting with the material (but may be continuing out of respect for outside providers). Such problems can be mitigated by engaging regularly with participants for feedback to ascertain comprehension, tracking non-verbal cues, and taking pauses to ensure comprehension. Furthermore, because some words do not directly translate, it may be necessary to create new terms that signify a similar meaning in the local context. See more below regarding language involving measuring impact.

Minimize mental health stigma

Stigma against mental health is a potential obstacle to effectiveness. In particular, simply convening people in order to offer psychological support can discourage participation. Integrating trauma-healing programs into other social support services through a local partner organization may be important to avoid stigma. Furthermore, stigma related to the disclosure of sexual violence, and associated issues (e.g. pregnancies, religious beliefs, or cultural practices) may prevent victims from seeking support. For example, in Sudan, in the Darfur internally displaced persons camps, treating victims for sexual violence was extremely difficult because of the penalties for sexual activity before marriage under Sharia law. The Sudanese government attempted to require NGO aid workers to register all sexual assaults; however, any resulting "illegal" pregnancies out of marriage could result in imprisonment, spousal abandonment, and other serious consequences. Minimizing risk requires the understanding of such legal and cultural practices, adherence to a strict confidentiality protocol, careful participant selection, and program delivery that offers protection against such risks of harm.

Ensure accessibility

Access for the most vulnerable needs to be considered in any service program design, where travel is expensive or impossible due to the impact of the disaster (including safety and security concerns, disrupted public transportation systems, and a lack of accommodations), where those who are most impoverished have few or no resources for participation in formal programs, and where disabilities and injuries need to be accommodated. It is also important to consider the need for child care among parents, making room for caretakers or inviting participants to trade responsibilities with each other. Finally, it is important to consider the timing of programs to ensure they do not interfere with regular household needs; work; accessing food, water, medical care or other aid services; market days; school times; and the need to travel in daylight for safety. In all cases, programs should be designed with a participatory approach, drawing from local ideas and needs

Chapter 8

before attempting to solve complications. As much as possible, bringing programming to participants where they live at little to no cost will reduce obstacles to access and ensure the broadest impact.

Facilitate transferability

Working with low-tech and easy-to-learn techniques that are transferable allows for spread and use in under-resourced areas. Working where mental health infrastructure is lacking, where there are few mental health workers, or where mental health workers are also traumatized, as is likely after war or disaster, necessitates methods that do not require a one-on-one therapeutic relationship to deliver over time. Program providers must be prepared to work in locations without power or sanitation facilities, or in otherwise suboptimal conditions. For example, inside locations may be dark, unstable, and subject to weather and climate issues (e.g. heat, humidity, flooding, the noise of severe weather). Mind-body practices that require few props, technology, electricity or other material support are distinctly advantageous.

Provide immediate efficacy

Immediate efficacy where people can feel the impact from a practice in a single session, allows for buy-in even without an understanding of the science behind the method. It further makes it more likely that participants will want to learn more, practice on their own, and share with others.

Consider long-term support

Continual support should be considered to ensure there is adequate time to learn a method and benefit from its practice over time. There tends to be an emphasis on "moving forward" in reference to trauma, yet healing from trauma is not a linear path. Short-term interventions can bring profound pain and turmoil to the surface, only to leave that individual more vulnerable if access to continued care and support is limited.[33] When dealing with the aftermath of trauma, there must be a commitment to ongoing care, for oneself and community, sustainable over many years if meaningful healing is to take place. It is important to consider how best to teach participants to maintain the practice on their own, conduct regular convenings, and build local capacity for continued services after the recovery work is complete.

Customize impact measurement methods

Measuring impact may require customized methods in foreign cultures or with disadvantaged populations. Programs can utilize surveys with a sample group of participants to establish a baseline and periodically assess changes in trauma symptoms using tools such as the PTSD Checklist for DSM-5 (PCL-5), which is directly downloadable from the National Center for PTSD website (ptsd.va.gov). Working in a foreign language requires translation into the foreign language and then back translating by another party to ensure accuracy. Understanding the limits of language or the capacities of participants is important in accurately assessing impact. For example, in Haiti, the local language does not allow for a sense of gradation between "never" and "always" or between "none" and "the worst" in assessing the frequency and severity of symptoms. In these cases, using a five-part Likert scale is not effective. One alternative is to convert a standardized test to a visual analog scale, which uses a line to denote symptom frequency and severity between the two extremes. The 10 cm line for each question is drawn on the paper survey. Participants are asked to make a mark on the line at the point that best describes their experiences. The length of the line from one end to the mark can then be quantified as a score, and compared between questions on baseline and endline assessments.

Using mind-body practices among populations of mass disaster and conflict

The field of trauma healing in disaster and conflict scenarios is characterized by vast needs and an array of promising initiatives. There remains widespread need for more sustained and more holistic interventions to address the particular needs of underserved individuals and communities in the wake of crises. Mind-body programs provide one of the best alternatives for care in these particular and sensitive situations.

Yoga for complex trauma survivors

Alison Rhodes

I am not going to have resolution, but yoga helped give me a sense of peacefulness and a place. — Complex trauma survivor

Introduction

While PTSD is a useful construct for capturing the symptoms associated with many types of traumatic exposure, it falls short in capturing the deleterious effects of prolonged or repeated exposure to trauma, especially when that exposure begins in childhood and when it is of an interpersonal nature.[1] Examples of this kind of trauma exposure include childhood emotional, physical, and sexual abuse, severe neglect in childhood, prisoners of war, concentration camps, human trafficking, and domestic violence. Ultimately, these are conditions where individuals face extreme powerlessness, humiliation, deprivation, and loss of control over their own lives and bodies.

Survivors who face such trauma suffer in all dimensions of their being—mind, body, and spirit. They struggle to function effectively and to be present in their lives. Although there is currently no official diagnostic category that captures the range of symptoms following prolonged trauma exposure, the constellation of symptoms that emerge from such traumatization are well documented and researched and are referred to as *complex trauma*, *complex PTSD*, or *DESNOS* (disorders of extreme stress not otherwise recognized).[1,2]

Symptoms of complex trauma

Symptoms of complex trauma cluster around six interrelated problem areas:[1,3,4]

1. ***Regulation of affect and impulses***. Survivors of complex trauma frequently have difficulty modulating emotional reactivity (e.g. persistent dysphoria, explosive anger), and often turn to maladaptive methods to cope with overwhelming emotions such as self-injury, suicidal ideation, and substance abuse.

2. ***Memory and attention***. Chronic traumatization commonly leads to alterations in attention, memory, and consciousness including amnesia, dissociation, and/or depersonalization.

3. ***Self-perception***. Feelings such as shame, guilt, and self-blame tend to be prominent, leading to low self-esteem and self-worth.

4. ***Interpersonal relations***. Complex trauma survivors often have difficulties with trust and intimacy and struggle in their relationships with others; those who have experienced childhood abuse in particular are more predisposed to re-victimization.

5. ***Systems of meaning***. Many survivors experience feelings of hopelessness or despair, a loss of sustaining faith and/or long-held belief systems.

6. ***Somatization***. Many experience recurrent or multiple medical conditions; these bodily problems may relate to actual physical harm caused by the trauma or they may be psychosomatic reactions such as unexplained numbness or pain in the body that have no apparent organic cause.

Chapter 9

They also include the physical manifestations of the impact of chronic arousal of the autonomic nervous system (e.g. gastrointestinal distress, fatigue).

As with uncomplicated PTSD, the range of symptoms associated with complex trauma cohere around self-regulatory problems, though to a more severe degree. As Cloitre and colleagues explain, "Understanding the effects of trauma as the result of disturbances or vulnerabilities in self-regulatory capacities is useful as it creates conceptual coherence to the multiple, diffuse, and apparently contradictory symptoms of complex PTSD. Disturbances in self-regulation account for both overactivation and deactivation/avoidance in emotions and interpersonal behaviors."[5(p. 2)] It is important to note that these problem areas overlap with, yet go beyond the symptoms of PTSD; this is why we see complex trauma survivors carrying a myriad of concurrent diagnoses along with PTSD, such as anxiety disorders, mood disorders, substance use disorders, ADHD, personality disorders, and beyond.[6,7]

Prevalence of complex trauma

Rates of complex trauma are difficult to quantify given that it has not been recognized as a distinct disorder in current diagnostic classification systems. However, we can begin to gain a sense of the number afflicted when we examine rates of PTSD as well as the rates of childhood trauma exposure. As mentioned earlier in the book, the lifetime prevalence of PTSD is approximately 7% in the American population.[6,7] Although men are more likely to be exposed to a traumatic stressor, women are significantly more likely to develop PTSD (11.7% vs 4.0% among men).[6,7] Moreover, among those who develop PTSD, 40% experience chronic symptomology regardless of whether they seek treatment.[8] Finally, among those diagnosed with PTSD, 84% have at least one additional psychiatric diagnosis, including (but not limited to) depressive disorders, anxiety disorders, and personality disorders.[8]

It is the nature of the trauma that most accounts for the different gender rates of PTSD, the intractability of the disorder in many people, and the likelihood of comorbid conditions.[1,9] A large proportion of the individuals suffering from PTSD have been exposed to chronic trauma, often beginning in youth. A survey of 17,000 HMO members (the Adverse Childhood Experiences (ACE) study) showed that more than a quarter of adults in the United States have experienced some form of serious maltreatment during childhood (e.g. abuse, neglect, witnessing family violence), and that there is a direct relationship between this exposure and longer term mental and physical health.[10-12] Adverse childhood experiences tend to co-occur, and the more ACEs a person has experienced, the more likely they are to experience such problems in adulthood.[10,12,13]

Research also shows that women are more likely than men to experience recurrent interpersonal trauma perpetrated by intimates, often beginning in childhood, such as sexual abuse.[8] Moreover, women who experienced childhood maltreatment tend to experience multiple types of trauma across their life spans including sexual assault, physical assault, emotional abuse, neglect, and domestic violence.[13,14] In both men and women, treatment unresponsiveness and complexity in symptom presentation are correlated with earlier onset of trauma exposure and with chronicity of exposure.[1,5,15]

In sum, we see that a substantial proportion of individuals who are diagnosed with PTSD are suffering the effects of complex trauma. Additionally, there are a large number of adults who may not meet criteria for PTSD yet suffer with a range of mental and physical health problems associated with their chronic trauma exposure. The fact that so many experience chronic symptomology even after seeking treatment for PTSD or other trauma-related conditions speaks to the need to continue to advance treatment approaches that will be effective with this population.

Limitations of current treatment approaches

As was touched on in previous chapters, talk therapies—many of which emphasize cognitive reframing, memory processing, and/or exposure and desensitization—are often ineffective for PTSD, because they (1) do not attend to the role of the body in recovery processes; (2) do not sufficiently address self-regulatory deficits; and (3) often activate brain regions associated with intense emotional responses which in turn deactivate speech areas, thus decreasing one's ability to translate experiences into language.[16] Rather than desensitize the person to the trauma trigger as intended, for at least some people, exposure therapies can overwhelm and activate (often worsening) the very symptoms the treatment aims to reduce.[17–20]

The above scenario is particularly the case for complex trauma survivors, many of whom have never developed the internal resources to modulate their distress (due to very early trauma exposure) or else have lost these resources over time and are thus unable to stay affectively present through the treatment. For example, a dissociative response to exposure treatment would yield such treatment ineffective because it allows the survivor to avoid the stimuli and removes any opportunity for habituation.[20,21]

Psychobiology of complex trauma

It is essential to understand and address the brain and body's role in complex trauma responses in order to effectively treat the self-regulatory problems that underlie survivors' symptoms. As described in detail in Chapters 3 and 4, the same neurobiological dysregulation that underscores PTSD is at work in cases of complex trauma. Additionally, complex trauma survivors are coping with the residual effects of unresolved ANS responses to prior trauma. Of particular importance is the "freeze" response in complex trauma. Because of the chronic and inescapable qualities of the traumatization this population experienced, many survivors are stuck in states associated with the dorsal vagal response that was activated during their trauma exposure. So, in addition to being emotionally flooded in response to trauma reminders, many survivors are chronically dissociated and thus shut down to any present moment experience. As a result, they may under-respond to real threats, such as by remaining in a hostile relationship, and/or lack awareness of basic needs, such as hunger or the need for rest.

However, dissociation does not account for all of the struggles complex trauma survivors have in attending to their needs; for many, a history of being denied things essential for healthy development also contributes to these problems. These include physical necessities like food, shelter, and clothing and also emotional needs like attunement and love, especially from caregivers upon whom they were dependent. In order to maintain the connection with a caregiver who is not meeting their basic needs, the child comes to feel shame for having those needs and feelings, and ultimately stops seeking for those needs to be met. Thus, there is a pattern of deprivation that many complex trauma survivors will continue with into adulthood related to this chronic shame state where they do not feel deserving of care from themselves or anyone else.

Furthermore, in cases where caregivers were abusive or neglectful or failed to be relatively consistently attuned with the child, or in cases where trauma outside the home may have disrupted the formation of healthy attachments with caregivers, self-regulatory capacity is negatively impacted. Indeed, recent research has shown that brain systems involved in affective regulation are formed through healthy dyadic (pair) attunement with attachment figures. Thus, chronic traumatic experiences early in life would undermine the development of one's ability to successfully process emotions, modulate stress, and self-soothe.[22]

To summarize, what we commonly see in complex trauma survivors is a challenge of being embodied, of knowing how they feel and what they need in a consistent way. The burdens of their trauma history make it challenging to engage effectively in their lives; they tend to overreact to situations that are safe or underreact to situations that demand a higher level of engagement. In order to address these issues, survivors must improve their ability to accurately interpret bodily sensations, their surroundings, and their experiences through increased ability to stay present with mindful attention. Additionally, they need to learn to tolerate and modulate distress (such as when triggered) through healthy self-soothing mechanisms that help calm their nervous systems when flooded and through strategies to increase attention and energy when dissociated. They also need to learn to practice basic self-care, which begins with a felt awareness of their physical experience and learning to make choices that attend to whatever they are experiencing with an attitude of non-judgment and kindness.

Benefits of yoga for survivors of complex trauma

Yoga has the capacity to address many of the issues plaguing survivors of complex trauma. For many of the survivors that I have worked with, yoga was one of the first times in their lives that they set aside time and space to pay attention to themselves and work on making choices based on self-care. Yoga also taught them much needed skills to self-soothe. However, like any other treatment modality, yoga may be challenging for complex trauma survivors. In this chapter, I share the research evidence on yoga for complex trauma survivors that came out of the Trauma Center of Justice Resource Institute, which has successfully run a yoga program for complex trauma survivors for well over a decade.[23,24] I also present a composite case vignette based on this research. I worked with the Trauma Center's research team on their randomized controlled trial[25] and the related long-term follow-up study,[26,27] and also taught Trauma-Sensitive Yoga classes at the clinic.

Review of the literature

The Trauma Center's yoga program, referred to as Trauma-Sensitive Yoga (TCTSY), was developed by trauma-informed clinicians and yoga teachers. The approach emphasizes gentleness in forms and teaching style, creating a sense of safety for traumatized students, and opportunities for the yogis to make choices for their own bodies (see references 23 and 28 for a more detailed account of Trauma-Sensitive Yoga). After many years of success in offering group classes for both men and women at the Trauma Center, as well as small group lessons at residential treatment facilities for traumatized adolescents, the Trauma Center carried out the first large-scale randomized controlled trial (RCT) of yoga for women with chronic PTSD.[29] This was followed by several other quantitative and qualitative studies, most of which were related to the original RCT. These studies are discussed below, starting with the quantitative studies before diving deeper into the personal experiences of the participants as described in the qualitative studies that follow.

Quantitative studies

In the original RTC, 64 women, all of whom had histories of exposure to prolonged trauma, were randomly assigned to a treatment group, which participated in 10 hour-long weekly sessions of trauma-informed yoga, or a control group, which participated in supportive women's health education classes at the same frequency and dosage. Most of the women had experienced some form of childhood maltreatment (e.g. 77% experienced physical abuse; 87% experienced emotional neglect) and the majority also experienced trauma in adulthood such as serious accidents, sexual violence, and life-threatening illnesses. On average, participants endorsed experiencing at least eight types of traumatic experiences during their lifetime. In addition, they had all been living with PTSD (as well as many other comorbid mental and physical health problems related to their trauma histories) for at least 12 years at the start of the study. The study findings included significant reductions in PTSD symptom severity, greater improvements on measures of depression, and greater decreases in engagement of negative tension reducing activities (e.g. self-injurious behaviors) among those who participated in yoga. Furthermore, 52% of participants in the treatment group no longer met criteria for PTSD as compared with 21% of participants in the control group.

After completing their participation in the RCT (following an interlude ranging from 9 months to 2.75 years), 49 of the original study participants took part in a follow-up study where information was gathered on traumatic symptomology as well as on the frequency of continuing yoga practice since completing the RCT.[27] This study further reinforced the earlier findings that practicing yoga was associated with improvements in PTSD symptomology and depression. Another key finding from this study was that the more frequently participants practiced yoga in whatever setting—whether home practice, yoga in the wider community, and/or Trauma-Sensitive Yoga classes at the Trauma Center—the greater the benefits.

Building on the prior research, the Trauma Center recently carried out a treatment feasibility study of a 20-week Trauma-Sensitive Yoga protocol for women with chronic, treatment-resistant PTSD (n=9).[30] Results showed that this more intensive format, which included a longer period of weekly classes as well as assignment and monitoring of home practice, led to significant reductions in PTSD and dissociative symptoms. The symptom reductions appeared to go beyond what has been demonstrated in treatments of less intense and shorter durations, showing promise for this longer duration, more frequent format.

Qualitative studies

Two qualitative studies were also carried out at the Trauma Center to better understand participants' experiences of yoga and its potential role in their recovery. In the first study, West and colleagues[31] interviewed all 31 participants who had completed the yoga treatment in the original RCT conducted by van der Kolk et al.[29] It was found that, in line with the RCT quantitative findings, the women experienced improvements in their trauma symptoms after 10 sessions of yoga. The women reported positive changes that went well beyond symptom improvement toward experiences of personal growth, which the authors synthesized in themes of "gratitude and compassion, relatedness, acceptance, centeredness, and empowerment" (p. 182).

The second qualitative study was a phenomenological study that I carried out with all of the participants in the follow-up study[27] who had experience with yoga (n=39) to further understand their experiences of healing through yoga over time.[26] This study articulated a core experience for the participants of what it meant for them to heal through yoga after complex trauma over time as a multidimensional process of "claiming peaceful embodiment." In contrast to states of shame, pain, sadness, anxiety, rage, fragmentation, and numbness that dominated the women's experiences prior to yoga, the women spoke of a greater sense of control over their emotional and mental states. They could be more present in their lives, and increasingly experienced positive changes in how they related to their bodies and their identities more generally; their ability to tolerate and express emotions; their relationships with others; and their priorities, sense of meaning, and/or outlook on life.

The interviews mentioned above revealed themes that were common to both qualitative studies.[26,31] Here, however, here I present quotes from my own research.

Chapter 9

First and foremost, participants revealed significant changes in their relationships to their bodies. As one participant stated:[26(p. 250)]

> Just inhabiting my own skin is a major step forward. It allows me to be in my life now ... I think the practice of being more in tune with my body and being able to develop some tools to control my internal energy and the calmness that can come is significant.

The positive changes in the women's felt experiences of their bodies empowered changes in behavior. Notably, they began to practice self-care off the yoga mat. This included becoming aware of and attending to basic needs:

> I've always been content to not think about myself at all. I live in my head and my eyes and don't think about anything below my chin. Yoga did make me start thinking more about—even when I'm not in yoga class—thinking about the chair underneath me or what I'm seeing or smelling or what is going on around me, more tune in the world. It had a huge impact because I was just so good at ignoring all the physical sensations before that, and now I've started to realize that they are important. It's important information if you are hungry, tired, or in pain.

There were also significant changes in the women's relationships to their emotions. They saw their yoga practices enabling more reflectiveness, less reactivity, and improved intentionality around emotional well-being:

> Instead of having an emotional outburst you realize there is a place to process it. Yoga is a process to open you. It's not abrupt—jump up and down, lose 10 pounds. It's not jarring. It's a slow step-by-step deliberate process to make you open. You connect that same thinking to your emotional health. You realize it's a process and you say okay this got on my nerves and maybe I should process that, what's behind it. Suddenly I think it applies to everything else you do.

They also reported greater ability to create safe interpersonal boundaries. The women articulated having previously engaged in harmful relationships or focusing more on pleasing others than taking care of themselves. As they began to become more in tune with their own needs and feelings, and value themselves more, they were empowered to be able to say "no" when it came to pushing their limits:

> I don't want my boundaries to be violated again so I'll put up a boundary and say no to someone—versus just numbing out one way or another ... I just feel more comfortable making myself a priority and thinking that I am important ... It has made me adamant that I'm not going to compromise that for anyone and I will not put that on the back burner or ignore my own needs anymore.

Moreover, they expressed a sense of hope—hope for their futures, hope that they would continue their journeys of healing, and hope and belief that they were good people and capable of living better, more enjoyable and more meaningful lives. This was a turning point for many of the women, as without the belief in the possibility of positive change, there is little room for actual change to occur. With this hope came a sense of self-efficacy and empowerment:

> I think [yoga] helped more than a lot of other things. I did talk therapy for 10 years before yoga. I think [talk therapy] helped, but maybe I just was not as engaged in my own recovery at that time. Now I am really trying and really working the program so to speak. I'm just more active in the process. Maybe it's all those things about feeling more empowered personally that have made me more active in saying I want to do something about this.

While yoga offered substantial opportunities for healing, the path was not always easy. For some women, yoga was an enjoyable experience from the start, a time when they felt strong, calm, and more present. For others, especially those that struggled with dissociation, there was a period of becoming more aware of difficult body sensations—pain, discomfort, anxiety and so on.

Many participants also described flashbacks being triggered in yoga. Often there was a process of working through the struggles of increased body awareness and eventually experiencing the positive dimensions of yoga.

The case study that follows is a composite based on the interviews I carried out to further illuminate the processes of recovery through yoga after complex trauma and some of the challenges those I interviewed faced. Quotes come directly from the participants, but some details have been disguised in accordance with the consent process and clinical requirements.

CASE STUDY Amanda

Amanda is a 40-year-old, white, heterosexual, single female who experienced emotional and sexual abuse as a child. She also witnessed domestic violence, and was sexually assaulted in her early 20s. Amanda carried diagnoses of PTSD, major depressive disorder, and panic disorder, and reported significant challenges in attending to basic needs. For instance, it was a real struggle for Amanda to shower daily, not only due to difficulty paying attention to her own body but also because she had been sexually abused in a bathroom on numerous occasions. She also did not eat with a healthy frequency and stated that she was often unaware of feelings of hunger. Further compromising her health were sleep difficulties caused by her hypervigilance and chronic nightmares.

Amanda reported regular experiences of dissociation and chronic shame states. She described herself as a perfectionist, was often hard on herself, and regularly sought external validation of her self-worth. She struggled with chronic suicidal thoughts and for a period in her teens and early 20s she engaged in self-injurious behaviors, including cutting and burning herself.

Amanda had been in talk therapy on and off for over 15 years when she participated in the yoga group in the Trauma Center's 10-week RCT.[29] Her yoga practice was somewhat sporadic after the study—she would attend classes at the Trauma Center regularly for a couple months and then stop for a couple months. She also practiced some yoga forms at home on occasion and with her current psychotherapist who has some experience in yoga.

Amanda had never tried yoga before the study trial, but had heard about its many benefits and hoped it might help with her ongoing trauma symptoms. However, initially her experience in yoga was very challenging. As she explained, "It was difficult to start at first, just to get acquainted with my body, especially after dealing with trauma. So, starting it at first, I didn't like doing yoga." At first it was common for her to have many negative bodily experiences in the classes including pain, discomfort, and flashbacks, and on one occasion, she experienced embodied fear to the point that she screamed out in class. "It was really hard, and I wasn't expecting the reactions that I had during the classes," she said.

Certain yoga forms, especially those where she was lying supine on the floor, with her legs open

Chapter 9

Consider duration, pace, and class size

The group classes at the Trauma Center for adults are an hour long. However, benefits can be derived in clinical settings by doing a yoga form here or there, or engaging in a brief sequence during the session. With adolescents we have seen a shorter format (usually about 15 minutes) work well.[32] Additionally, with adolescents we have found that dyads and triads (twos and threes) are preferable to larger classes.[32]

Smaller groups tend to work better than bigger groups for adults, and individualized work can also be very beneficial. Complex trauma survivors have articulated a preference overall for a gentle, slow practice.

Nurture a healing alliance

Trauma-informed yoga teachers ideally embody many of the qualities of a good therapist, including being present, engaged, welcoming, approachable, and flexible (in terms of making changes). At the same time, teachers must respect the limits of their professional qualifications by referring students to a licensed mental health counselor (if they are not one themselves) to process through any personal issues that may be drawn to the surface during yoga and disclosed to the teacher. To further facilitate safety, it is helpful if the teacher does not move around the room too much and practices asana with the students on his/her own mat. Similarly, it is generally recommended to avoid offering physical assists, which can be experienced as invasive and triggering.

Choose your words carefully

Another key issue to attend to is choice in language. Emerson[28] explains that the commonly used term "pose" can be triggering for complex trauma survivors given that some have histories of being forced to pose in sexually exploitive ways and given that posing speaks more to how the asana practice looks than to how it feels. Teachers are encouraged to prefer the term "form" (as is used in this book); this phrasing aims to emphasize connecting with feeling, as opposed to trying to do something "correctly" or "better." And it has been found that the terms "relax" and "relaxation" can be highly triggering for complex trauma survivors and therefore they are avoided.

Use a language of inquiry, grounded in bodily experience

Prioritizing a language of inquiry[28] further helps survivors connect more to their internal experience and make choices based on what they are experiencing. This includes keywords such as "notice," "curiosity," "allow," "try," "when you are ready," "you are welcome to," "if you like," etc. Phrasing such as this invites students/clients to notice what they are feeling in the present moment and practice self-care by making choices for their own bodies.

Encourage curiosity, choice, and self-care

Overall, choice emphasized through language is aimed at creating an atmosphere of curiosity and self-care that allows survivors to "take effective action" (e.g. make themselves feel better) over placing demands on one's body.[28] I once worked with a survivor who felt very vulnerable with her arms extended wide in Warrior II form. Through experimentation, she found that by placing her hands on her hips she felt strong, and she really enjoyed that experience.

Giving verbal cues for modifications can also provide opportunities for students to become curious about their experience and explore taking effective action. For instance, during a standing forward fold, a teacher might say, "You are welcome to explore this form with your hands on the ground or you are welcome to experiment with placing blocks under your hands."

Consider clients' readiness for potentially triggering forms

It is helpful initially to avoid yoga forms that are likely to be more triggering such as those that focus on the pelvic area (e.g. Happy Baby). The goal may be to develop more comfort in potentially triggering forms, but it must be done at the client's own pace.

At the close of classes, Trauma-Sensitive Yoga teachers will provide a range of options for the final resting form, in addition to the classic Savasana (which can be quite challenging for some). These include, for instance, sidelying, seated on the floor or in a chair, or any other form that allows the client to access some sense of ease. Modifications of any form are always presented as equally good options—no one form is better than another. Offering the choice of practicing in a chair or opting out of any form is encouraged.

PART 3

East meets west: the theory and guidelines of Sensory-Enhanced Yoga®

Sensory-Enhanced Yoga®: healing trauma through the koshas 10

What is most compelling about the kośas is that they offer us a paradigm through which we can feel and investigate the interpermeating nature of the mind, body, breath, and energy as it manifests in the here and now. — Michael Stone[1(p. 99)]

Up to this point, we have discussed yoga from the Western scientific perspective and provided objective research evidence to support the assertion that yoga is one of the best adjunct treatments for PTSD. Describing what yoga actually *is*, however, can only be undertaken from the perspective of its traditional Eastern origins. This chapter re-introduces yoga from the ancient yogic perspective of the kosha model which provides the foundation for the Sensory-Enhanced Yoga program. This discussion will lead directly into the **Transdisciplinary Model for Post-Traumatic Growth** and the definition, purpose, and guiding principles of **Sensory-Enhanced Yoga**. The program synthesizes Western theoretical concepts with traditional Eastern yogic philosophy to produce a cogent practice model for healing symptoms of combat stress, PTSD, anxiety, or other unresolved trauma or ANS conditions.

A path to self-awareness and integration

Yoga is a mindfulness-based practice that has evolved over the past 5,000 years or more, and has its roots in ancient India. The word "yoga" is derived from the Sanskrit word *yuj* ("yoking"). Its most common contemporary translation is "union" which has most frequently been interpreted to mean the union of mind, body, and spirit. Whether or not yoga is a religion (a common question) depends upon the type of yoga practiced, as yoga is a very broad term that encompasses many different styles. The vast majority of these styles are secular, though some are still grounded today in Hinduism and/or Buddhism—the religious cultures from which the practice evolved. There are also styles that are explicitly Christian as well as styles that are marketed more as fitness programs, including in school systems in the US.[2]

Yoga has easily moved beyond its Eastern cultural origins because the practice helps to bring one home to oneself, wherever one is located on this planet, and whatever one's faith or lack thereof. Patanjali, author of the *Yoga Sutras* (circa 400 CE), writes in Yoga Sutra 1.2: *Yoga is the cessation of the fluctuations of the mind.* By clearing the mind of the clutter created by the sensory world and our resulting conditioning, a person comes to better understand their own true nature, which can ultimately draw them closer to their own faith if they have one. However, the practice of yoga does not inherently involve devotion to a god or savior. Father Tom Ryan writes:[3(pp. 18,19)]

The experience of many in intercultural encounters is that when something of value is discovered in another philosophy or worldview or religion, it sends you back with fresh eyes and renewed appreciation for what is analogous to that in your own faith tradition which before you took for granted.

The classical tradition of Yoga represents a valuable gift from India to the world, and what makes it particularly precious is that it can be used selectively

Chapter 10

the *Niyamas*, or observances, and are briefly listed in Table 10.2.

It is thought that Patanjali positioned these yogic dos and don'ts prior to the asana (forms) and pranayama (breath work) limbs because working at the physical and energy levels can draw out emotions, and one needs to know how to handle these emotions in an ethical manner when they arise. Thus, the ethical guidelines provide a top-down wisdom-based approach to managing potential emotional abreactions (purging of emotional tensions) that may be elicited from the bottom-up effects of the yoga movements and breath work, in addition to more generally guiding our actions in our everyday lives.

Those suffering from PTSD, combat stress, or other deep emotional wounds tend to be at greater risk for developing negative attitudes and/or false beliefs that may perpetuate their symptoms. In the case of PTSD specifically, these can generally be sorted into two major categories: *"the world is dangerous"* (hyperarousal) and/or *"the world is meaningless"* (dissociation). There are often others, e.g. *"I can't trust you"*; *"I don't care about you"*; *"my life will never get better"*; *"my mind can never heal"*; *"no one cares about me"*; or *"it is too late to change"*, any of which can lead someone to compromise their ethics. In particular, those who feel their life has hit rock bottom and they have nothing more to lose may be less apt to restrain their impulses.

Or, it may have been a breach of personal ethics that led to the emotional wound in the first place. For instance, the breach may have occurred due to pressure from an authority figure or as a result of conditioning, such as is the case with the "battle-mind mentality." A prime example of that is the "moral injury" many of our service members have suffered, which has recently made headlines in the media and was discussed in Chapter 5. According to Litz and colleagues,[5] moral injury is "an act of serious transgression that leads to serious inner conflict because the experience is at odds with core ethical and moral beliefs." The core belief here is *"It is my fault and I am a bad person."*

Moral injury shares PTSD-like symptoms (such as intrusions, avoidance and numbing) but also includes symptoms of shame, guilt, demoralization, self-handicapping behaviors, and self-harm.[6] Hyperarousal is not considered a symptom of moral injury; thus, as mentioned in Chapter 5, moral injury and PTSD are two different but related conditions (Figure 10.1). However, one can certainly suffer from both. War zone events that may contribute to moral injury include (but are not limited to) mistreatment of enemy combatants and acts of revenge, incidents involving civilians, and within-rank violence such as military sexual trauma or friendly fire.[6]

Individuals suffering from moral injury require very special care. Due to the depth and complexity of the injury, we cannot simply ask a service member to forgive themself for transgressions made while in

Table 10.2 Yamas and Niyamas

Yamas (things not to do)	Niyamas (things to do)
Ahimsa (nonviolence)	Saucha (cleanliness)
Satya (truthfulness)	Samtosha (contentment)
Asteya (non-stealing)	Tapas (self-discipline, perseverance)
Brachmacharya (non-excess) i.e. of sensual pleasures, including sexual energy	Svadhyaya (study of one's self) i.e. self-awareness; self-knowledge
Aparigraha (non-possessiveness; non-greed)	Ishvara pranidhana (devotion) i.e. surrender of the fruits of one's practice to a higher power

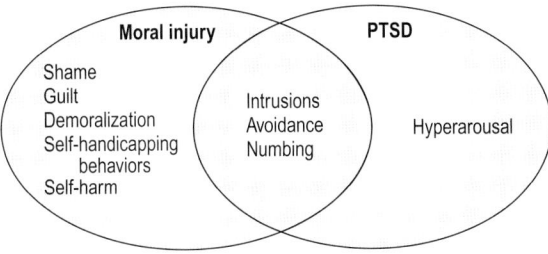

Figure 10.1
Symptom overlap between PTSD and moral injury. Based on the article "Moral injury in veterans of war", by Shira Maguen and Brett Litz[6]

the military. Some trauma experts who are also veterans have warned that reciting affirmations on self-forgiveness may backfire. We also cannot address moral injury using strategies to reduce hyperarousal, as moral injury is shame-based, not fear-based:[6] addressing hyperarousal will not address the shame. However, as with all deeply held emotions, the moral injury is carried in the body, and will likely remain there until it is safely released from the body, and not simply through an act of intellectual rationalization. Yoga and breath work combined with careful languaging—together with professional counseling—can help to safely release these difficult emotions and thoughts and allow space for more positive attitudes and beliefs to take hold.

Guiding treatment principle: *New beliefs and attitudes more easily take hold when we first prepare the body to receive and accept them.*

Anandamaya kosha (bliss body)

The *anandamaya kosha*, known as the "bliss body," is a transcendent state of consciousness characterized by a feeling of deep peace, joy, and love, achieved when we are "one" with the experience of being fully immersed in what we are doing. It is often discussed in the context of a deep state of meditation but can also be experienced when actively engaged in a task to the point where the person loses their sense of separation from it. Unlike the vijnanamaya kosha, which steps back from an experience to witness it, at the level of the anandamaya kosha you do not witness the bliss, you *are* the bliss. You are not "doing" skiing, you are skiing *itself*. Once you stop to contemplate it, you are no longer experiencing the anandamaya kosha but have instead dropped back down to the vijnanamaya kosha, as the witness.

Truth to tell, there are many interpretations of the anandamaya kosha. A few modern scholars[7] have aligned it with the concept of the "peak experience" coined by the psychologist Abraham Maslow, who described it as an event which typically occurs in the context of "doing." He felt these experiences were more likely to occur in people who had reached a state of "self-actualization," having fully met their physiological needs, safety needs, love and belongingness needs, and self-esteem needs.[8]

In the original source, the Taittiriya Upanishad itself, the anandamaya kosha is described in sometimes conflicting ways, including akin to the state achieved when we are in a deep, dreamless sleep, which we all experience regardless of our stage of psychological development. This is explained in the English interpretation of the Taittiriya Upanishad written by Swami Sharvananda:[9(p. 74)]

It is called Anandamaya Kosha inasmuch as while in that deep sleep state the Jiva is not conscious of any change, modification or multiplicity which give rise to the sorrows of life; he enjoys a kind of serene peace, even the individualized consciousness is absent there, so with it also the feeling of limitation. Moreover, in the scale of subtlety, it is but one step removed from the Supreme Brahman.

Though described as similar to a deep sleep state, the anandamaya kosha is not devoid of emotion: "Love

Chapter 10

is its head, joy its right wing; delight is its left wing; bliss is the trunk (self); Brahman is the tail, the support."[9(p. 71)] Also in the same text: "This Anandamaya is the enjoyer of all fruits of action and hence has it been said to be formed of bliss."[9(p. 74)] Here, bliss is tied to action but appears to be described as a state that occurs as a consequence of "doing" rather than during the process of "doing" as implied by Maslow's "peak experience."

With respect to PTSD it seems apropos to describe the bliss body as *both* a state of optimal being and a state of optimal doing, particularly since PTSD is a mental condition in which an impairment in occupational functioning, i.e. doing, is a diagnostic requirement. States of "being" and "doing" usually do go hand in hand and relate to the concepts of spirit and self-empowerment, respectively. As both an occupational therapist and yoga therapist whose domain of concern is helping people achieve both happy and productive lives, I must look at trauma through this wider lens. This is reflected in the fifth guideline to practice.

Guiding treatment principle: **Self-empowerment is born on the wings of the spirit rising from the mind-body connection.**

Table 10.3 depicts a healing process through the koshas for those individuals who have PTSD and fall into the hyperarousal/reliving/re-experiencing subgroup or the hypoaroused/dissociated subgroup, as defined by Bremner[10] and Lanius.[11] Many people who have been traumatized will experience symptoms from both categories, along a continuum or even simultaneously.[12–14] For example, it is common to experience intrusive thoughts of the trauma and at the same time experience poverty of thought as it relates to the typical "mental chatter" that occurs as people go about their daily lives. In a similar vein, a person may be hypersensitive to certain types of sensory input, such as sound or visual stimuli, at the expense of registering other types of input, such as bodily sensations—or conversely be preoccupied by internal bodily sensations at the expense of noticing what is happening around them in the environment. And we are wired biologically to disconnect from the body when being "in" the body feels unsafe. You will notice that the guiding principles for treatment are the same for both subtypes of PTSD.

Sensory-Enhanced Yoga®

Thus, we have arrived at the very heart of the book, the description of the Sensory-Enhanced Yoga program, including its underlying theoretical model and guidelines for practice. This program is closely informed by the kosha model and all of the information presented in previous chapters. The program is intended for use in clinical practice by occupational and physical therapists; clinical psychologists, counselors, and social workers; yoga therapists; and related mental health professionals who serve individuals who have experienced trauma or high stress and/or who suffer from related conditions such as high anxiety, ADHD, sensory processing disorder, bipolar disorder, or mixed anxiety-depression.

Sensory-Enhanced Yoga program definition and purpose

Definition: Sensory-Enhanced Yoga incorporates carefully selected sensory input, breathing techniques, and language into yoga practice, within the context of a safe container, in order to address issues related to hyperarousal, hyperactivity, hypervigilance, dissociation, and/or sensory sensitivities.

Purpose: The purpose of Sensory-Enhanced Yoga is to help individuals manage (and hopefully eventually resolve) these symptoms and be able to self-regulate, that is, conduct their daily lives in a calm, centered, focused, and productive manner.

Sensory-Enhanced Yoga®: healing trauma through the koshas

Table 10.3 Healing trauma through the koshas

Kosha	Hyperarousal/re-experiencing	Hypoarousal/dissociation	Guiding principle
Annamaya kosha *Physical body*	Lost sense of bodily safety	Lost sense of bodily connection	A sense of safety is essential for healing
Pranamaya kosha *Energy body*	Hyperarousal	Hypoarousal	The most direct and powerful way to self-regulate is through control of the breath
Manamaya kosha *Mental body*	Sensory sensitivity Rigid movements Intrusive thoughts	Low registration Dissociated movements Poverty of thought	Yoga can promote effective sensory, motor, and cognitive processing of traumatic experiences and thus aid healing
Vijnamaya kosha *Wisdom body*	"The world is a dangerous place" In the case of moral injury: "It is all my fault and I am a bad person"	"The world is a meaningless place"	New beliefs and attitudes more easily take hold when we first prepare the body to receive and accept them
Anandamaya kosha *Bliss body*	Too hypervigilant to relax into joy	Too numbed out to feel joy	Self-empowerment is born on the wings of the spirit rising from the mind-body connection

Important note: This table is simplified as many trauma survivors have symptoms from both columns. For example, individuals who have the dissociative subtype of PTSD often have intrusive thoughts of the traumatic event along with the poverty of thought (disrupted mental chatter) that often accompanies a dissociated state, while those who do not have the dissociative subtype are a lot less likely to experience poverty of thought.

The program is designed to help participants meet the following goals:

- Effectively manage stress before it leads to emotional dysregulation and/or inappropriate behaviors.
- Develop emotional resiliency, that is, the ability to rise to meet a challenge or threat, as well as easily calm once it has passed.
- Decrease hypervigilance and overreaction to sensory input (e.g. visual, crowds, touch, noise, movement).
- Improve quality of sleep and energy level to support wellness and enhance daily productivity.
- Decrease intrusive thoughts by learning to become present through breath and body awareness.
- Enhance their sense of self-worth and personal empowerment.

Sensory-Enhanced Yoga is founded on a treatment model that synthesizes theoretical concepts and research findings from the fields of occupational therapy, trauma psychology, neuroscience, and traditional Eastern yogic philosophy. The yoga sessions skillfully apply therapeutic tactile, proprioceptive (muscle) and vestibular sensory input, breathing practices, and language, within the context of a trauma-informed asana yoga practice to foster a sense of safety, calm, and tranquility throughout the entire bodymind. Special care is taken to help students coordinate movements with the breath, which is especially powerful in reducing hyperarousal and drawing the mind back into the body and the present moment.

The movement and breath work help to safely release body-stored tensions, trauma, and negative attitudes, thus preparing the body to more readily respond to positive suggestions and guided meditations, which are also incorporated into the program. These verbal elements of the program promote a sense of self-worth and personal empowerment, which support health, well-being, and achieving one's goals. Thus, the program promotes healing from both the bottom-up, using the *power of the body to influence the mind*, and the top-down, *using the power of the mind to influence the body*. Great care is also taken to create a "safe container" for students, both physically and psychologically, in which healing can occur. Students' abreactions are welcomed and responded to skillfully and with compassion, and appropriate precautions are followed when working with trauma survivors.

The ***Transdisciplinary Model for Post-Traumatic Growth*** and the ***Guiding Principles of Sensory-Enhanced Yoga*** guide the implementation of a Sensory-Enhanced Yoga program. These are discussed in the remainder of this chapter.

A Transdisciplinary Model for Post-Traumatic Growth

Figure 10.2 presents a theoretical framework for addressing mind-body health and quality of life for those who suffer from combat stress or PTSD. It summarizes the underlying theory for Sensory-Enhanced Yoga through a wide lens, showing how carefully designed mind-body modalities may help one heal from PTSD, regain a positive outlook, and develop a sense of self-empowerment that will facilitate successful re-engagement in valued occupational activities and roles in society. When used within a therapeutic setting, mind-body modalities should ideally be presented in concert with an articulated plan for meeting client-set goals in order to capitalize on the person's physiological readiness for psychological change.

I originally designed the Transdisciplinary Model for Post-Traumatic Growth to explain the likely reasons why the Iraq Yoga Study protocol worked and the treatment implications. I more recently added the kosha language at the top of the model after it was already fully developed. This model was written entirely from a Western science perspective, incorporating research and concepts from the fields of occupational therapy and trauma psychology, before I even realized how well it fit in with the kosha model. Many experts have identified and developed important concepts for healing trauma and I simply wove them together, effectively recreating the (ancient) wheel. As we delve into the model, I hope to impress upon readers that some of the perceived discrepancy between Eastern philosophy and Western science is simply due to the language barrier and that Western science is quickly validating what the ancient yogis have theorized all along. A brief summary of the model is presented below, following which I will introduce the ***Guidelines for Practice***.

To promote healing in PTSD, we need to help the individual **safely reconnect to the body, aka the annamaya kosha**, and to accomplish that, we need to help the person to **self-regulate**. We can do this pretty effectively through the use of carefully selected sensory input and breathing techniques designed to rebalance the autonomic nervous system (at the level of the ***pranamaya kosha***), as described earlier, and by helping to release trauma-based muscular tension. These techniques must be provided within a "safe container," which is a term used in trauma work

Sensory-Enhanced Yoga®: healing trauma through the koshas

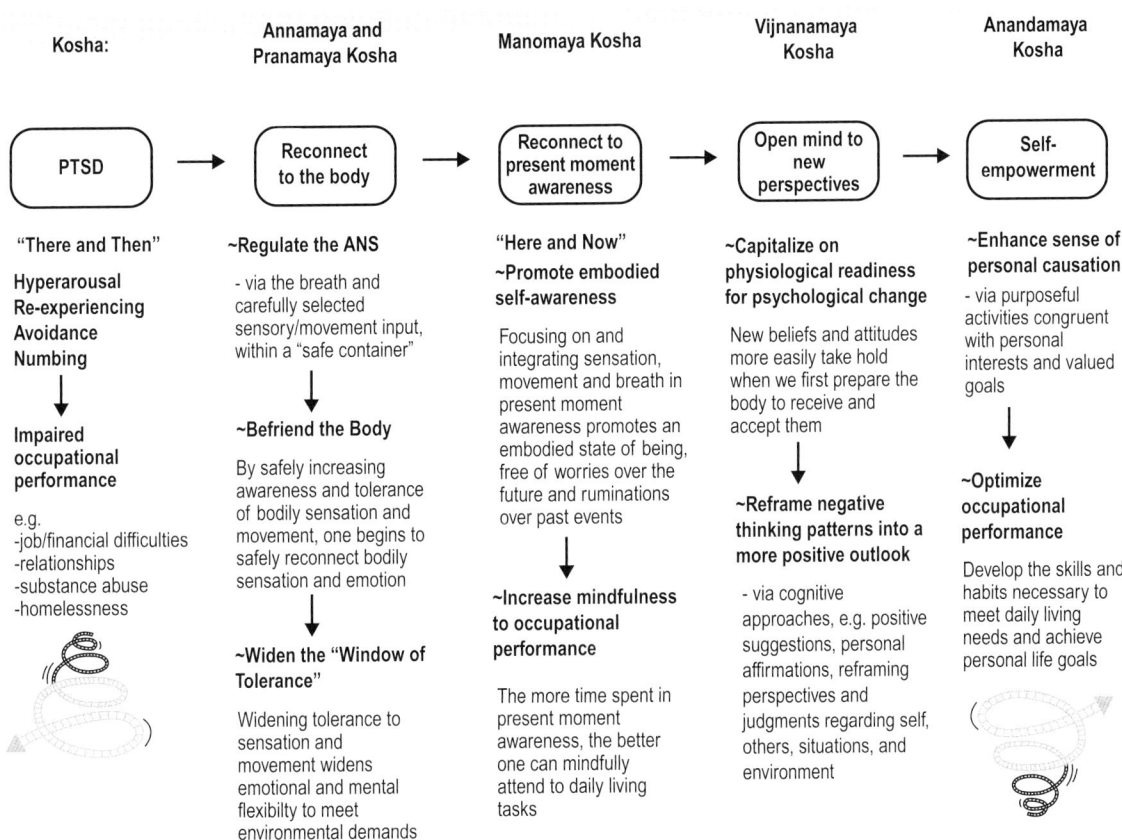

Figure 10.2
Transdisciplinary Model for Post-Traumatic Growth (by Lynn Stoller, MS, OTR/L, C-IAYT ©2012–19)

that means attending to the environmental qualities of the setting as well as the interpersonal relationship between therapist and client. We cannot guarantee safety for our clients but we can control the variables that influence it (see Chapter 11).

By safely increasing awareness and tolerance of bodily sensation and movement, one begins to **safely reconnect bodily sensation and emotion—at the level of the manomaya kosha, or mental/emotional body.** This helps to develop the emotional and mental flexibility to more effectively adapt to social and environmental demands.

Focusing on and integrating sensation, movement and breath in *present moment awareness* promotes an embodied state of being, free from worries over the future and ruminations over past events. The more

121

Chapter 10

time spent in the here and now, the better one can mindfully attend to daily living tasks, and the more value these tasks will hold for the individual.

Through this process, the mind becomes more open to new perspectives—at the level of the vijnanamaya kosha, or wisdom body. New beliefs and attitudes more easily take hold when we first prepare the body to receive and accept them. For example, it is more difficult for someone who is wound up tight with anxiety or slumped over in depression to take a counselor's advice to heart. Talk therapies may thus be more effective when paired with yoga and combining top-down and bottom-up approaches within yoga—such as through Sensory-Enhanced Yoga—can be especially therapeutic.

Re-framing negative thinking patterns into a more positive outlook helps to promote a sense of self-empowerment, which is associated with the bliss body, or anandamaya kosha. It is by working through the other layers that we achieve an optimal sense of well-being *and* an optimal sense of well-doing. This can be further promoted through a variety of purposeful activities congruent with personal interests and valued goals. Through this process, one develops the neurophysiological readiness and the intrinsic motivation to address the skills and habits necessary to meet daily living needs and achieve personal life goals, finally returning the traumatized individual back home from war (or whatever horror the person is stuck in) and into a fully engaged life in society.

Guiding principles of Sensory-Enhanced Yoga for self-regulation and trauma healing

The five guiding principles listed below are closely informed by the Transdisciplinary Model for Post-Traumatic Growth.

1. ***A sense of safety is essential for healing.*** The hyperarousal symptoms of trauma are rooted in an unresolved fight–flight reaction that occurred in response to a serious safety threat. In order to resolve these symptoms, it is necessary to restore a sense of safety within the body. Toward this end, great care is taken to create a "safe container" for students within the Sensory-Enhanced Yoga classes. Among the variables to consider are the setting and timing of classes, choice of asanas and other techniques, and the interaction between the yoga instructor and the yoga participant. Classes are conducted at a quiet time and in a quiet place to reduce the possibility of disturbance by other people in the building. Efforts are made to reduce visual clutter and environmental noise as much as possible to promote calming. If music is used, instrumentals are chosen which are soothingly melodic and/or have a slow, even rhythm. High pitched or low threatening sounds are particularly avoided. Special care is taken before introducing any scents (such as incense) into the environment as olfactory nerves synapse directly on the emotional center of the brain (amygdala) and can potentially trigger hyperarousal or re-experiencing symptoms.[15] Instructors recognize and avoid presenting yoga forms that promote a sense of vulnerability in particular individuals, such as certain wide-legged yoga forms (e.g. bound-angle), or in certain cases, even lying flat on one's back in a group setting. They also help to foster the student's sense of control in the session, through the use of invitational language and by presenting choices. Instructors offer physical assists very judiciously (if at all) and always ask first. If used, they employ a firm, "whole hand" touch rather than a light feathery touch.

2. ***The most direct and powerful way to self-regulate is through control of the breath.*** Respiration is the only function of the autonomic nervous system that humans typically have control over. All other functions of the ANS (heart rate, blood pressure, sweating, eye dilation, digestion, and so on)

are involuntary. Yogic pranayama (breathing) techniques have been shown to facilitate sympathetic or parasympathetic activation, depending upon the technique used.[16] Sensory-Enhanced Yoga instructors choose pranayama practices that bias the autonomic nervous system toward parasympathetic (rest and digest) rather than sympathetic (fight/flight) dominance, in order to reduce symptoms of hyperarousal and thus potentially the re-experiencing symptoms. They also encourage their students to coordinate yoga movements with the breath (such as by inhaling when moving upward, toward the center, or expanding the chest and exhaling when moving downward, folding, twisting, or away from the center), and to move slowly enough to allow fuller diaphragmatic breaths rather than quick, shallow breaths, which also help to activate the parasympathetic nervous system. Mindfully coordinating movements with the breath links the mind and body in present moment awareness, promoting a fully embodied experience. During static forms, students may be cued to direct the breath into the area(s) being stretched, which often helps to release muscular (sometimes trauma-held) tension and can produce a calming effect. Students are also given opportunities to explore the effects of certain mudras (ancient yogic hand gestures) that are carefully selected for their postulated effects on the bodymind, especially including the breath and the autonomic system.[17]

3. **Yoga can promote effective sensory, motor, and cognitive processing of traumatic experiences and thus aid healing.** Sensory-Enhanced Yoga incorporates principles from sensory integration theory and neurorehabilitation into the yoga sessions to maximize the innate benefit of yoga for reducing symptoms of trauma or extreme stress. Yoga sessions are especially designed to provide enhanced proprioceptive (muscle) input, deep touch pressure, some slow rhythmical movement, carefully selected pranayama (breathing) techniques that promote calming, and a series of asanas that are chosen to balance the nervous system toward a more relaxed and steady state. Generally speaking, a session will have a greater predominance of forward bends, twists, and/or forward inversions and will take special care to provide effective counter-forms to balance the potentially arousing effects of backbends. Backward inversions (with head strongly tipped backwards) are either avoided altogether or presented with extreme caution. Balance forms promote sensory integration on many levels and are especially powerful for helping to improve focus, bringing the mind back to the present moment.

4. **New beliefs and attitudes more easily take hold when we first prepare the body to receive and accept them.** When a person is struggling with anxiety, a trauma, depression, or other difficult situation, the mind often develops negative thinking patterns which can become reinforced over time in a downward spiral, leading to an increased sense of hopelessness. This negative mindset often expresses itself in the body in a myriad of ways *and* is further reinforced by that expression. For example, anxiety is frequently accompanied by an increase in heart rate and muscle tension, while depression tends to be accompanied by lethargy and fatigue. Mind states also affect, and are further reinforced by, the manner in which one holds and moves the body, such as through protective posturing (e.g. hunched shoulders, aversive gaze, stiff movements). By helping to release these body-stored emotions, and by calling the mind back to the present moment, yoga clears space to allow new positive beliefs and attitudes to take hold. Sensory-Enhanced Yoga capitalizes on this opportunity by pairing positive suggestions with specific asanas that embody their essence in order to bring the power of the thought into

Chapter 10

the full mind-body experience. These suggestions are carefully worded to increase awareness of and validate the practitioner's own observations.

5. ***Self-empowerment is born on the wings of the spirit rising from the mind-body connection.*** People cannot function well in life when their spirit has been broken by trauma. In many cases, everyday tasks become more of an effort and there is no motivation to create or pursue long- or short-term goals. When the spirit plummets, so too does the sense of self-empowerment. But when we address the trauma by carefully choosing and integrating bottom-up and top-down approaches, as described by the other guidelines, we provide the right conditions for the spirit to lift again. Life regains meaning and motivates the person to re-identify and pursue interests, hobbies, dreams, and goals. Occupational therapists, licensed mental health professionals, and certified yoga therapists are especially qualified to facilitate the life re-engagement process using the tools of their respective trades. Many grassroots organizations working with limited resources and staffed mostly by volunteers have also been highly effective in empowering both individuals and entire communities. Building partnerships between various professions and organizations can help form the necessary referral networks—essentially safety nets—to ensure that those in need are fully supported along their journey to reconnect body, mind, and spirit and to find renewed meaning in their lives.

Summary

This chapter provided an overview of the Sensory-Enhanced Yoga program and the ***Transdisciplinary Model for Post-Traumatic Growth,*** which provides its foundation. This model synthesizes the ancient kosha model with current treatment concepts from the fields of trauma psychology and occupational therapy in order to support clinical decision-making when working with traumatized individuals. The remaining chapters of Part 3 will provide detailed information on each of the guidelines and then in Part 4 we will put the whole practice together.

Guideline 1
A sense of safety is essential for healing

The first task of recovery is to establish the survivor's safety. This task takes precedence over all others, for no other therapeutic work can possibly succeed if safety has not been adequately secured. — Judith Herman[1(p. 159)]

Establishing a sense of safety is widely considered to be the first essential task to promote healing from trauma.[2-4] In yogic philosophy, a sense of safety has been traditionally linked with the **annamaya kosha,** since without a physical body a person cannot survive. In discussing her three stages of trauma recovery (safety, remembrance and mourning, and reconnection with ordinary life), Herman writes, "[In] the course of a successful recovery, it should be possible to recognize a gradual shift from unpredictable danger to reliable safety, from dissociated trauma to acknowledged memory, and from stigmatized isolation to restored social connection."[1(p. 155)] And from Porges: "In other words, any intervention that has the potential for increasing an organism's experience of safety has the potential of recruiting the evolutionarily more advanced neural circuits that support the prosocial behaviors of the social engagement system."[4(p. 273)]

Yet, as Burstow points out, there are two problematic assumptions underlying the concept that a "sense of safety" should be used as a measure of one's level of healing from trauma: (1) "the world is essentially benign and safe, and so general trust is appropriate," and (2) "people who have been traumatized have a less realistic picture of the world than others."[5(p. 1298)] Burstow raises the issue that for many people of minority races and for "psychiatric survivors" the world is actually not a safe place, so their world view is *not* distorted, and that those who have not been traumatized are "walking about with a certain cloak of invulnerability," (p. 1298) editing out the risks as they go about their lives.

Safety is a relative concept

We must therefore acknowledge that safety is a relative concept, influenced by time, space (including circumstances), and perception. For example, there is no doubt that I sit in relative safety in my comfortable suburban home as I type these words, certainly much more so than a soldier on foot patrol, a refugee in a detention camp, a person in prison, or a wife in an abusive relationship. Yet it is never too far from my mind that two of the most powerful leaders in the world are currently bragging about the size of their nuclear buttons. This potential threat, from thousands of miles away, presents in my body from time to time as a free-floating anxiety, most perceptibly upon first wakening in the morning as my body takes its first "safety" reading of the day.

This type of potential threat affects us all, layered on top of any safety threats closer to home, which vary from person to person. We cannot possibly know all of the calamities that could potentially befall us in any given moment; it is our **perception** of threat that influences our bodily reactions. My concerns are not necessarily the same as those of my friends.

Chapter 11

Our sense of safety also varies moment to moment, again affected by perception. Some people are nervous drivers, acutely aware of potential dangers on the road; others drive to work on autopilot, hardly aware of any threat to safety. People may feel safer or less safe at work or at home, depending upon their personal circumstances. Likewise, some may feel safer in yoga class, even while deployed to the front lines, or returning to an abusive household or unsafe neighborhood following class. Conversely, they may feel *less* safe, aware that things may be brought to the surface during yoga that they have been pushing back from their minds outside of class.

We may have little influence over students' personal situations outside of the yoga class, but how we present our yoga session will have a strong influence on how safe our students feel during that time, and if a feeling of safety and relaxation is sufficiently soaked into their bodyminds during class, they may walk out of class with an enhanced **perception** of safety in their lives. There are cases when this goal may be too incongruent with the reality of life or circumstances,[5] but we can nevertheless provide a pocket of time in which the autonomic nervous system has a chance to learn to relax and feel safe for the moment. As Porges[4(p. 250)] points out, "The human nervous system evolved efficiently to shift between conditions of safety and danger." It is in this manner that we promote greater **resilience**, that is, the ability to rise to meet a challenge and the ability to calm once the challenge has passed—thus mastering a sense of safety within the context of time and space.

Three things to consider

When considering the concept of safety in a yoga session, we need to concern ourselves with three things:

1. What is the student's perception of safety within the environmental setting, and how can we modify the setting to positively influence that perception?
2. What is the student's perception of safety with respect to their relationship with us (the teacher or therapist), and how can we modify our behavior and/or attitude to positively influence that perception?
3. What is the student's felt sense of safety (or lack thereof) regarding being in his or her body, and how can we modify the practice to positively influence that perception?

When providing yoga to traumatized students, the ideal is to design an optimal environment, to embody the qualities of a good therapist when welcoming and working with the student(s) within that environment, and then to help the student(s) gradually and safely reconnect with their bodymind within this healing soup of conditions. But an ideal environment is not always available, such as in a war zone, prison, or refugee camp. So again, it is helpful to consider the concept of safety in relative terms: a yoga tent within a forward operating military base; a yoga room within a prison setting; a special space set aside in whatever difficult environment the person finds themselves in and which, over time, they begin to associate with healing and which inspires them to let down their guard for even just moments of time.

Create a healing space

We need to create a space for practice that allows students to deeply heal. This is often referred to as creating a "safe container." We modify the environment to reduce stimuli that may reinforce hyperarousal or hypervigilance or possibly trigger an abreaction (see the sections on sensory precautions and triggers below). We also remove any objects or symbols which could be construed to promote a certain religion or culture, such as statues of Buddha or Hindu gods or goddesses, or artifacts of Western religions for that matter. (If the class does intend to

Guideline 1
A sense of safety is essential for healing

merge religion and yoga, that should be explicitly stated prior to students joining the class.) We create a space that is psychologically safe by interacting with our students in a manner that respects boundaries and which welcomes whatever arises in them as well as our own reactions to it, so that we can respond to the situation with self-awareness rather than fear. To do this, we need to be grounded. If the student has an emotional catharsis, we support the person in an authentic, trusting, and unconditionally accepting manner to allow it to complete the process and serve as a healing experience. We communicate to our students our confidence that he or she has the inner resources that will allow them to process their trauma the way they need to process it. However, we do not play the role of a counselor unless we *are* a licensed counselor; instead we refer on if the student starts to confide personal issues beyond the domain of our licensed profession.

Above all, we place the students—not the instructor or therapist—in full control of their own experiences. We do this by encouraging students, in every yoga session, to listen to their own bodyminds and to get out of a yoga form or stop a breathing or meditation practice if it causes discomfort or distress, and also by giving them a *choice* in every aspect of the yoga practice. As Emerson and Hopper[6] have emphasized, this is especially vital when working with individuals who have been traumatized.

Consider class segregation

As a general rule, survivors of trauma will especially benefit from trauma-informed yoga classes that are designed specifically for them and are closed to the public. For example, segregated classes designed exclusively for active duty military personnel and veterans often foster close-knit communities in which each member feels deeply supported. The students learn to develop a deep trust among one another that feels safe enough to reveal their inner feelings without fear of being judged in a negative manner. Sometimes the veterans decide to open the class up to their significant others, which creates a different dynamic but can lead to wonderful, supportive friendships among the couples and provide a shared bonding experience for the veteran and their partner, which is often therapeutic in itself. In fact, a few veterans have expressed that they felt more comfortable coming to class when accompanied by their spouse or significant other. However, the decision to open the class up to significant others is best left to the trauma survivors themselves, and it should never be a requirement.

In the case of sexual trauma, it is especially helpful to segregate the genders to foster a sense of safety, while remaining cognizant of the fact that sexual trauma can be perpetrated by someone of the same gender. This includes segregating female veterans from male veterans, as a high percentage of female military personnel have experienced sexual trauma and may feel uncomfortable in a room with men, especially in vulnerable positions. Of course, it is important to be sensitive to the fact that men can experience military sexual trauma as well. If it becomes known that a male or female student has experienced sexual trauma, whether in a mixed gender class or not, the teacher should consider offering a spot in class where there will be no students positioned behind them when assuming yoga forms such as a Standing Forward Fold, Table, or Down Dog.

If it is a specialized class for sexual trauma (or even if not), positioning the mats in a circle so students are facing the center of the room may be advisable. Also, all yoga classes should ensure sufficient space between students. Yoga mats should not be placed one directly behind the other, and likewise there should be ample space between mats if placed side by side to avoid awkward wide-legged Forward Bends when facing the long edge of the mat.

Chapter 11

Promote safety in the bodymind

Once the environmental and interpersonal factors are addressed, the therapist can begin to help the student foster a sense of safety in the body, or as van der Kolk put it, "befriend the body."[7,8] Van der Kolk points out that, "In order to change, people need to become aware of their sensations and the way that their bodies interact with the world around them. Physical self-awareness is the first step in releasing the tyranny of the past."[8(p. 101)] Attending to bodily sensation is a hallmark of a mindful yoga practice. However, with trauma survivors, this process needs to proceed in a careful manner in order to avoid becoming inundated by these sensations. Rothschild[9] has famously used the analogy of a pressured soda bottle to drive this point home: the safest way to release the pressure is to open and close the cap in a slow, cautious, and intentional manner so as to prevent an explosion.

How does this translate to yoga practice? For one thing, it is clearly not a good idea to present a hip opening series to a group of women who have been sexually traumatized, though hip openers might be ever so slowly introduced as part of the healing process. I recommend that any yoga form that includes a hip opener be presented with an alternate choice that does not open the hips. For example, you might present the choice of a standard Seated Forward Fold (with both legs outstretched and parallel to each other) *or* a one-legged seated forward fold (see Dynamic Head to Knee, Chapter 17). Additionally, a blanket can be offered to all participants during more vulnerable yoga forms such as Bridge or Dynamic Head to Knee, a solution taught to me by Annie Okerlin, founding director of the Exalted Warrior Foundation (see Figure 13.17 in Chapter 13 for an example). Use of a blanket not only fosters a sense of safety within the practice but also provides neutral warmth to the body, which promotes calming and the release of muscle tension—and this could be the stated intention.

Many experts feel that yoga straps should be avoided in classes designed for sexual trauma survivors or survivors of other types of interpersonal violence that may have potentially included bondage. Though I have not personally witnessed hesitation in using a strap, the belief does seem intuitive. Certainly every yoga class designed for trauma survivors or even for the general community should present yoga straps as a **choice**, not a requirement—and it should be called a yoga strap (or assistive band), not a belt. All yoga forms and moves performed with a yoga strap can also be easily performed without one, and this should be stated. However, banning yoga straps from a program altogether would eliminate an opportunity to experience a particularly rich form of proprioceptive input that can promote a felt sense of embodiment in a sensorially comfortable and integrating manner (via inhibitory gating mechanisms). One expert on our faculty offers the **choice** of using a yoga strap during the third week of her class series for sexual trauma survivors. She has mostly used the yoga strap for arm stretches, which all of her students have appeared to greatly enjoy. However, one person was triggered when the yoga strap was offered for leg stretches, which are also strong hip opening stretches in a more vulnerable position when done on a yoga mat; thus, it is recommended that these leg stretches not be included in a class for sexual trauma survivors. These stretches have been very well received by male military veterans, though, so are included in this book so as not to deny others the benefit of the therapeutic sensory input. Another therapist offered lightweight, flowing women's scarves (the indoor-type) in lieu of straps to her class for domestic violence survivors, which were very well received by the group and still provided the same type of sensory input. Observing and soliciting feedback from our students can help us make the best decisions with regard to these types of quandaries.

Some of the yoga forms that appear to be innocuous can actually be challenging for people who have been

Guideline 1
A sense of safety is essential for healing

traumatized. For example, while many look forward to the moments when they are invited to simply rest supine on their mats, this position can feel particularly vulnerable for those who have PTSD. Again, offering choices is important, such as Crocodile in which the person is prone rather than supine, with the chest raised a bit and the head resting on the forearms (see Chapter 17). Other options include Child or a sidelying position. Some people may simply choose to remain seated during times when others are lying on their mats, because it feels safer to them.

Among the most obviously vulnerable yoga forms are Happy Baby and Reclined Bound Angle. On occasion I will present Happy Baby in a generic veterans yoga class but when I do, I first offer an alternative choice such as fully crossing one thigh over the other and holding onto the feet while stretching the knees downwards toward the floor and away from the body and/or hugging the knees into the chest. If appropriate, I may then offer the choice to continue with the stretch they are in or try uncrossing their legs and holding their feet (without asking them to separate their legs—if they want to they will on their own). In a similar vein, a restorative backbend over a bolster with legs straight and parallel is a good alternative choice for a restorative reclined bound angle with legs apart. Beginning with the restorative backbend with legs together, you might add, if it seems appropriate, "you may continue here or, if you like, bring the soles of your feet together and release your knees downward towards the floor". This latter example can be performed while covered with a blanket (for the entire two-part series). This is a gentler way to introduce a hip opening yoga form to individuals who may have experienced sexual trauma, when they eventually appear ready. But I would first start with hip openers in standing (the least vulnerable position), then sitting, and eventually in table and reclined positions—or not at all, depending on the particular student. It is not a "goal" that must be achieved.

One thing to keep in mind when offering yoga students choices in positioning is that someone is likely to take you up on the alternative offer, and when they do, you need to be prepared to instruct them in what to do next! This takes some advanced planning and choreography so the person who decided to assume Crocodile isn't just lying there the whole time while you are moving others through supine leg stretches. I have been there before ... offering "any position that feels comfortable" and then wondering how the next moves are going to work for everyone. In the example just provided, I simply would not offer that combination; instead, I might offer the choice of doing the leg stretches on the mat or sitting in a chair. Earlier in the session, during the initial centering—which involves listening and working with the breath rather than movement—is where I would offer the choices of reclining in supine, prone, or sidelying (or sitting in a chair).

Observe sensory precautions

As we saw in Part 1, people who have PTSD often exhibit sensory overload in the nervous system that contributes to hyperarousal and hypervigilance. We can help to reduce these symptoms and thus improve the perception of safety by observing the following sensory precautions:

- *Choose a quiet time and place for class so the students do not bump into people who are arriving or leaving from other classes in the building.* A small, quiet yoga studio or church hall is far more conducive to a healing yoga practice for trauma survivors than a busy fitness gym. Having said that, certain trauma population groups (such as emergency responders) are more familiar with working out in gyms than attending a yoga studio and may thus be more willing to try a yoga class held in a fitness setting, which tends to reinforce a sense of masculinity. If this is the case, carefully choosing a quiet time of day and a more isolated

Chapter 11

room location can help to offset the pitfalls of a large gym setting.

- **Reduce visual clutter and environmental noise as much as possible, as this can reinforce hyperarousal.** Also consider street noise coming through windows. You might consider installing heavy drapery in such settings to help muffle the sound. In fact, any setting that has windows should have some drapery, which should be closed during class during the darker hours of the day. One veteran I worked with chose to attend a class I was teaching in the next town over rather than the one I taught in his own town, generally stating he liked the ambiance better. Soon afterwards it dawned on me that we had been practicing yoga with no draperies on any of the windows, in the middle of winter when it was pitch black outside, which created a "practicing on stage" effect since anyone in the parking lot could see the whole show! The situation was quickly corrected.

- **Eliminate any "mysteries."** Robin Carnes, co-founder of Warriors at Ease, shared that she always made a point of orienting newly returned soldiers to the yoga room at Walter Reed Medical Center. She would explain that a certain door was locked and unused and where it led to and would also open each and every large cabinet door to show that no one was hiding inside any of them. Similarly, there can be unusual sounds, such as from plumbing pipes, heating systems, someone working in an adjacent room, a creaky staircase, or window breezes causing drapery cords to bang against the wall. It is best to point out the source of these sounds when they occur to reduce any fearful reactions.

- **Always ask first before assisting veterans in the yoga forms, and if you receive permission to assist, always employ a "firm touch," using the whole hand, rather than a light or feathery fingertip touch.** The setting may influence whether and to what degree physical assists are used. For example, at a polytrauma center or other clinic or hospital setting, therapists may need to physically assist clients in some of the yoga forms due to their physical limitations or conditions. Though many of these clients may be used to being touched, it is still important to ask first. In contrast, during my classes for fairly able-bodied veterans in my local community, I avoid touching students in order to maintain strong boundaries and to avoid what could potentially be experienced as an invasion of space, particularly when the goal is to help veterans get into their own embodied state of mind.

As soon as you touch a student, body and mind become separated: whatever level of bodymind integration had been achieved will be disrupted as they switch back on the thinking, judging mind. Physical assists may also give the recipient the impression that they are performing a yoga form incorrectly and that there is a right and wrong way to do yoga. It also reinforces the idea that the teacher is an authority figure, taking the onus of control away from the student. Also, traumatized individuals are at greater risk of experiencing sensitivity to touch than the general population. Finally, one must keep in mind that the purpose of a yoga class for self-regulation and trauma healing is to especially support psychological (and brain re-balancing) as opposed to physical goals. We are not looking for perfect alignment in the yoga forms, though safe alignment is imperative. Careful verbal instruction and demonstration—repeated if necessary to the entire group (vs singling a student out)—will usually meet the latter criteria.

Thus, the choice to provide assists requires careful consideration of the context in which the yoga therapy is provided (and its boundary norms), the level of trust between the therapist and student, the purpose for the physical assist, its potential effects on other goals of therapy, as well as the student's level of comfort with

Guideline 1
A sense of safety is essential for healing

touch and desire to be assisted. Also keep in mind that self-imposed sensory input is much more easily tolerated and integrated than sensory input imposed by others.

- Be careful with olfactory input (smells), as olfactory nerves synapse directly on the amygdala and can cause hyperarousal. Smells can carry strong emotional associations, positive or negative, and we usually do not know what those are for a given person. Some people are also sensitive to smells; in fact, one study suggested that 30.5% of the US population find scented products on others to be irritating.[10] In a recent Australian study (n=1098), 55.6% of asthmatics and 23.9% of non-asthmatics reported adverse health effects from scented products,[11] while in a parallel US study[12] (n=1136), 34.7% of the population reported health problems when exposed to such products. People have experienced respiratory, mucosal, and/or neurological symptoms, including migraine headaches, when in proximity to a person wearing fragrances.[12] These studies did not discriminate between pure essential oils and other types of perfumed products, most of which contain added chemicals. Based on these studies, it is suggested that teachers ask participants to refrain from wearing scented products to yoga class, and that they do not use air fresheners in the room.

Aromatherapists also caution that advanced training is essential for the use of pure essential oils—for example, there are over 40 types of lavender and not all have calming effects. The training may be worth it, however, as the evidence base is building to support the use of aromatherapy for the treatment of a variety of health conditions including anxiety, stress, and depressive disorders.[13-21] Given the earlier caveats, it is suggested that essential oils not be used in group yoga sessions and only aromatherapy-trained therapists use scents in private therapy sessions, when invited to do so by the client.

- ***Music can be calming or alerting.*** Meditation music in particular was shown to reduce state anxiety in a group of 70 Indian army recruits as compared to controls.[22] If music is used, it is recommended that you choose instrumentals with a slow, even rhythm, or soft melodic music (e.g. Native American flute, acoustic guitar, or soft piano music). In accordance with polyvagal theory,[4] avoid high-pitched chimes, sudden loud sounds, or low "Peter and the Wolf"-type sounds that can arouse the ANS. When in doubt, warn the class in advance that you will be using a particular sound at a specific point in time, and invite feedback from the participants. In addition, songs with words can distract a person from the mental process of entering an embodied state. Many CDs developed for yoga classes include Asian instruments or sounds that may remind combat veterans of the places in which they fought; it is best to avoid those if teaching a class for veterans or active duty military personnel.

Introduce the Inner Resource

Another technique that helps to build a "safe container" is the ***Inner Resource***, developed by Richard Miller as a component of his Integrative Restoration (iRest®) program, which has been used at military and veteran facilities around the country. The Inner Resource is a somatically felt state of well-being produced by the pure, present-moment awareness of the unchanging qualities of "being" itself. Initially, people tend to find it easier to access this state using sensory imagery, though this is simply a portal to the Inner Resource and not the Inner Resource itself. Miller emphasizes the importance not only of developing the imagery but also of letting it fall away in order to rest in the feeling state itself (iRest Level 1 manual, Chapter 3, with permission).

Chapter 11

The Inner Resource script begins by helping the student(s) draw into their mind a full, detailed, sensorial image of a place, person, or other sensory experience that helps them feel safe, secure, and at ease. It may be a place the person has visited in the past, such as a favorite vacation spot, a childhood home, a special room, or a beautiful landscape. Or, it could be someplace the person has never experienced but saw on TV, in the movies, or created in the mind. Or it could be a person or a pet that helps the person to feel calm and secure. Or it could be a smell, sound, taste, or tactile experience, such as the smell and taste of Grandma's apple pie, the sensations of floating on a raft on a lake on a hot sunny day, or the sound of Mom's calming singing voice—which may then draw up the sensory experience of a person and place. It is traditionally presented near the beginning of a yoga class, so that it can be accessed if the need arises during the practice. Though there may not always be sufficient time to fully present the Inner Resource, it is especially helpful to do so whenever there is a new student in attendance. Once the students are familiar with the script, it can be sufficient sometimes to simply remind them that they can draw on their Inner Resource any time they feel the need to foster a sense of safety and comfort.

Below is one example of an Inner Resource script that comes from the iRest tradition. (Advanced training is suggested to use the techniques skillfully—please go to www.irest.org to learn more.)

> Take time now to develop your Inner Resource ... a feeling of well-being in your body where you feel totally at ease and secure ... You might imagine a special, peaceful place that you've visited ... or a beautiful scene from a movie ... or a place entirely in your imagination ... one that makes you feel safe, relaxed, and comfortable. It could be in an outdoor setting, or in a special room, or may be the image of a special person or pet that helps you experience the feeling of well-being in your body ... Allow your senses to come into play ... the sights ... sounds ... smells ... and tastes ... or other resources that evoke the feelings of deep peace ... comfort ... and ease .... Then allow these images to completely fade away while you remain with the felt sense of well-being in your body ... a Being aware and awake to Itself ... this is your Inner Resource ... [long pause] ...
>
> ... During practice, or during your daily life, should you feel distressed, you can return to your Inner Resource and feel at ease, secure, and comfortable.

Avoid common triggers

Fostering a sense of safety also requires attending to other aspects of the environmental setting, to reduce the potential for triggering flashbacks or states of dissociation. A trigger is a troubling reminder of a traumatic event, and may consist of just about anything: people, places, noises, music, images, candles, smells, tastes, objects, emotions, animals, scenes in movies or TV shows, dates or other time events, tones of voice, body positions, bodily sensations, words (e.g. sandbag, surrender, eye socket, corpse), colors (e.g. orange, which has brought up images of agent orange) or even weather conditions. Individuals with PTSD typically avoid triggers that they are aware of, which can significantly affect daily functioning and result in leading a more restricted lifestyle.[23]

For example, a person may avoid malls or large social gatherings, noisy places, certain smells (or situations that involve them), firework displays, and so on. They may also actively modify their living environment, for example keeping the window shades down at home or drowning out sounds using "white noise" such as fans, background music, etc. In more extreme cases, individuals with PTSD may assume a bunker mentality by bolting the doors and/or rarely leaving the home. This is not uncommon: several people have approached me looking for help for a sibling who had

Guideline 1
A sense of safety is essential for healing

returned home from the war in Iraq or Afghanistan and rarely left their bedrooms. Society is not aware of these individuals: they are not seeking help and they are not on the street holding signs asking for money; they are often living with family members, invisible to the rest of us.

Triggers can be difficult to anticipate. In a yoga class, it is helpful to try to eliminate the most common triggers (e.g. vulnerable body positions, loud noises, busy environments, certain words that have alternative meanings in a combat situation or in the sex trades); however, it is usually impossible, as well as unnecessary, to eliminate everything that has ever been a trigger for someone. After reducing or eliminating the most common triggers, the best approach is to simply be observant to the verbal and bodily reactions of your students in yoga class, such as a hesitancy to assume certain yoga forms or commenting on certain words, and, if reasonable, make adjustments for that particular class.

Effectively manage emotional abreactions

It is also important to be observant for signs of dissociation and flashbacks, both of which were described in Chapter 2. Flashbacks tend to be more obvious than states of dissociation and can involve acting out the trauma. I once attended a yoga class during which a male student acted out an entire combat scene. Possible signs of dissociation include staring off into space, talking to oneself, grimacing or other facial expressions that do not match the present situation, twitching, self-soothing behaviors such as rocking, missing conversation or being slow to respond, darting eyes or far-away gaze, memory lapses, flat affect, over- or underactivity.[24] In contrast, outpourings of deep mourning are healthy reactions and are best allowed to unfold and process through the system. Flashbacks and dissociated states may or may not be triggered by something happening in the present moment.

How to handle flashbacks and dissociated states

"*Grounding techniques*" are considered to be the most important techniques for helping someone handle dissociation or flashbacks. These techniques are designed to help the person come back to their present surroundings by engaging the senses. There are two basic types: sensory awareness techniques and cognitive techniques. **Sensory awareness techniques** use the senses to draw the person back into their body and present surroundings. **Cognitive techniques** involve asking questions to orient the individual to place and time. Both of these techniques are demonstrated below.

Babette Rothschild[25] discusses the importance of developing "dual awareness" of the *experiencing self* and the *observing self,* concepts she learned from van der Kolk et al.[26] When someone is having a flashback, they are completely immersed in the experiencing self, and the observing self needs to be re-awakened. Some ideas for doing that are provided here:

- Go over to the person, and using a firm but soothing voice, ask the person to sit up and look around the room.
- If it seems that touch would be helpful, *ask* them if you can touch their shoulder or arm (to help with grounding and so they know you are there to care for them).
- Ask the person to:
  — describe objects or other details in the room, such as the color of the walls
  — press their feet into the floor or stomp the feet
  — rub the mat, rub their hands together, or rub another object, such as a piece of ice.
- The following questions and statements were suggested by the military yoga group Warriors at Ease, for use if appropriate to the situation and at appropriate points in the process:

Chapter 11

"I'm right here, I'm right here with you, I'm sticking with you the whole way."

"Where in your body do you feel this right now?"

"Where are you experiencing sensation? Can you describe the sensation to me?"

"Perhaps this experience can be a helpful part of the healing process."

"You have the resources and support to allow this process to unfold and complete."

"It takes time to heal and process all that's happened—that is natural, that is normal."

"You're among friends; you're in a good place now."

"If you feel yourself feeling a bit overwhelmed, you can go back to your Inner Resource."

"Tell me about your Inner Resource—can you describe it to me, what does it look like, what sounds are in it, is there anyone there with you?"

"Can you just be aware of this experience right now without trying to fight it for a few moments?"

When the person's **observing self** is again on-line, Rothschild recommends using the following flashback halting protocol, which she says is usually quickly effective. This is intended for use in clinical settings or for self-use but could be adapted for a yoga class setting **only under the supervision of a mental health professional**.

Rothschild's flashback halting protocol[25]

The client says the following, filling in the blanks and following the directions:

Right now I am feeling _____ (describe emotion)

And I am sensing in my body _____ (describe bodily sensations)

Because I am remembering _____ (name trauma by title but give no details)

At the same time, I am looking around where I am now in _____ (the actual current year)

Here _____ (name the place where you are)

And I can see _____ (describe some of the things you see right *now*, in *this* place)

And so I know _____ (name of trauma, by title only, again) is not happening now/anymore.

A recent brain imaging study suggests that putting feelings into words can reduce emotional reactivity by activating the right ventrolateral prefrontal cortex (RVLPFC), which in turn activates the medial prefrontal cortex, which inhibits the amygdala.[27] Thus, labeling emotions and their associated bodily sensations may reduce their potency.

Try to avoid having the person leave class

It is important to make every effort to ensure the person who just experienced a flashback is fully grounded before they leave the class. You can invite them to sit at the side of the room, so you can check on them later to be sure they are okay. However, under no circumstances should you restrain the person from leaving if they are intent on doing so. If the person's actions pose a dangerous threat to themselves or others, seek help from a qualified person at the facility or call 911. If the class is being held in a community setting, such as a yoga studio, it is especially helpful to invite a mental health professional to join the class for free who can provide mental health support for the teacher or therapist should challenging situations crop up, or conversely, serve as a support to students if questions pop up that are outside of the teacher or therapist's professional licensure to address. Obvious choices are a Vet Center counselor if it is a class for veterans; a trauma or domestic abuse center counselor if it is a class for people who have survived sexual or domestic assault; or a church counseling

Guideline 1
A sense of safety is essential for healing

pastor if the class is being held on church grounds. At a minimum, an arrangement should be made with a mental health professional to serve as a contact person by phone if needed.

Suicidal remarks

If a student makes a suicidal remark, inform them that you take it seriously. Listen attentively, supportively, and without placing blame as you gently ask probing questions such as the following: "Is this something you have been thinking about a lot? Are you afraid for your own safety? Have you thought about how you would take your own life?" Through sensitive questioning and listening, you can determine whether they have a plan, a time frame, and access to methods for taking their life (such as a weapon or pills). It may seem counterintuitive and frightening to invite people to talk about suicidal thoughts but it is necessary for assessing the level of seriousness of the threat. Also, offering the opportunity to talk about the feelings can reduce the risk of acting on them. The Mayo Clinic (January 2018) suicide guidelines echo this philosophy.[28]

If a person responds to your questions in a way that leads you to believe they are suicidal, do not leave them alone—wait with them until there is a mental health professional or a family member to help them. If the person asks you to not tell anyone, explain that you can't make that promise if you think their life is in danger. If the situation happens in an organizational setting such as a VA hospital, you can call or walk them to their mental health professional if they are working in the same facility. If it occurs in the community or some other place in which you do not have access to a mental health professional, ask the student if they have a counselor and/or family member you can call to help them. As a best practice, all yoga students should fill out a student information form that includes emergency contact information before beginning the yoga class. If you can't locate a mental health professional or emergency contact person, you should call the national emergency number or suicide hotline (see Box on helplines).

> **Personal Crisis Helplines**
>
> **US:** Call 911 or the National Suicide Prevention Lifeline at 1-800-273-TALK (1-800-273-8255). To reach the Veterans Crisis Line, use that same number and press 1.
>
> **UK:** Call 999 or the European Emergency Number, 112. The Samaritans (www.samaritans.org) suicide hotline number in the UK is 116 123.
>
> **AUS:** Call 000 or Lifeline Services at 13 11 14.

Despite the above recommendations, we do not always know how we will react if such a situation actually arises. A statement such as "I don't know how I can go on living like this" can be taken as an off-the-cuff, innocuous remark about a temporary life situation and not as a literal statement; however, people have taken their lives soon after making such a remark so it is important to clarify its meaning. More strongly worded remarks of suicidal ideation can feel disorienting and surreal for the listener and can even be blocked from consciousness if they threaten the safety of their own psyche. We can't help our clients feel safe if what they are telling us makes us feel unsafe. We need to have the presence of mind to do the right thing to handle the situation. Yoga techniques, especially the breathing and grounding practices, are among the best tools to help us with that. So as you help to ground your student in such crises, remember to ground yourself as well.

Chapter 12

3. It can be helpful to start breath work by linking the breath to movement and by gently and continually refocusing your attention to the sensations of bodily movement and breath. This helps activate the sensory parts of the brain (insula, sensory cortex), thus shifting energy away from the incessant neuronal loops causing the intrusive thought or images. Incorporating some of the sensory enhanced techniques discussed in the next chapter into the breath work can facilitate the process, such as dynamically moving in and out of yoga forms that involve heavy work to the muscles (e.g. Down Dog; Chair) or using a yoga strap during the movements, such as when performing the Sensory-Enhanced Moon Salute.

4. Accept that your brain may be double-tasking for a while during your breathing practices, playing the "film show" in the background while you simultaneously focus on sensation, movement, and breath. Eventually the film will fade and pause here and there but you won't know it for a while because if you check to see if you are still thinking about it, well, there it is. But the fact that you had to check tells you that you're making progress! When the memory has fully resolved itself, it will have an entirely different quality to it. You will enjoy complete concentration on your activities and if the memory comes up it will be because you voluntarily generated it. And because it has been resolved, that will occur very infrequently.

5. Even if resolution takes a few very long years, making peace with the situation and the process you are undergoing is well worth it because once you are at the other end of this harrowing tunnel, you will have many years left to fully enjoy all of life's blessings in a way that you will never take for granted again.

If the intrusions are a significant life problem, please seek professional help in managing them in addition to trying mindfulness strategies.

Many studies have been conducted on the effects of yogic breathing practices, the vast majority showing benefits in healthy individuals as well as for managing various clinical conditions.[2] Saoji et al.[2] recently reviewed studies on breathing practices showing positive changes in neurocognitive, psychophysiological, respiratory, biochemical, and metabolic functions. Unsurprisingly, most breathing practices demonstrated highly significant effects on autonomic functions, since for most people, the breath is the only function of the autonomic nervous system that is under voluntary control. All other functions (e.g. heart rate, blood pressure, digestion) are involuntary. Thus, the breath provides us with a potent portal to the ANS which in turn has a huge influence over the entire nervous system. In Saoji et al.'s study, the vast majority of yoga breathing practices produced a parasympathetic shift in the balance of the ANS, while high frequency breathing techniques such as Kapalabhati produced a sympathetic shift. They reported that, in general, yoga breathing practices can be considered safe when done under the supervision of a teacher professionally trained in the techniques, though further studies are warranted.

There are many breathing practices used for specific therapeutic purposes in the field of yoga therapy, but this book presents only a few, specifically those that have been found to be very helpful for those who are recovering from trauma. As you will have already guessed, these are ones that activate the parasympathetic nervous system. These practices are also very helpful for people who are under a lot of stress, even of a common, everyday kind. They are very safe and can be easily learned by health professionals to share with their clients, though it is highly recommended that additional training be sought by exploring one of the many trauma-informed yoga programs that have been highlighted in this book, including the Sensory-Enhanced Yoga Institute, or by a yoga therapy

Guideline 2
The most direct and powerful way to self-regulate is through control of the breath

training program that has been approved by the International Association of Yoga Therapists. The program I graduated from, Joseph Le Page's Integrative Yoga Therapy program, provides a thorough training in dozens of breathing practices for particular uses. The Mind~Breath~Body program developed by Richard Brown and Patricia Gerbarg (see Chapter 8), is another highly recommended program for advanced breath work training.

In this chapter, we will be discussing concepts developed within Eastern culture that are unfamiliar to most Westerners; however, when presenting the practices to trauma survivors it is recommended that Sanskrit and other non-English terms be avoided and the language of Western science preferred. Otherwise, the practices may be received as too esoteric or even feel threatening to someone's religious beliefs even though devoid of actual religious content. In fact, many of the concepts of ancient yogic science are now supported by Western scientific evidence and are simply packaged in a different language. Furthermore, many yogic scholars in India are embracing modern science just as quickly as yoga is spreading in the Western world, so the gaps between the two cultures are rapidly narrowing. I will discuss some traditional yoga concepts in this chapter to help the reader gain a better perspective of the original purpose of breathing practices in yoga and how they relate to current scientific knowledge.

What is pranayama?

As with yoga forms, breath practices are traditionally performed to prepare the mind for meditation and are an integral part of yoga practice. Many people have heard the term "pranayama" in association with breathing practices, but what exactly does it mean? Pranayama is actually the science of controlling, channeling, and expanding the life force, or **prana**. Tony Briggs explains:[3(p. 6)]

Many people are aware of the theory in modern physics that matter and energy are just different manifestations of the same thing. So one way to look at the body or body-mind is as a cloud of energy—a cloud of energy so concentrated that it's visible. Prana is just another word for that energy. Prana is the energy that moves the universe, or that is the universe.

While the term **prana** is unfamiliar in modern science and unmentioned in Western medicine, it is certainly discussed in Western physics, though in different language. We know that everything in the universe is made of molecules consisting of combinations of atoms, which in turn are made of positively charged protons, neutral neutrons, and negatively charged electrons. We also know there is an enormous amount of space between these energy particles (each atom is said to consist of more than 99.9999% space!). Thus, contrary to outside appearances, we are not actually solid but are literally a (human) "form" of energy. Everything in our bodies—nerves, blood vessels, tissues—is made of these subatomic electrically charged particles, which attract and repel each other, producing all of the processes in our bodies, including the process of breathing. This is prana.

According to the ancient yogic texts, **nadis** are channels through which prana flows. *Nadi* can be defined as a river, or when used in a biological context, as a pulse, vessel, or nerve, and indeed, some modern Indian yoga scholars have associated the ancient concept of nadis to gross anatomy. For example Khedikar and colleagues recently wrote "the flow of axoplasm and also the endoplasm within the axon and cell body of a neuron must be considered while interpreting the meaning of the term 'nadi'."[4(p. 109)]

However, there are others who believe that nadis are not related to gross human physiology at all but are energy currents that support that physiology.

Chapter 12

According to Swami Satyananda Saraswati:[1(p. 36)]

The word nadi means "flow". In this sense, nadis are subtle flows of energy, just as electricity, radio waves and laser beams are subtle flows. Nadis relate to the energy body and should not be confused with nerves, which relate to the physical body.

So which of the above is true? If there is only one Law of Physics, not two, then it would make sense for the gross and subtle energies to be interrelated. We know that the field of energy that holds our atoms together in human form creates electric fields within it, such as the oscillating brainwaves discussed in Chapter 4. Furthermore, just as a streetlamp lights up the surrounding neighborhood and not just the street, we now know that the "neighborhood" surrounding neurons is impacted by their energy—*and vice versa*—by **astrocytes**, a type of glial cell in the brain that surrounds neurons and is now believed to contribute to thought processes.[5–7]

Recent findings by Bellot-Saez and colleagues[7] show that astrocytes **tune neural oscillations at both the cellular and network levels** via their role in clearing potassium ions from the extracellular milieu (i.e. by sweeping the neighborhood outside the neurons). In the periphery of the body, a process involving yet another type of glial cell at gap junctions has been proposed to explain the metaphysical energy theory of the chakras.[8] Whatever the term nadi originally meant, Western physics has ascertained that energy flows through the body in **both** gross and subtle ways, and that the gross can affect the subtle, and vice versa—there is a connection between the two, just as all subatomic particles are connected in the universe. Therefore, it makes sense when considering the life force (prana) that we include the nerves, the blood vessels, energy of digestion, and all other biological processes, as well as the energy that is both emitted from these processes and affects these processes.

The traditional purpose of breathing practices is to correct this flow of energy in the body, which can be negatively affected by diet, lifestyle, injuries, trauma, and so many other factors. Some ancient yogic texts report that there are 72,000 nadis in the body including three primary nadis: **Shushumna**, which runs down the midline of the body, and **Ida** and **Pingala**, which wind around it in a curved fashion, forming balls of energies, referred to as chakras, where they intersect. Ida, which starts and ends on the left side, is associated with calming, cooling, feminine, lunar qualities, while Pingala, which starts and ends on the right side, is associated with energizing, warming, masculine, solar qualities.

Nadis, hemisphere dominance and the ANS

Khedikar et al.'s[4] double-blind, peer-reviewed article on the relationship of the nadis with the human nervous system provides interesting food for thought. Their hypothesis that nadis are correlated with nerves was presented earlier. They also proposed that the three primary nadis—**Shushumna**, **Ida**, and **Pingala**—are associated with the spinal cord, left sympathetic trunk, and right sympathetic trunk, respectively. They pointed out that though the sympathetic trunks are structured similarly, "the two cerebral hemispheres show different functions upon their activations,"[4(p. 113)] which they compare to descriptions of the characteristics of Ida and Pingala nadis. They also explained how each of these sympathetic trunks curves in to meet the spinal cord similarly to how Ida and Pingala are said to curve in and out from Shushumna.

Just as modern Western science has revealed that each cerebral hemisphere controls the opposite side of the body, Eastern yogic science states that Ida, which controls the left side of the body, is connected to the right hemisphere, while Pingala, which controls the right side of the body, is connected to the left hemisphere.[1] However, this is believed to be due to a different mechanism in the ANS, since the majority of these fibers innervate the ipsilateral vs contralateral

Guideline 2
The most direct and powerful way to self-regulate is through control of the breath

hemisphere.[9–12] As the theory goes, the SNS causes vasoconstriction and thus decreased blood blow in the ipsilateral hemisphere, resulting in vasodilation and parasympathetic activation of the opposite cerebral hemisphere.[12] Since ANS processes are more strongly activated in the right hemisphere,[13] Ida Nadi can thus be said to correlate with the parasympathetic nervous system and Pingala Nadi can be said to correlate with the sympathetic nervous system (Table 12.1).[1,4]

The nasal cycle, breath, and the brain

Pranayama practices designed to balance Ida and Pingala typically involve breathing through the left, right, or alternate nostrils. According to the traditional theory, breathing through the left nostril activates Ida, breathing through the right activates Pingala, and alternate nostril breathing balances both of these energies (although it may emphasize Ida or Pingala depending upon the exact method). According to Swami N. Saraswati, these ancient yogic practices developed due to the "phenomenon of alternating flows,"[1(p. 99)] now referred to in mainstream medicine as the **nasal cycle**, which is accompanied by sympathetic vasoconstriction in the nostril exhibiting dominant airflow and parasympathetic congestion in the non-dominant nostril. This type of biorhythm is called an **ultradian rhythm** as it occurs more than once per day. Lin and Danahey confirmed this phenomenon in a recent Medscape article:[14(p. 8)]

The nasal cycle is an additional feature of normal nasal physiology. This cycle causes turbinate hypertrophy to periodically alternate between the two sides of the nose, causing periodic unilateral obstruction approximately every three hours.

Kahana-Zweig and colleagues explained:[15(pp. 1–2)]

Nasal airflow is greater in one nostril than in the other because of transient asymmetric nasal passage obstruction by erectile tissue. The extent of obstruction alternates across nostrils with periodicity referred to as the nasal cycle. The nasal cycle is related to autonomic arousal and is indicative of asymmetry in brain function.

There have been a number of research studies investigating the relationship of the nasal cycle and brain activity. Werntz et al.[12] demonstrated a direct relationship between cerebral hemisphere activity and the ultradian rhythm of the nasal cycle, i.e. the hemisphere **contralateral** to the nostril receiving more airflow showed greater EEG activity. This relationship occurred across occipital, parietal, and central regions (i.e. all regions tested) and in general across the alpha, theta, delta, and beta frequencies. Price and Eccles' review[16] determined that it appears evident that there is a connection, but claimed there is a debate regarding how the process works or its significance. They proposed that the process works via brainstem oscillators which "flip-flop," creating dominance on one side while reciprocally inhibiting the other side, and also suggested that nasal airflow may influence brain activity by activating the trigeminal nerve.

Earlier papers proposed a model for hypothalamic regulation of the lateralized rhythms of all ANS functions as a generalized ANS-CNS rhythm.[17–20(p. R962)] Shannahoff-Khalsa and colleagues produced extensive evidence that "either a common pacemaker or mutually entrained pacemakers regulate the autonomic, cardiovascular, and neuroendocrine systems, via the hypothalamus."[19] These researchers presented a very interesting model for how the hypothalamus via its internal rhythms might control the ANS-CNS rhythmic coupling and how the other ultradian rhythms of the body are tightly coupled to this generalized ANS-CNS rhythm.[18,20] Unfortunately, this model was not reviewed by Price and Eccles.[16]

Chapter 12

Table 12.1 Concepts of nadis compared with the nervous system*

	Ancient science of yoga	Modern neuroscience
Source of energy	Nadi	Neuron
Main energy channel	Shushumna	Spinal cord
Energy channel location and direction	Vertically, along the midline of the body	Vertically, along the midline of the body
Parallel channels on lateral sides of main channel	**Ida and Pingala** Ida and Pingala surround Shushumna along its length on the left and right sides, respectively	**Left and right sympathetic trunks** Two sympathetic trunks surround the spinal cord along its length, on the left and right sides
Where these parallel channels intersect each other	Chakras Just happen to align with nerve plexuses	Nerve ganglions
Nostril activated	Ida: left nostril Pingala: right nostril	Left sympathetic trunk: left nostril Right sympathetic trunk: right nostril
Channel associated with PNS activation of the right cerebral hemisphere	Ida	Left sympathetic trunk
Channel associated with SNS Activation of the right cerebral hemisphere	Pingala	Right sympathetic trunk

*Based on Kedikar SG, Erande M, Shukla DV. Critical comparison of yogic nadi with nervous system. Journal of Indian System of Medicine. 2016;4(2):108–13. Available from: https://www.researchgate.net/publication/317664235_Critical_comparison_of_Yogic_Nadi_with_Nervous_System [accessed 7 October 2018].

Parallel to the yogic idea of a **parasympathetic–right hemisphere** connection through Ida Nadi, Schore[13] argued that it is the **right** hemisphere that is predominantly involved in regulating stress- and emotion-related processes and that, specifically, it is the **right** orbital and medial prefrontal cortices, especially the **vmPFC**, that provide the top-down cortical regulation of the sympathetic nervous system through their projections to the hypothalamic autonomic centers, which in turn project to the arousal centers in the brainstem and the spinal autonomic structures and related peripheral organs. He further explained that the right hemisphere has a wider range of arousal tolerance at both the high and low ends as well as a wider range of positive and negative affect than the left hemisphere, but that this is severely restricted in people experiencing dissociated states.

Schore's description of the medial prefrontal cortex being right lateralized for ANS processes raises another question as to whether the default mode and

Guideline 2
The most direct and powerful way to self-regulate is through control of the breath

central executive networks are each lateralized to opposite hemispheres. There is evidence that most of the DMN regions involved in processing autonomic information exhibit parasympathetic predominance whereas most task-positive networks involved in ANS regulation exhibit sympathetic predominance.[21] However, relegating the DMN and CEN to separate hemispheres would be incorrect since each of these networks is composed of paired, bilateral brain structures. Nonetheless, Stillman and colleagues'[22] statistical modeling of the default mode network produced clear evidence that nodes within the DMN have stronger connections within the same hemisphere compared to across hemispheres, suggesting that the DMN is wired in a way that could at least make it *possible* for the nasal cycle to increase activation of the left *or* right DMN structures at one time.

Future research is needed to move beyond conjecture regarding the relationship between the DMN (or CEN), ultradian rhythms, and cerebral hemispheres. Even so, it is conceivable that working with breath practices designed to rebalance Ida and Pingala—or, to use Western language, the right and left hemispheres respectively, through manipulation of the ANS—could be one way to help to rebalance the triple brain network discussed in Chapter 4. By increasing activation of the parasympathetic nervous system in the right hemisphere (Ida Nadi), we may be able to free the insula from the clutches of the amygdala, thus normalizing the salience network so it can once again assume its role as the switchboard operator between the default mode and central executive networks.

Lending support to the idea that working with the breath can affect brain networks gone awry, Heck and colleagues[23] produced evidence from both animal and human studies that cortical rhythms are modulated by respiration. According to this research group, respiration-locked synchronization of neuronal activity across large areas of the cerebral cortex, which is also seen in a common EEG pattern during meditative states, could be responsible for the calming effect of controlled, slow, deep breathing.[23-25] They also suggest that respiration likely had a role in modulating cortical rhythms since mammals first evolved, as the early mammals had proportionally large olfactory bulbs and strongly relied on the sense of smell to survive. An EEG study also showed inter-hemispheric beta coherence during meditation practice that included forced alternate nostril breathing.[23,26]

Effects of unilateral and alternate nostril breathing

A great many studies have been conducted on the effects of breathing through the left or right nostril and alternate nostril breathing. However, we do not have space here to examine them all and the interested reader is referred to, for example, references 15 and 27–32. A few examples follow:

- A study[27] of the effects of unilateral and alternate nostril breathing found that systolic and diastolic pressure decreased following alternate nostril breathing; systolic and mean pressure decreased after left nostril breathing; and systolic, diastolic and mean pressure significantly increased following right nostril breathing.
- Twenty yoga-trained individuals were studied before and after they performed nine rounds of each of six different breathing techniques; each technique was performed on a different testing day, totaling six days of testing. Respiratory rate was maintained at five to six breaths per minute. Study findings included an overall *decrease* in heart rate and blood pressure following each of the three **left** nostril initiated breathing patterns (inhale L/exhale L; inhale L/exhale R; L initiated alternate nostril), whereas there were *increases* in these parameters as well as shortened reaction

Chapter 12

times following the ***right*** initiated breathing patterns. Normal breathing produced insignificant changes. They suggested that the nostril used for inhalation determines the main effect of unilateral and alternate nostril breathing.

- In a study[29] conducted with geriatric patients, both unilateral left nostril breathing and unilateral right nostril breathing produced a decrease in both heart rate and blood pressure parameters, but left nostril breathing produced these effects more strongly.[30]

Triple network models and nadis are complicated concepts but if we distill everything down, we are still left with the simple idea that activating the parasympathetic nervous system and deactivating the sympathetic fight–flight system is how one reduces hyperarousal in PTSD. All of the studies lead us back to what we already know: that we need to reduce hyperarousal to get the brain networks to function properly again following trauma; that the way to do that is to rebalance the ANS; and that the most powerful way to regulate the ANS is through control of the breath.

Pranayama practices for trauma survivors

When presenting breath practices to trauma survivors, we need to start where they are. The breathing pattern of many traumatized individuals reflects sympathetic dominance, and this is often readily observed during yoga therapy sessions or even during everyday interactions with them. Oftentimes, their breath is quick and shallow, and stuck high in their chest. This breath pattern was not only originally caused by the sympathetic "fight–flight" reaction, but is also self-reinforcing. Breath counting practices that are timed by an outside force (the yoga teacher) can be counterproductive if the person's natural breathing pace cannot slow down enough to match the teacher's directions. Thus, if an external pacing cue is to be used, it is important to identify a client's baseline pace first before gently nudging them toward a slower, deeper breath.

We want to increase parasympathetic nervous system activation, which is demonstrated by cardiac vagal tone. This can be measured by respiratory sinus arrhythmia (RSA) and by heart rate variability (HRV).[33] HRV is simply the beat-to-beat variation in heart rate, while RSA refers to the natural fluctuations in heart rate associated with the breathing cycle. Since HRV mostly varies due to RSA, the terms are often used interchangeably and reflect the complex interactions between parasympathetic and sympathetic nerve fibers as well as other factors.[34] Normally, the heart rate quickens during inhalation and decreases during exhalation. Carl Lugwig first discovered this phenomenon in the 1800s through his study of the dog.[34] Singh et al. provided a clear explanation of this process:[35(p. 195)]

> *During inhalation intra-thoracic pressure lowers due to the contraction and downward movement of the diaphragm and the expansion of the chest cavity. Atrial pressure is also lowered as a result of this, enabling more blood to return to the heart. As more blood enters the heart, the vasculature and atria expand, triggering baroreceptors which act to suppress vagal tone, and, subsequently, heart rate increases.*
>
> *During exhalation, the diaphragm relaxes, moving upward and decreases the size of the chest cavity, causing a subsequent increase in intra-thoracic pressure. This increased pressure inhibits venous return to the heart and thus less atrial expansion and activation of baroreceptors occurs. As these baroreceptors are no longer acting to suppress vagal tone, heart rate decreases.*

So, contrary to intuition, a variable heart rate is a ***good*** thing. Heart rate variability reflects the combined sympathetic and parasympathetic tone

Guideline 2
The most direct and powerful way to self-regulate is through control of the breath

on heart rate. High HRV is an indicator of increased parasympathetic tone in normal subjects and has been shown to be negatively associated with heart rate.[36] Van der Kolk[36] verified in a controlled study that hatha yoga can significantly increase heart rate variability in normal subjects. Furthermore, numerous studies cited by Russo et al.[37] have confirmed that heart rate variability and respiratory sinus arrhythmia are maximized at approximately six breaths per minute. Slow breathing approximating six breaths per minute causes an increase in venous return, which is further supported by diaphragmatic breathing since the diaphragm increases efficiency of venous return through its physical connection with the inferior vena cava.[37–39]

In order to bias the ANS toward parasympathetic dominance, we need to *slow* and *deepen* the breath. Slow, rhythmic, diaphragmatic breathing is one of the most effective techniques to produce a calmer and more relaxed state of mind. According to Stephen Elliot,[40] developer of the **Coherent Breathing Method**, breathing frequency and breathing depth influence (and reflect) the SNS and PNS, respectively (Figure 12.1). He explained, "the analysis assumes an underlying sympathetic bias, this bias resulting from the physical and emotional stress and strain of life" (Elliot, personal correspondence, May 2013).

The Coherent Breathing Method was fully described by Gretchen Ki Steidle in Chapter 8; she has used it extensively and successfully in her work with displaced populations and victims of mass disasters to help people self-regulate following trauma. The method is taught by pacing the breath to an external auditory cue to slow down and smooth out the breathing process. Steidle learned the technique from her colleagues, Patricia Gerbarg and Richard Brown, who described its effects:[41(p. 5)]

Once coherent breathing has shifted a patient out of the sympathetically driven defense mode and into the more parasympathetic social engagement mode, it becomes easier to engage in any form of therapy, to be more open and trusting, and to cognitively process whatever is discussed in treatment. In addition, if overwhelming emotions arise, the breath practice can be used for self-regulation during sessions.

To further explain why the technique works, Gerbarg and Brown[41] point to Streeter et al.'s[42] hypothesis that slow breathing practices could release GABA from the prefrontal cortex and possibly the insula to the central nucleus of the amygdala, thus modulating the amygdala's hyperactivity. Studies have been conducted combining coherent breathing with Iyengar yoga practices, which found a significant decline in depressive symptoms[43] and suicidal ideation,[44] as well as increased thalamic GABA levels and increased heart rate variability in depressed individuals.[41]

Pranayama practices can bias the ANS in different directions depending on various factors, particularly rate of respiration. Sharma et al.[45] compared slow and

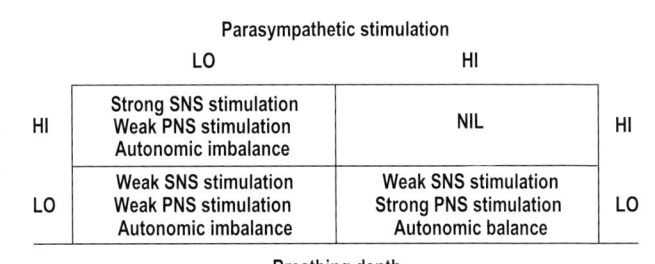

Figure 12.1

Relationship between respiration and the ANS (Elliot, *Coherence*,[40] adapted with permission)

fast pranayama practices and discovered that only the slow practices reduced heart rate and various blood pressure measurements, among other cardiovascular indicators. Russo et al.[37] conducted a review of studies on slow breathing in humans and concluded that these practices have (positive) "effects on respiratory muscle activity, ventilation efficiency, chemoreflex and baroreflex sensitivity, heart rate variability, blood flow dynamics, respiratory sinus arrhythmia, cardiorespiratory coupling, and sympathovagal balance."[37(p. 298)] These researchers explained that these results represent an increase in parasympathetic and a decrease in sympathetic activation of the nervous system.

The Sensory-Enhanced Yoga method only uses pranayama practices known to bias the nervous system away from sympathetic dominance and towards parasympathetic dominance; therefore, no vigorous breathing practices are presented. Though other calming pranayama practices exist, the slow breathing practices presented in this chapter are among the most common and most effective and include the diaphragmatic breath, the complete Yogic Breath, alternate nostril breathing, Ujjayi Breath, and Sitkari Breath. The main point to remember is, **the slower and deeper the breath, the more it will bias the ANS toward parasympathetic dominance**. It is important to consider this concept during active movements as well. In the popular vinyasa types of yoga that emphasize rigorous movement flows from form to form, the breath often has to speed up to keep up with the movement, which only further stimulates the fight–flight response. One of the major keys of a healing practice for PTSD is to allow the natural breath to guide the pace of the movement, and not vice versa.

How to incorporate breath work into asana practice

T. K. V. Desikachar, the son of the "father of modern yoga", Śrī T. Krishnamacharya, wrote in *The Heart of Yoga*, "The first step of our yoga practice is to consciously link breath and body. We do this by allowing every movement to be led by the breath as we practice the asanas. The correct linking of breath and movement is the basis for the whole asana practice. The simple exercise of raising the arms on an inhale and lowering them on an exhale helps us find the rhythm of combined breath and movement."

General principles for how to incorporate the breath during static and dynamic yoga forms are outlined below. Be sure to tell your clients that if a breath pattern is not working for them, they are free to reverse the inhalation and exhalation or let go of any control of the breath.

Principle 1

Coordinate movement with the breath in dynamic forms, choosing whether to inhale or exhale based on the natural tendency of the body. For example, the natural tendency is to exhale on a forward fold because the breath is literally being squeezed out of the lower abdomen, whereas backbends open up the front of the body inviting air to be drawn in due to the reduced air pressure in the lungs. Thus, in yoga we generally:

- inhale→ when moving upward, toward center or expanding the chest
- exhale→ when moving downward, folding, twisting, or moving away from the center.

Principle 2

Move slowly, pacing your movement with the breath.

- Many people do the reverse, speeding up the breath in an attempt to keep up with the pace of movement, which often fails and only serves to reinforce hypervigilance.

Principle 3

Ideally use the **diaphragmatic breath** throughout the yoga practice to activate the PNS and inhibit the SNS fight–flight system.

Guideline 2
The most direct and powerful way to self-regulate is through control of the breath

- To establish this takes time and can be easier initially when practiced in supine. If this is too difficult, just use it during short segments and at other times let go of all control of the breath and simply use your natural breath.

Principle 4

When in static forms, direct the breath into the areas being stretched.

- When in a *forward fold*, breathe into the back to accentuate its expansion.
- When in a *backbend*, direct the breath into the front of the chest and the heart center.
- During a *lateral bend*, breathe into the ribcage that is being stretched, feeling the small muscles expand between the ribs on the inhalation and release on the exhalation.
- When in a *twist*, lengthen the spine with each inhale and maintain that length as you perhaps move a tiny bit further into the twist on the exhalation (only when you sense some space to do so).
- Even *breathe into areas where the lungs don't stretch*! Send your breath into your hamstrings during leg stretches, or any other area of your body where you feel any muscle restriction from the stretching or discomfort from chronic pain or tension. The mind works in mysterious ways, and oftentimes the suggestion of breathing into these areas somehow invites those muscles to soften and release. The insula processes both breath and visceral sensations and may be responsible for this effect.

Recommended Breathing Techniques

The following breathing techniques are those most recommended by the Sensory-Enhanced Yoga Institute to promote healing from trauma, anxiety, or related conditions.

Breath awareness

Sovik[46–48] has suggested that the most important breath technique is simply to watch the breath flow in and out of the body since it takes some time to become familiar with the flow of one's breath. There are neurological benefits to watching one's natural breath as well. Spontaneous quiet breathing is associated with coordinated neural activity within the medulla, pons, midbrain, amygdala, anterior cingulate, and anterior insular cortices.[49] Furthermore, Zelano and colleagues' study findings suggest "air plumes that periodically enter the nose at the rate of quiet breathing may elicit slow and rhythmical neuronal oscillations that propagate throughout limbic brain networks".[50(p. 12463)] So there is actually a lot going on up in the brain when lying on the yoga mat doing nothing but sensing the breath flow in and out. A breath awareness script is incorporated into the **Initial centering** script in **Chapter 16**.

Diaphragmatic breath

The diaphragmatic breath is the most important structured breathing practice for activating the PNS. When learning diaphragmatic breathing, Sovik[46–48] suggests to "simply relax" at the end of the exhalation to allow inhalation to begin naturally on its own, and similarly to relax at the end of the inhalation to facilitate a smooth transition to exhalation. This makes great sense as a learning strategy for many people, but since the word "relax" can sometimes cause a hyperaroused person to feel more tense in their knowledge that they "*can't* relax", it may be wise to substitute the phrase "release all effort" when using this technique to teach diaphragmatic breathing to those healing from trauma. To perform this breath:

- Lie comfortably on your back and take a moment to make any adjustments you need to make so that you feel completely supported without effort. Begin to observe your breath … just notice how your breath is right now, without any need to

Chapter 12

change it … noticing whether it is constricted or relaxed … deep or shallow … What parts of your body move as you breathe? … Does your breath "catch" at any point along the way? … (pause)

- Now we will begin to draw the breath down into the belly. You may wish to place a weight (sandbag) or your hands on your belly, which can invite the muscles of your belly to soften … Release the muscles of the throat … and inhale through the nose, drawing the breath all the way down to the lower lungs … feeling your abdomen gently rise on the inhale … and sink back towards the spine as you exhale … allowing your breath to do all of the work … without any muscular effort …
- At the top of the inhalation, simply release all effort; the exhalation will begin naturally on its own … At the end of the exhalation, again release all effort … the body will naturally inhale …
- Continue to take several more breaths, inhaling and exhaling through the nose … slowly … smoothly … letting your breath flow naturally without exertion.

Complete Yogic Breath

After at least a minute or two of established diaphragmatic breathing, gradually lengthen and expand the breath:

- On your next inhale, when the lower lungs are full and the abdomen is fully expanded, continue to inhale, filling up the entire lungs … expanding the chest … and feeling the ribcage expand in all directions …
- Gradually exhale from the top of the lungs to the bottom. If you like, slightly contract the abdomen at the end of the exhalation to release more air.
- Perform 4–10 complete breaths and then return to the more gentle diaphragmatic breath.

Alternate nostril breathing

Alternate nostril breath (nadi shodhanam) calms the nervous system by balancing the sympathetic and parasympathetic nervous systems. The slowing and deepening of the breath during this practice contributes to the calming effect. The practice is often used prior to meditation as it helps to still the mind; many people naturally go into a meditative state immediately following the practice. Be especially careful of your body posture when you perform this practice as this has been shown to affect both nasal flow and dominance. This practice is generally performed in a sitting position but can also be performed in supine using the **alternate body breathing technique** (see next section), which does not involve physically blocking the nostrils with the hands.

- First blow your nose with a tissue if you need to do so. (Avoid the practice if you have a cold or flu.)
- Assume a comfortable upright sitting position with a straight spine (including neck), and rest your left hand on your lap.
- Begin by establishing diaphragmatic breathing, feeling the belly gently rise and fall with each breath.
- Bend the index and middle fingers of the right hand to the palm, and position your right thumb gently on the side of the right nostril to prepare for alternate nostril breathing.
- Inhale and exhale through both nostrils, then *gently* close the right nostril, and *begin the practice by first inhaling through the left nostril.*
- Release the thumb from the right nostril, <u>gently</u> press the left nostril with your ring finger, and *exhale through the right nostril.*
- Inhale through the right nostril, switch fingers, and exhale through the left nostril. This completes one round.
- Continue in this fashion, exhaling and then inhaling through the same nostril, then exhaling

Guideline 2
The most direct and powerful way to self-regulate is through control of the breath

and inhaling through the other nostril, slowly and deeply, evening out the inhalations and exhalations.
- Complete nine (or more) rounds, ending by exhaling through the left nostril.
- Then lower your hand to your knee and gently breathe through both nostrils.

This approach has been shown to increase parasympathetic activation.[28] Students should be encouraged to breathe slowly and deeply (the study results were produced at five to six breaths per minute).

A classic approach that mixes left-initiated and right-initiated alternate nostril breathing is to perform three sets of three rounds each of the above method with a short rest between the rounds, beginning the second round by inhaling first through the right nostril and the third round by inhaling first through the left nostril. This is a better method if you want a more equal balance between SNS and PNS activation.

People with low or high blood pressure should seek the advice of a fully certified yoga therapist before engaging in any alternate nostril breathing technique.

Alternate nostril body breathing

This is a wonderful practice to perform in supine, but you can also perform it sitting in an upright position, observing the postural precautions listed for the standard alternate nostril breathing practice. If lying supine, make sure the body is aligned straight and not leaning to one side or the other. Though the nostrils are not blocked off with the fingers as they are with alternate nostril breathing, oftentimes the breath will naturally switch sides during the practice.

Begin with breath awareness followed by the diaphragmatic breath. Then:

- You may continue with the diaphragmatic breath, or, if you like, you may follow my instructions for alternate nostril body breathing.
- Imagine you can inhale your breath in through the sole of your left foot, palm of your left hand, and left nostril, all the way up through the left side of your body.
- As you exhale, imagine the breath moving down through the right side of the body and out through the sole of the right foot, palm of your right hand, and right nostril.
- On your next inhalation, sense the breath moving in through the sole of your right foot, palm of your right hand, and right nostril, all the way up through the right side of your body.
- As you exhale, imagine the breath moving down through the left side of the body and out through the sole of the left foot, palm of your left hand, and left nostril. This completes one round.
- Continue in this manner, exhaling then inhaling through one side of the body, followed by exhaling then inhaling through the other side of the body.
- Complete at least nine rounds.

Ujjayi Breath

With this breathing technique, the glottis of the throat is slightly constricted to produce sound and sensation, though both the inhalation and exhalation are performed through the nose. The sound, which should just be audible to the practitioner, is similar to a light snoring sound or the sound you hear inside a sea conch shell, and facilitates the ability to focus on the breath. This breath is classically used during challenging yoga forms as it fosters endurance while holding a yoga form. It is energizing in an empowering sense, but in calming and grounding way.

First establish the diaphragmatic breath. Then:

- You may continue with the diaphragmatic breath, or, if you like, you may follow my instructions for the Ujjayi Breath. (Then explain, as above.)
- It is often easier to learn how to tighten the glottis by starting with the mouth open, and

Chapter 12

whispering, "**haaaa**" as you exhale. You might imagine steaming up a mirror with your breath. Go ahead and try that, and notice the sensation of the tightening of the throat muscles.

- When you are ready, close the lips and see if you can maintain the tightening of the glottis as you breathe in and out. Avoid tightening the glottis too strongly. The practice should produce a soft sound, only heard by you.
- Breathe slowly and deeply, evening out the breath between the inhalation and exhalation.
- Practice for three to five minutes (or for the duration of a particular yoga form). Please come out of the breathing pattern at any time and perhaps return to the diaphragmatic breath, if Ujjayi becomes uncomfortable for you.

Sitkari Breath

This breath is calming and cooling and is included also because of the deep touch pressure it provides to the palate when using the method below (there are many variations). Pressure to the palate is known to be calming. Just ask any baby who sucks their thumb! Occupational therapists have developed techniques for providing deep touch pressure to the upper hard palate to reduce sensory defensiveness.[51,52] Sitkari Breath is a way to produce this sensory input in the context of a calming breathing practice.

- Sit in any comfortable seated position, maintaining an upright spine, including the neck.
- Establish the diaphragmatic breath.
- Press the top front portion of the tongue (or tip) against the anterior bony hard palate, behind the top front teeth. (*Alternatively, fold the tongue over so the lower surface of the tongue is pressed against the upper hard palate. The folded tongue should not come forward between the teeth.*)
- Lightly touch the teeth together, keeping the lips slightly apart.
- Inhale slowly through the mouth, making the hissing sound of "ssssss" as the air flows in between the teeth.
- Then close the lips and exhale slowly through the nostrils.
- Repeat this breath for at least nine rounds.

Precautions for breathing exercises

- If you have any health issues related to the heart or lungs or if you are pregnant, seek approval from your doctor before engaging in structured breathing practices.
- The breathing practice should feel comfortable; if it feels forced or strained, come out of it.
- Fast breathing techniques such as kalabhati or bellows breath should be avoided by those who have PTSD, anxiety, or a related SNS-biased condition, and by those who have high blood pressure.
- Do not encourage holding of the breath as it can cause anxiety, thus reinforcing hyperarousal.
- Avoid extra-calming breathing exercises (such as left nostril initiated practices) if you have low blood pressure.
- Always remind your yoga class participants that they may come out of the breathing exercise at any time.

Guideline 3
Yoga can promote effective sensory, motor, and cognitive processing of traumatic experiences and thus aid healing

Trauma memory is as much in the sensory receptors, in the skin and in the muscles as it is in the brain.
— Alan Fogel[1(p. 259)]

As van der Kolk[2] has emphasized, trauma is stored in every cell of the body and must be safely released by the body for complete healing to occur. Trauma can express in the genes of our cells (e.g. see Yehuda et al.[3]) as well as the functioning of our organs, which are controlled by the autonomic nervous system. Trauma is also stored in our muscles, as reflected in our posture and movements,[4,5] which in turn affect our emotions and attitudes.[6] Thus, to help traumatized individuals heal, we need to help them clear out the trauma-related memory imprints not just from the "mind" but from the entire "bodymind", as the separation of body and mind is simply a mirage. These memory imprints present as obstacles along the path to experiencing the peaceful, clear-minded existence that every human being deserves. Thus, this guideline to practice speaks to the need to process trauma through the sensorimotor (bottom-up) and cognitive (top-down) channels that influence emotional well-being, and which, when blocked, keep an individual from the blissful experience of present moment awareness, i.e. the power of **now**.

The scope of this guideline is very broad and encompasses the next guideline as well (see Chapter 14). In that chapter, you will learn about the top-down elements that are incorporated into a Sensory-Enhanced Yoga practice, such as positive suggestions and guided meditations. But here we present sensory-based practices designed to influence the brain from the bottom-up. These practices have been successfully used in sensory-based occupational therapy treatments for decades, thanks to the insightful work of Jean Ayres,[7] founder of sensory integration theory and treatment. However, Sensory-Enhanced Yoga differs from a traditional sensory integration program in several ways, an important one being that, in our program, sensory-based practices are intertwined with mindfulness practices, drawing in a powerful top-down component to the bottom-up practices which is particularly therapeutic for rebalancing brain networks in PTSD. Specifically, we will discuss the therapeutic application of specific types of sensory input within the context of yoga for the purpose of healing trauma as well as related ANS conditions including high stress and anxiety, attention deficit disorder (ADD), and bipolar disorder.

Since we will be talking a lot about the processing of bodily-based sensation, we will need to introduce more neuroanatomy, namely, the neural pathways that transmit somatosensory and vestibular information to the brain. These pathways converge on and influence the functioning of the thalamus (as well as certain other structures). In turn, the thalamus, according to Nakajima and Halassa's hypothesis, "controls functional connectivity within and across cortical areas."[8] Yet keep in mind that the cerebral cortex also has a huge influence on the thalamus and dynamically manipulates its excitatory and inhibitory processes such that "the cortex can serve as a dynamic activity-dependent gatekeeper of its own sensory input."[9] In fact, according to Crandall et al.,[9] the descending axons from the cortex to the thalamus outnumber the ascending axons by 10:1. So clearly, the thalamus and cerebral cortex work very closely together and more collaboratively than we had

Chapter 13

previously thought, further supporting the idea that combining top-down (mindfulness) and bottom-up (sensory-based) practices would be the most powerful approach for addressing PTSD, anxiety, or related mental health conditions.

Developing a witness mentality

One powerful way that yoga draws the mind back to present-moment awareness is through "witness consciousness", which Kabat-Zinn, founder of Mindfulness-Based Stress Reduction (MBSR), defined as "paying attention in a particular way: on purpose, in the present moment, and non-judgmentally."[10(p. 4)] In most yoga classes, and certainly those that follow the Sensory-Enhanced Yoga methodology, participants are encouraged to notice sensation as they move through the yoga forms and attune to their breath, and to step back and observe them as a witness when sensations get too strong, so as not to get caught up in them. Learning to step into, as well as step back from, sensation, mindfully, is an important skill for healthy embodiment. Sensory-Enhanced Yoga provides additional therapeutic sensation to attend to, which can be even more effective in drawing one's mind to the present moment, particularly for those who suffer from intrusive thoughts or who feel uncomfortable with the usual sensations in their bodies (which therapeutic input can cancel out through sensory gating mechanisms). A simple seated meditation can be overwhelming for many of these individuals, but a short, seated meditation immediately following a session of yoga asana and breath work can be more accessible, as the bodymind has been prepared for it—especially if the yoga session includes a sufficient threshold of *therapeutic* sensory input to attend to for those whom subtle input is not enough.

This process of drawing the senses inward to engage in non-judgmental attention to bodily sensation theoretically helps to strengthen the neural inhibitory mechanisms necessary to rebalance the networks of the brain.[11,12] In Chapter 4 we saw that intrinsic sensory hyperactivity tends to occur in the somatosensory cortex, visual cortex, and precuneus of those who have PTSD, which then forward along this excessive sensory excitation to medial prefrontal cortex structures, resulting in the flooding of information to these brain regions.[13,14] The inhibitory techniques presented in this chapter are designed to improve sensory processing in the thalamus so the information is not passed along unfiltered to the sensory and visual cortices and precuneus, creating a "traffic jam." The thalamus can then more effectively co-engage with higher brain structures to influence the brain networks that have been altered in PTSD. Kerr et al.[15] suggested that in standardized mindfulness practices this process occurs through attention-controlled modulation of sensory alpha wave activity (via attention to sensation) and then spreads throughout the entire brain, and that this process can reduce ruminative thoughts.

Sensory-Enhanced Yoga combines sensory and mindfulness-based practices to enhance this process. We know that certain types and applications of sensory input can inhibit the sympathetic (fight–flight) branch of the autonomic nervous system, reduce sensory over-responsivity, and facilitate self-regulation.[7,16,17] The following types of therapeutic sensory input are included in the program:

- deep pressure touch
- enhanced proprioceptive input
- slow rhythmical linear movement
- neutral warmth.

Many yoga styles emphasize one or two of these sensory modalities. For example, B. K. S. Iyengar emphasized active static holds that provide strong muscle sensation (proprioceptive input), passive static holds (often providing deep touch pressure input) using props such as bolsters to achieve a particular

Guideline 3
Yoga can promote effective sensory, motor, and cognitive processing of traumatic experiences and thus aid healing

bodily alignment or other therapeutic goal, as well as combinations of the above.[18] Thus we could say that Iyengar exploited the benefits of therapeutic deep touch pressure and enhanced proprioceptive input in his style of yoga. Iyengar directly taught many students who subsequently became famous in their own right, including Judith Hanson Lasater, whose restorative yoga forms incorporate the use of yoga sandbags to provide enhanced deep touch pressure.[19,20]

Other styles have emphasized slow, rhythmical repetitive movement, the best known being the Viniyoga style popularized in the US by Gary Kraftsow, who learned it from T. K. V. Desikachar. Some of these rhythmic flows stimulate the vestibular apparatus while others do not; the ones that do incorporate movement of the head through space. Though Kraftsow does not mention the benefits of vestibular input in his most famous book, **Yoga for Wellness**, we can easily choose flows from this rich resource that will provide the inhibitory effect in the nervous system we are looking for.

While Iyengar and Desikachar seem to have evolved their styles in completely different directions, they each learned these styles from the "father of modern yoga", Śrī T. Krishnamacharya. (In fact, Desikachar is the son of Krishnamacharya while Iyengar is Krishnamacharya's brother-in-law.[18,21]) The story I was told is that Krishnamacharya individualized his approach when working with each of them, based on their individual health needs. Thus, by individualizing the practices, Krishnamacharya could be seen as the father of yoga *therapy*.

Krishnamacharya also mentored another famous yogi, K. Pattabhi Jois, founder of the Ashtanga vinyasa yoga style (see: https://sharathjois.com/biographies/k-pattabhi-jois/), but the nature of Jois' health needs led Krishnamacharya to suggest a more active style of movement sequences, connected with the breath. While Sensory-Enhanced Yoga does not recommend quick yoga movements for people healing from trauma, such as the jumping or bouncing of an Ashtanga yoga class, it does incorporate sequences such as Sun and Moon Salutations (see Chapter 18) and emphasizes movement with the breath (as does Viniyoga). It is interesting to consider that Sensory-Enhanced Yoga may not be a new way of thinking after all but rather a re-synthesis of the separate elements of Krishnamacharya's yoga style back into a unified paradigm of thinking for the purpose of healing trauma. In other words, we need to consider what effect(s) we are looking for in the bodymind and decide what combination, dosage, and qualities of sensory input will help us reach a therapeutic threshold to achieve that effect.

Let us now discuss each of these modalities in turn.

Deep touch pressure

Temple Grandin, an American professor of animal science, created the "hug box" for people on the autism spectrum, based on her own experience of the condition. She articulates well the therapeutic benefits of deep touch pressure:[22]

Deep touch pressure is the type of surface pressure that is exerted in most types of firm touching, holding, stroking, petting of animals, or swaddling. In contrast, light touch pressure is a more superficial stimulation of the skin, such as tickling, very light touch, or moving hairs on the skin. In animals, the tickle of a fly landing on the skin may cause a cow to kick, but the firm touch of the farmer's hands quiets her. Occupational therapists have observed that a very light touch alerts the nervous system, but deep pressure is relaxing and calming.

There are two major somatosensory (body sensation) pathways from the spinal cord to the

Chapter 13

brain that we need to concern ourselves with in order to effectively apply this modality: the spinothalamic and dorsal column medial lemniscal (DCML) pathways (Figures 13.1 and 13.2). Both of these pathways converge in the ***ventral posterolateral nucleus*** of the thalamus, where the net sum of excitatory impulses from these pathways determines whether the current sensory landscape of the body will have an overall arousing or calming affect on the nervous system.

The spinothalamic pathway (Figure 13.1)

The lateral tracts (including the spinothalamic tract) are functionally interconnected with the reticular formation.

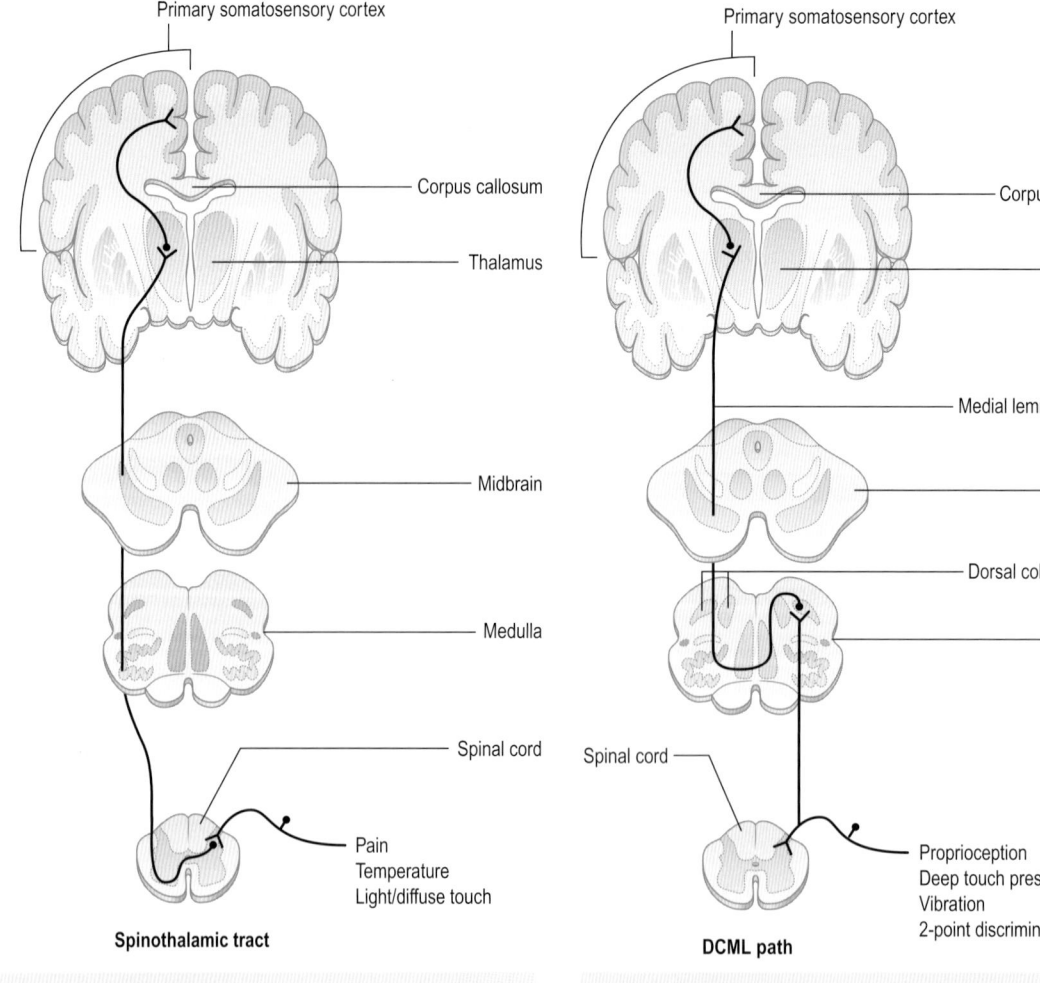

Figure 13.1
Spinothalamic pathway

Figure 13.2
Dorsal column medial lemniscal (DCML) pathway

Guideline 3
Yoga can promote effective sensory, motor, and cognitive processing of traumatic experiences and thus aid healing

The spinothalamic pathway transmits:

- pain
- temperature
- superficial pressure
- light/diffuse touch

to brain areas critical for arousal (reticular activating system; RAS), emotional tone (limbic system), visceral control (hypothalamus), and subconscious recognition of input (thalamus). It facilitates the sympathetic fight–flight branch of the autonomic nervous system (ANS).

The dorsal column medial lemniscal (DCML) pathway

Transmits:

- proprioception
- deep touch pressure input
- vibration
- tactile discrimination information

to the thalamus, and from the thalamus to SI, SII, Area 5, Area 7, and the limbic structures.

This is a major system we are trying to activate in Sensory-Enhanced Yoga classes. Experts have long hypothesized that the reason deep touch pressure and proprioceptive input helps to produce calming is due to the DCML pathway overriding the spinothalamic pathways.

The "**sensory homunculus**" (Figure 13.3) shows the relative amount of cerebral cortex surface given over to processing the different sensory inputs of the human nervous system. The image represents the sensory cortex (aka somatosensory cortex). Hands, feet, and oral areas are strongly represented in the sensory homunculus due to the much greater number of neurons and dendrites. Therefore, touch pressure to these areas can have a powerful inhibitory affect to the ANS. Pressure can be deep, such as weight-bearing through the hands and feet in Downward Dog, or it can involve more subtle

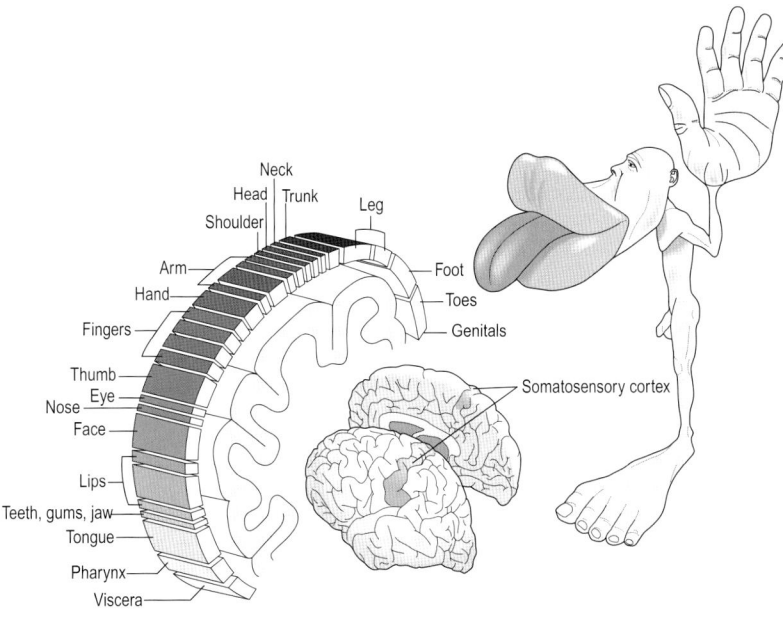

Figure 13.3

The sensory homunculus

Chapter 13

pressure, such as pressing palms together in the Namaste prayer position, which is also calming and grounding.

Ways to embed deep touch pressure into a therapeutic yoga class

Deep touch pressure can be provided through the use of yoga props, such as bolsters, sandbags (which we call "weights" to avoid the military connotation of the word sandbag), and/or blocks; by offering yoga forms that naturally place pressure on various body parts (often through weight-bearing) such as the hands, feet, and various parts of the torso, e.g. back, shoulder blades, or belly; by performing certain mudras (hand gestures), such as Adhi, Ishvara or as mentioned, Anjali mudra (see Chapter 14); or by presenting a breathing technique that places pressure on the hard palate (Sitkari Breath, see Chapter 12).

For years, OTs and other neurorehabilitation specialists have known that pressure to the hard palate is very calming to the nervous system, and they use various methods to provide deep pressure to the palate, even for adults. The Sitkari Breath (see Chapter 12), also known as the cooling breath, which is relaxing to the nerves and calming to the mind, uses the tongue to place pressure on the roof of the mouth.

Examples of deep touch pressure using props

- Bolsters provide comforting deep pressure when used in restorative forms, and can be used in conjunction with other props such as blankets, blocks, straps, and yoga weights (see the Restorative section, below).
- A 10-pound soft yoga weight can be placed:

—*on the belly* (such as during diaphragmatic breathing)

—*on the feet* (such as during Legs Up the Wall)

—*across the upper sacrum*, such as during Restorative Child

—*over the backside of the body*, such as during Restorative Twist

—*on the forehead* (see the Mental tension reliever restorative form in this chapter).

Other spots have been used as well. Many students enjoy having two weights placed on their bodies, such as across the upper buttocks/lower back and vertically along the spine, forming an inverted "T" (see Figure 13.5). (The bags are bought unfilled from yoga supply stores and can be filled with play sand from a home building supply store. The sand tends to be moist when first purchased so allow at least a week or two to thoroughly dry it out before filling the bags.)

- The wall of the room can be used to promote a sense of "grounding", such as by placing a foot (or feet) on the wall during spinal balance, a reclined symmetrical stretch, or during a single leg raise in supine position.
- Eye pillows can provide comforting pressure to encourage the muscles surrounding the eyes to soften and release.

Examples of deep touch pressure using the body (weight-bearing)

Yoga forms can provide pressure **through the back**, such as in Knee to Chest; **through the hands**, such as in Downward-Facing Dog, Plank, or Upward-Facing Dog; **through the belly**, such as in Crocodile or Baby Cobra, **through the feet**, such as by pressing the feet away from each other in Warrior II to enhance the sense of grounding, or **through the limbs**, such as Eagle. More examples are provided in Appendix B.

A small sampling of gentle restorative forms providing deep touch pressure

Most of the restorative forms described on the following pages (or variations thereof) can be found in at least one of references 18, 20, 24, and 25.[18,20,24,25]

Guideline 3
Yoga can promote effective sensory, motor, and cognitive processing of traumatic experiences and thus aid healing

When choosing yoga forms from books, you should consider the typical effects of the form as described by the author. Some are geared for depression, others for anxiety, and so on. For trauma healing, it is safest to choose the ones that are designed to reduce anxiety, as ones for depression are more apt to strongly expand the chest area and/or involve a deep backbend, which can reinforce hyperarousal. Having said that, a fully supported and gentle restorative backbend is much less apt to be anxiety inducing than unsupported backbends with the head tilted backwards, such as Camel. Many traumatized individuals are constricted across the chest and could benefit from gentle stretching in this area, yet we should not lose sight of the fact that they are protecting their heart centers for a reason. Thus, we start within the person's window of tolerance and gradually move them into more expansive yoga forms as they are ready to embody them. Additionally, we often offer a 10-pound yoga weight (or two) during some of the restorative yoga forms to enhance the calming effect.

Weighted Child (Figures 13.4 and 13.5)

- Kneel at the short end of the bolster with your knees straddled around it.
- Place a firm folded blanket between your buttocks and lower legs to support your body and help the knees stay comfortable.
- Place your hands on the floor on each side of the bolster and slowly walk the hands away from you until you are lowered onto the bolster. Turn your head to one side.
- Ask a friend to position a 10-pound weighted cloth bag across the top of the sacrum/lower back area to provide deep touch pressure, adjusting the sand evenly in the bag first (Figure 13.4).
- If desired, have your friend place another 10-pound weighted bag vertically along the spine, overlapping the first bag so both bags form an inverted "T". Make sure the strap of this bag is positioned as shown in the photo and isn't touching your back (Figure 13.5).
- Rest for approximately five minutes, or however long it feels good, turning your head at the halfway point.
- *Optional*: during set-up, position a block (at its middle height) under the head end of the bolster to angle it (Figure 13.5).

Figure 13.4

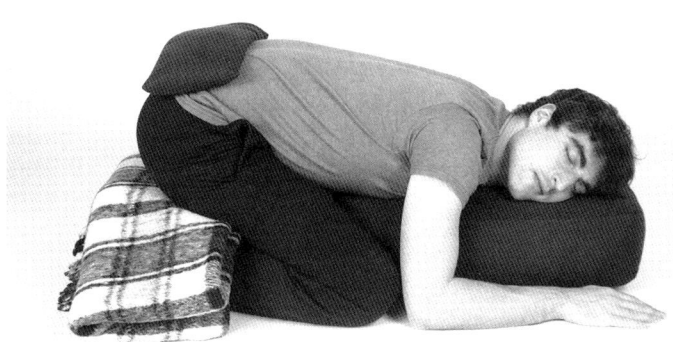

Chapter 13

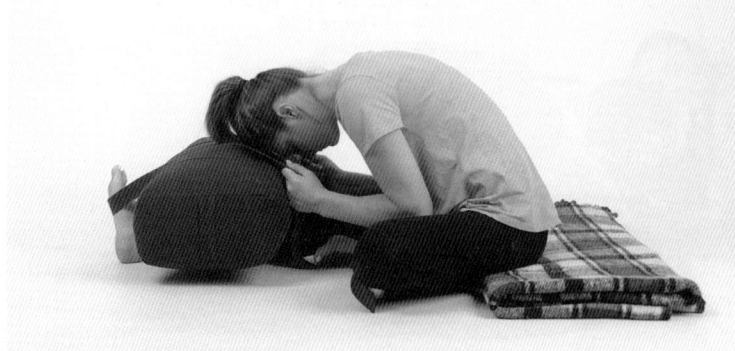

Figure 13.9

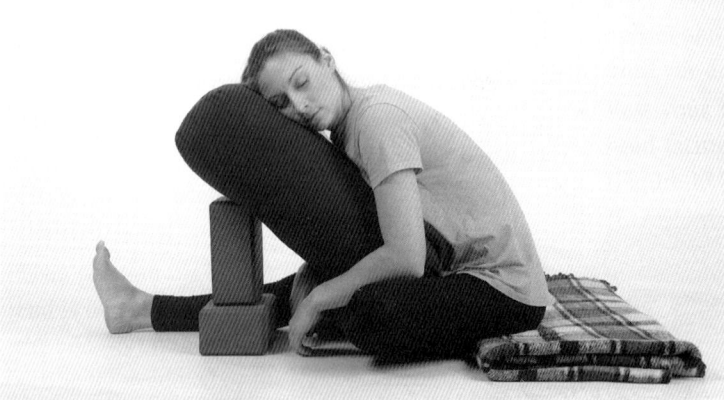

Figure 13.10

- Press your hands into the floor next to your hips, and take several breaths, lengthening up through the crown of your head with each inhalation and maintaining that length during each exhalation.
- Position the sole of your left foot against the inner surface of your upper right thigh.
- Position a yoga strap over the ball of your right foot and position the top end of the strap within reach on the floor for now.
- Ideally, perform a few rounds of Dynamic Head to Knee here, to prepare for the hold (see Chapter 17).
- Position a bolster widthwise on your lower outstretched leg.
- Lengthen the spine on an inhalation, and as you exhale, fold forward to rest your forehead on the bolster.
- Then hold onto the yoga strap with both hands. (With a shorter height bolster than shown, you may be able to hold the strap close to your foot with your arms outstretched.)
- Stay for at least 30 seconds, sensing your breath stretching the back of your body on each inhalation, and releasing muscle tension on each exhalation (Figure 13.9).
- Switch to the other side.
- *Modification*: see Figure 13.10 for a less deep forward bend that can work particularly well for someone who has tight hamstrings.

Guideline 3
Yoga can promote effective sensory, motor, and cognitive processing of traumatic experiences and thus aid healing

Restorative Backbend (Figures 13.11 and 13.12)

- Sit with your back facing the bolster, then slowly lie back over it (Figure 13.11).
- If the bolster places any stress on the lower back, move your buttocks further away from it.
- Rest your head on a folded firm blanket positioned horizontally over the bolster.
- Rest your forearms on the floor (or folded blankets) with palms naturally turned up.
- You may also wish to place a half-folded blanket under the lower part of the body for comfort, especially for the heels.
- *Optional*: position a block (at its 2nd height) under the head end of the bolster to angle it (Figure 13.12).

Supported Savasana (Figure 13.13)

- Lie down on the mat.
- Position a bolster horizontally under your thighs so both the buttocks and feet are comfortably resting on the floor.
- Partially roll a blanket just enough to comfortably support the neck without hyperextending it. (Chin should ideally be slightly tucked.)
- *For breath work, you may choose to place a weighted bag over your lower belly as shown to strengthen the diaphragm and naturally deepen the exhalation, which facilitates relaxation. See the Initial centering script in Chapter 16 for details.*
- Rest the arms on the floor, and stay as long as you like.

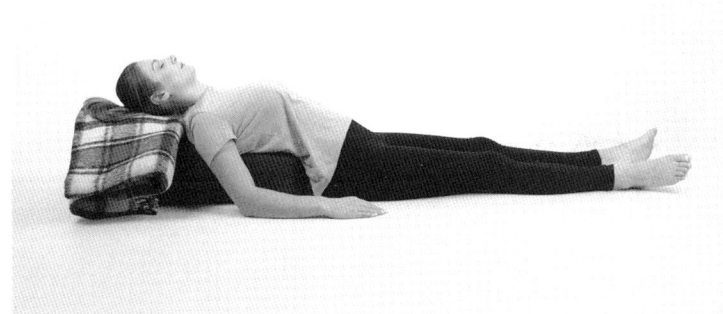

Figure 13.11

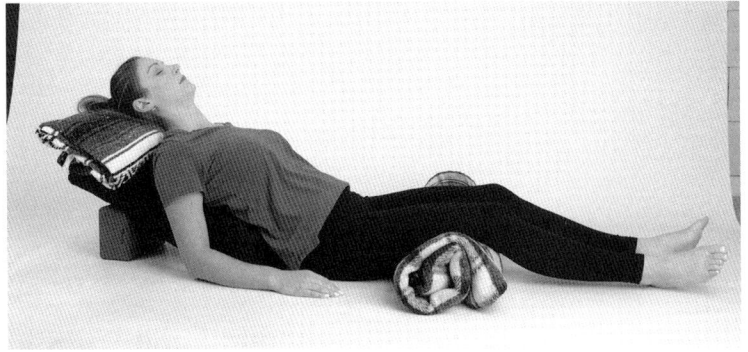

Figure 13.12

Chapter 13

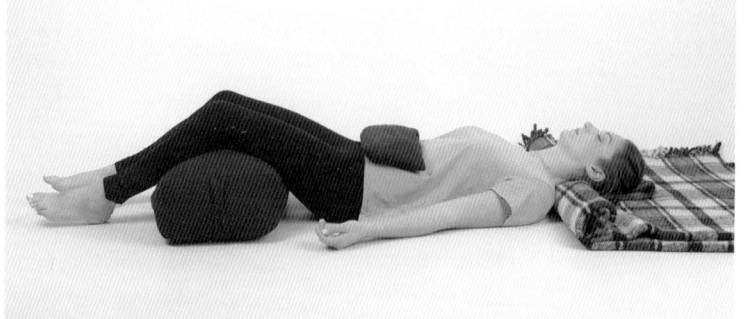

Figure 13.13

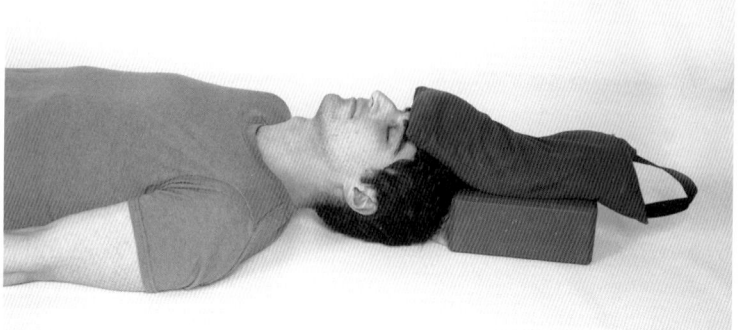

Figure 13.14

Mental Tension Reliever (Figure 13.14)

- Lie supine on a blanket or mat placed on a firm surface.
- Position a four-inch thick block behind the head at its shortest height with the short end against the crown of the head.
- Lay a 10-pound weighted cloth yoga bag over the block and forehead. (First adjust the sand inside the bag so the amount of weight on the forehead conforms to the student's wishes.)
- Rest for about five minutes.

Weighted Legs Up the Wall (Figure 13.15)

- Position a mat or blanket up to a wall.
- Sidesit on the mat/blanket as close to the wall as possible, so one of your hips is touching it.
- Slowly swing your legs up the wall as you carefully lower your back to the floor.
- If desired, place a folded blanket under your head.
- Ask someone to balance a weighted bag on the bottom of your feet (evening out the weight of the sand in the bag prior to placement); you will need their help to remove the weighted bag afterwards, too.
- Rest for about five minutes.

Supported Bridge (Figure 13.16 and Figure 13.17)

- Lie supine on the mat with a block close by and adjust your body so it is symmetrical.
- If desired, cover yourself and the block with a blanket (or ask someone else to cover you).
- Bend your knees and place your feet on the mat, close to your hips and hip-width apart (your shins should be vertical).
- Position your arms straight by your sides with your palms facing down on the mat, close to your heels.

Guideline 3
Yoga can promote effective sensory, motor, and cognitive processing of traumatic experiences and thus aid healing

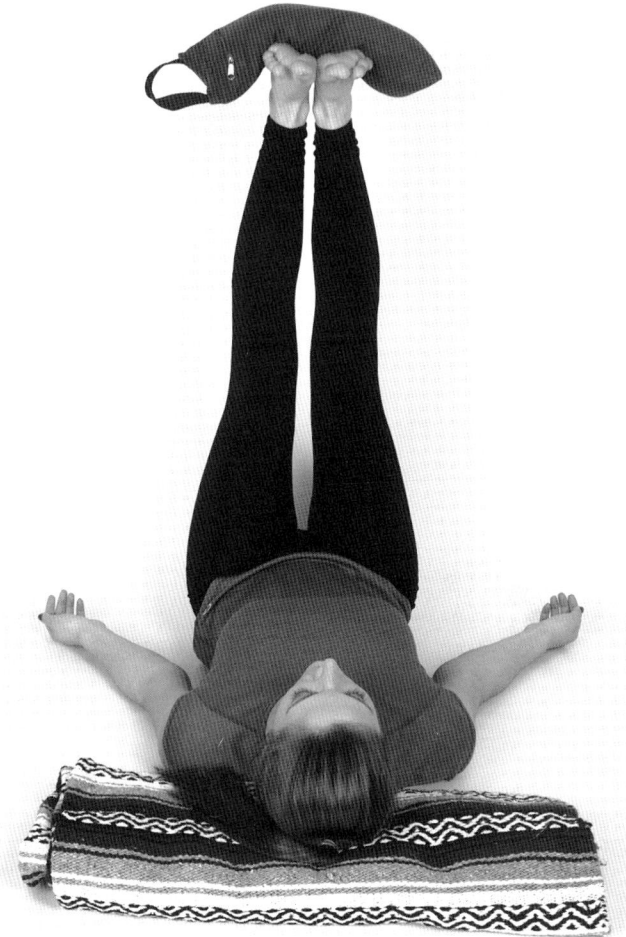

Figure 13.15

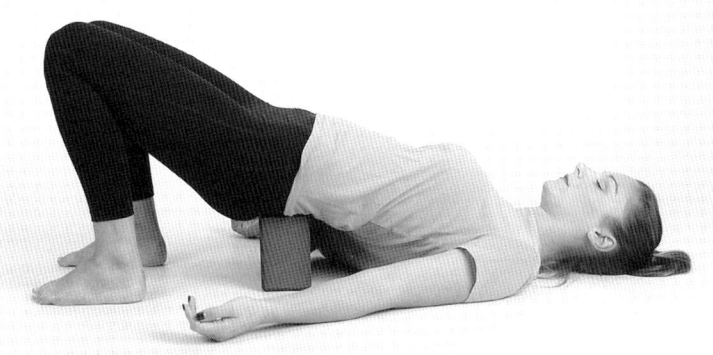

Figure 13.16

Chapter 13

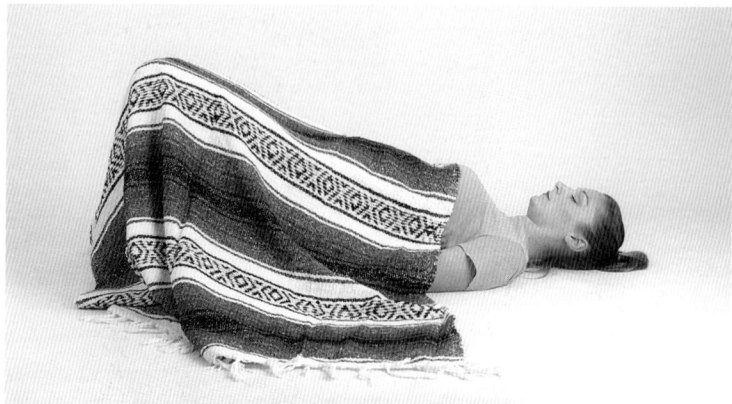

Figure 13.17

- On your next inhalation, *tuck your tailbone* as you press your lower back to the floor, engaging your abdominal muscles; as you exhale, slowly release your tailbone back down to the mat, allowing the natural lumbar arch to return to your spine.
- On your following inhalation, tuck your tailbone (engaging your abdominal muscles), lift your sacrum, and continue lifting one vertebra at a time off the mat, up through your lower back, and as you exhale, slowly and completely release your spine down to the mat, one vertebra at a time.
- Repeat this movement at least two more times, rising from the base of your spine upwards, lifting more vertebrae with each inhalation, and completely releasing your spine to the mat with each exhalation.
- When you lift high enough that you are supported by your shoulder blades, feet, and arms, lift up on your toes so you can position your block at its middle height (or whichever height works for you) under your sacrum (not under your lower back). Release your heels back down to the mat.
- Roll your shoulders underneath you and sense the expansion of the chest.
- Notice the grounding sensation of your feet pressing into the earth and your sacrum pressing into the block.
- Soften the belly to invite full deep breaths.
- Rest here for a couple of minutes or longer.
- After you remove the block, slowly lower your spine back down to the mat.
- Draw your knees to your chest (as a counterform, to loosen any tension in the lower back).

Restorative Crocodile in a Chair (Figure 13.18)

- Position two chairs facing the same direction, one in front of the other.
- Place a folded blanket over the back of the chair in front.
- Sit in the other chair and, if desired, position a weighted yoga bag across the top of your feet.
- Place your forearms on the blanket; rest your head on your arms.
- Stay as long as you like.

Enhanced proprioceptive input

Proprioceptive sensation is produced by receptors in muscles and joints. The muscle spindle is the major stretch receptor within muscles. Golgi tendon organs and joint afferents monitor stresses and forces at the tendons and joints. According to sensory integration theory, activities that provide enhanced

Guideline 3
Yoga can promote effective sensory, motor, and cognitive processing of traumatic experiences and thus aid healing

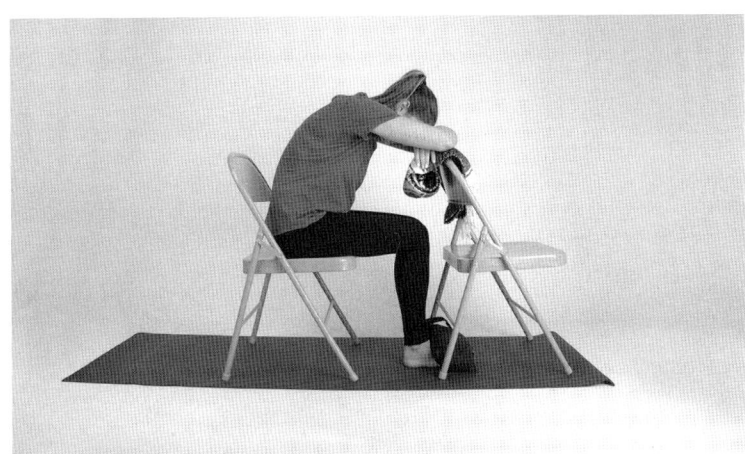

Figure 13.18

proprioceptive (muscle and joint) input are believed to decrease sensory sensitivity and improve self-regulation.[26,27] According to Mollo and colleagues,[28] this is hypothetically achieved by inhibiting sympathetic nervous system (SNS) activity and by increasing activation of the parasympathetic nervous system (PNS). Self-initiated proprioceptive input is frequently used therapeutically to help individuals "increase body awareness, improve motor coordination, help modulate arousal level, and aid in the processing of sensation through other sensory systems."[26(p. 109),28]

It is important to remain sensitive to the fact that trauma is held in the muscles (as well as all of the other tissues of the body) when presenting enhanced proprioceptive input to traumatized individuals. Although muscle and joint sensation is generally considered to be a very safe form of sensory input that is very integrating, there are some special considerations for trauma survivors. As you will recall, during the stress response, cortisol-, adrenaline-, and noradrenaline-infused blood is shunted to the limbs to assist in the fight–flight response. If the stress response is not adequately resolved, this excess energy is stored in the muscles, still ready to fight or flee, while the person remains in a frozen state of immobility. (One such muscle is the psoas; please see the special note in the box describing muscle elongation techniques, p. 166). This creates trauma-based muscle tension that can present in one's posture and movements, accompanied by psychological tension. As discussed in Chapter 11, this tension/pressure needs to be released slowly, so it is important to proceed thoughtfully when elongating the muscles and not ask people to over-extend their bodies into the full expression of a yoga form if they are not ready for it—and especially, do not go over to the person and overextend them yourself! Always start where the person is at, staying within their physical and psychological range of motion.

The box on p. 166 describes two effective muscle-elongation methods that can help to release trauma-held muscular tensions when performed correctly. It should be noted that muscles cannot actually stretch (see Ralph Stephens' excellent tutorial at https://yogainternational.com/article/view/why-you-cant-stretch-a-muscle). Following elongation, a muscle should be used actively and functionally, either on or off the yoga mat. This is particularly important for loose-jointed individuals who actually need yoga forms and movements that emphasize joint compression rather than joint traction to help hold themselves together (as Rothschild points out in her case study of Thomas in Chapter 19 of *The Body Remembers: Casebook*).[29]

Chapter 13

The Sensory-Enhanced Yoga program provides plentiful opportunities for joint compression through weight-bearing forms and through use of a yoga strap (for those individuals whom a strap is appropriate), which provides co-activation of muscles around the joints.

> ## Muscle elongation techniques used in the Sensory-Enhanced Yoga program
>
> 1. ***Repetition and hold.*** This method consists of dynamically moving in and out of a yoga form in coordination with the breath. A classic example found in most yoga classes is the Cat-Cow flow (see Chapter 17 for this and other examples). A leading pioneer in this approach is Gary Kraftsow.[30] Dynamically moving in and out of a form *with awareness* provides us with feedback regarding our movement habits, including our protective holding patterns and release valves, so that by the time we hold the form, we are likely to be in much better alignment than had we simply gone straight into it on the first breath. Also, muscles elongate further after contracting, due to the mechanism of reciprocal innervation between antagonistic muscles, thus drawing us deeper into the form with each repetition. Finally, trauma survivors may start out with more constrained movements and as they slowly become more embodied through awareness of sensation, movement, and breath, may begin to demonstrate greater range and ease of movement.
>
> 2. ***Maintained stretch.*** This method is used during static yoga forms or during the hold portion of a dynamic form when you meet up with a restriction in movement. A good example of its use is during leg stretches with a yoga strap. Ralph Stephens (see link on previous page) presents one of the best tutorials on this approach and it is how I was taught in my own yoga training. He instructs students to move the body part just until you feel the stretch, and then stop there and simply breathe and relax into it. After several seconds, the muscles will soften and you will sense space allowing you to move a bit further (even if just a little). Once again, stop and breathe into the stretch. You might undergo this process three or four times before the final range is reached for that session. In the words of Yee: "resistance ... pause ... breath ... space ... movement ... resistance".[31(p. 130)]
>
> ***A note about the psoas muscle.*** The psoas muscle is the largest hip flexor and is wired tightly to the SNS, as it is needed in order to run away during the fight–flight reaction. Due to its position in the body, when it contracts, it pulls on the diaphragm. It is this pull that causes us to make that short gasp when something frightens us. It contracts during activation of the SNS even if we are sitting down and not actively moving. Many trauma survivors have an especially tight psoas, which can affect diaphragmatic breathing, contributing to a shallow breath. There are several published yoga classes designed to release the psoas muscle (see, for example, the Yoga International website). Examples of yoga forms that stretch the psoas include Warrior I, Lunge, and Restorative Bridge (with a block). There is a common follow-up to Restorative Bridge where the legs are then completely stretched out straight rather than keeping the knees bent with the feet on the floor (while still on the block); however, this last stretch can be too much for a trauma survivor (not to mention psychologically disconcerting for a sexual trauma survivor). You may also notice a decreased stance during Warrior forms. Again, it is important to start where the person is. If you suspect a tight psoas, it is recommended that a certified yoga therapist or physical therapist be consulted for proper treatment.

Guideline 3
Yoga can promote effective sensory, motor, and cognitive processing of traumatic experiences and thus aid healing

Ways to increase proprioceptive input

Yoga naturally provides rich proprioceptive input; however, there are several ways we can enhance the proprioceptive qualities of a yoga session to boost its therapeutic effects. We can use yoga straps to increase the muscle activation (taking care to do so safely by not *over*stretching muscles); we can present yoga forms that offer heavy muscle work in static positions; and we can choose slower dynamic yoga flows that incorporate increased muscle loading, the latter of which also helps to modulate any hypersensitivity that may occur from the movement of the flow. When presenting yoga forms that include the use of a strap, it is a good idea to offer an alternative option, in case anyone in class has experienced bondage (see Chapter 11). Simply state "You can choose to do these movements with or without the yoga strap."

Some recommended muscle-loading yoga forms are listed below. It is particularly effective to bear weight on the arms, such as in Down Dog, or activate more muscles due to the awkwardness of the position, such as in Chair. Chapter 17 provides examples of how to use yoga straps and Chapter 18 examples of how to adapt yoga flows for enhanced proprioceptive input. Appendix B identifies the sensory qualities of selected yoga forms, which may also be helpful to you in planning your yoga sessions.

- Spinal Balance
- Downward-Facing Dog
- Down Dog to Up Dog Flow
- Modified Hare to Up Dog Flow
- Baby Cobra or Cobra
- Arm or Leg Stretches with strap
- Plank (chair version is shown in Chapter 18)
- Sphinx (not shown in this book)
- Bridge
- Extended Side Angle
- Raised Knee Lunge (not shown in this book)
- Warrior I and II
- Chair
- Victory Squat

Slow rhythmical linear movement

In 1954, Margaret Rood published a paper on her neurophysiological approach to the development of motor control.[32] Among the principles of her approach was the concept that, through the careful selection and use of sensory stimuli, the autonomic nervous system could be biased toward sympathetic or parasympathetic activation, which would influence muscle control accordingly.[32,33] She believed that it was the ***intensity***, ***frequency***, and ***rhythm*** (or lack thereof) of the sensory stimulus that determined whether it would have a sympathetic or parasympathetic effect. Among the sensory stimuli suggested to activate the parasympathetic nervous system were slow, rhythmic, repetitive rocking and slow rolling,[33] techniques which have been adapted for yoga in the Sensory-Enhanced Yoga program.

Jean Ayres[7] was strongly influenced by Rood when she developed her sensory integration theory and intervention program for children. It was Ayres' work that inspired me to enter the occupational therapy field in the first place and much later to suggest that slow rhythmic movements be integrated into the Iraq Yoga Study treatment protocol for active duty military personnel.

Though she believed passive rocking would inhibit the nervous system to a greater degree than active rocking (I would agree), Ayres stated that active participation can be encouraged to help modulate the vestibular effects if they are too inhibitory or excitatory, and that "organizing a response tends to balance the excitatory and inhibitory components

Chapter 13

of brain function."[7(p. 120)] Given the popularity of rocking chairs for stress reduction, which involve active movements, I wondered whether slow, *active*, rhythmic movements along the same planes advocated for passive linear movements would also produce a calming effect. If so, I surmised that incorporating such movements into the Iraq Yoga Study protocol for military personnel could potentially reduce symptoms of hyperarousal caused by living and working in combat conditions. Regarding the age disparity between children and full-grown military personnel, we now know that there is a lot of neuroplasticity even in the adult brain that was unknown when Ayres developed her theory of sensory integration. I will share with you some of the research that has since been conducted in this area, but first we start with some important background on the vestibular system itself.

The vestibular sense, embodiment, and sense of safety

The vestibular system is part of the labyrinth of the inner ear, and detects our head movement through space as well as its position relative to gravity. Thus it contributes to balance and to spatial orientation, and is the dominant sense that provides information about our movement through the environment, almost like a GPS system. The vestibular system consists of the utricle and saccule, known as the otoliths, and the three semicircular canals (Figure 13.19). They are attached

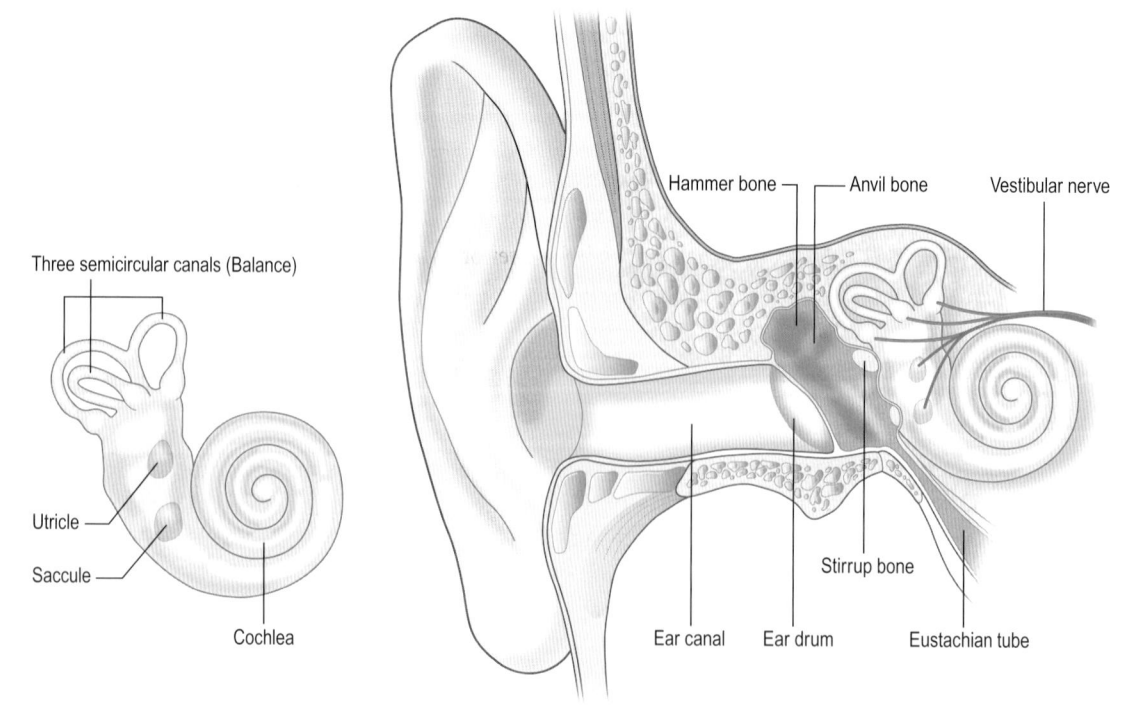

Figure 13.19
The Vestibular Apparatus

Guideline 3
Yoga can promote effective sensory, motor, and cognitive processing of traumatic experiences and thus aid healing

to the hearing apparatus (cochlea), also located in the inner ear. These structures are lined with hair cells and are also filled with fluid (endolymph). When the head moves, the fluid moves, displacing the hair cells, which sets off nerve impulses. The otoliths and semicircular canals respond to different types of vestibular input:

- The **otoliths** are gravity receptors and, as such, detect the position of the head in relation to gravity. They also detect linear movement through space. The otoliths consist of the *saccule*, which detects vertical movement, and *the utricle*, which detects forward and backward and side-to-side linear movements.

- The **semicircular canals** detect angular (or rotary) movement, such as spinning or rotating the head from side to side or doing somersaults.

The vestibular sense works closely with the proprioceptive sense to enable us to maintain balance and an upright posture. It is also closely involved with the visual system, allowing us to judge our motion in relation to the objects around us. Our sense of "grounding" is largely attributable to the vestibular sense as it detects our positional relationship to the Earth. When a person is feeling intense anxiety, it can be accompanied by a "floating in space" sensation due to the strong connections between the vestibular and autonomic systems. When this occurs, deep touch pressure and/or enhanced proprioceptive input will usually effectively modulate the sensations and help to psychologically "re-plant" the person back on the ground. The ungrounded feeling that can accompany anxiety may be at least partly due to decreased connectivity between the vestibular nuclei and insula, which was found in the dissociative subtype of PTSD (vs non-dissociative PTSD and healthy controls) in a neuroimaging study conducted by Harricharan and colleagues.[34] These researchers hypothesized that a weakened interoceptive sense would contribute to hypervigilance to evaluate one's safety in the environment.

Lenggenhager and Lopez[35] presented findings from various fields to support their hypothesis that vestibular input contributes "to aspects of the bodily self, such as basic multisensory integration, body schema, body ownership, agency, and self-location." A major theme of Part 2 of this book was on the importance of restoring a sense of embodiment in trauma survivors; therefore, studying the potential role of the vestibular system toward that goal would certainly be a worthwhile undertaking. Indeed, Harricharan et al.[34] pointed to the urgent need to conduct more studies on the vestibular neural circuitry of those who have PTSD to develop interventions that address decreased interoceptive awareness and disembodiment related to impaired vestibular function.

Vestibular pathways to the brain
Vestibular pathways to the cortex

Vestibular pathways project to numerous areas of the cerebral cortex, including the parieto-insular cortex, temporo-parietal junction, several areas of the somatosensory cortex, posterior parietal and medial superior temporal cortices, anterior and posterior cingulate cortex, and retrosplenial cortex.[36] The parieto-insular cortex of humans is believed by many scientists to be the homologue of the *parieto-insular vestibular cortex* (*PIVC*; vestibular cortex) in the monkey, though this area is still being defined in humans.[37,38] Frank and Greenlee[38] recently suggested that the human vestibular cortex consists of at least two separate areas, the PIVC and posterior insular cortex (PIC).

Neuroimaging studies have shown that the PIVC receives input from both the semicircular canals and otoliths and is involved in the perception of verticality and self-motion. It also has strong connections to the anterior insula, precuneus (a structure linked to "happiness"), lateral thalamus, among other important areas.[39] As we saw in Chapter 4, the anterior insula is postulated to hold a key role in switching between the central executive and default mode networks so it is noteworthy that vestibular stimulation can influence this brain structure. Also, the connection between the PIVC and precuneus likely explains the euphoria experienced by many people during rides at amusement parks (and to the automatic big smiles of my four-month old grandson when lifted into the air!).

Brandt and Dieterich[37] presented evidence showing that activation of vestibular cortex and certain other vestibular-related areas demonstrate a significant right-hemispheric dominance, which is particularly interesting considering the ANS is also a right-hemisphere dominant system. Though afferents from both the semicircular canals and the otoliths project to the anterior insula and posterior operculum (which covers the insula), these vestibular cortical regions activate differently in response to these two different types of vestibular input,[40] which could help to explain why different types of vestibular input have different effects on arousal, mood, and other factors underlying self-regulation.

Vestibular pathways to the hippocampus

Four main vestibular pathways have been identified that travel to the hippocampus, with study findings by Hitier et al. demonstrating "the fundamental role of vestibular inputs in integrating different maps of the same environment in the hippocampus."[36(p. 3)] Vestibular stimulation has been shown via functional neuroimaging to activate or deactivate the hippocampus and parahippocampal areas in humans.[36,41–46] What if we could devise a vestibular treatment that would help process traumatic memories through the hippocampus? Wouldn't that be something?

Lending support to this idea are studies that show an increase in REM sleep or certain REM sleep variables following vestibular stimulation.[47,48] REM sleep has been hypothesized to reflect the process of memory consolidation. For example, based on the results of their own (non-vestibular related) sleep study, Rauchs and colleagues suggested that "consolidation of truly episodic memories mainly involves REM sleep,"[49(p. 395)] though there is some debate in this area.[50] Pace-Schott et al.[51] pointed out that it often takes several months for the PTSD symptoms to fully develop and that during this time period insomnia, nightmares, and fragmented REM sleep are common and additionally predict the later development of PTSD symptoms. These researchers hypothesized a causal relationship between sleep disturbances and the full development of PTSD. Given all of the above, it would be highly worthwhile to investigate the effects of carefully designed vestibular stimulation on sleep and hippocampal memory consolidation with trauma survivors.

Vestibular pathways to the thalamus

At least four vestibular pathways project to the thalamus, and each vestibular nucleus projects to at least several thalamic nuclei.[36] First order relay thalamic nuclei receive only vestibular information, whereas second order relay thalamic nuclei receive multimodal information including somatosensory and visual inputs.[36] Many vestibular nerve fibers synapse on the same ventral posterior thalamic nuclei that receive information from the spinothalamic and dorsal column–medial lemniscal pathways, where much of the intermodal tactile, proprioceptive, and vestibular processing takes place,[52] though it also takes place in the inferior parietal lobe and insula.[34] Additionally, there is a strong interplay between proprioceptors and vestibular inputs in the vestibular nuclear complex in the brainstem and cerebellum.[53] In fact, the proprioceptive input generated from neck movements strongly attenuates the vestibular response from such movements[53] (otherwise, we would get dizzy every time we moved our head). Thus slow, rhythmic movements of the head are not invited into the "slow, rhythmic movement" club of

Guideline 3
Yoga can promote effective sensory, motor, and cognitive processing of traumatic experiences and thus aid healing

treatment strategies since we want the stimuli to reach the thalamus and higher brain centers, not get cancelled out at the lower levels.

Vestibular pathways to the cerebellum

The vestibular system also works in close coordination with the cerebellum to control postural adjustments and maintain balance (Gray, n.d.). The cerebellum encodes head and body signals to enable postural control and also sends ascending projections to—you guessed it—the posterolateral ventral nucleus of the thalamus,[54] where, not to sound like a broken record, much of the intermodal somatosensory information is integrated. Llinas and Negrello[55] explained that with regard to motion, the forebrain generates the strategies (the what, where, and when), while the cerebellum deals with the tactics (the how to), that relate especially to motor execution, timing, coordination, and compensation. Ayres reported that the cerebellum acts on descending pathways to "smooth and coordinate action and influence muscle tone."[7(p. 46)] She also wrote of the cerebellum, "Its close connection with the vestibular system, receiving information from and sending information back to the vestibular nuclei, requires that every reference in this book to vestibular function imply involvement of that portion of the cerebellum functioning with it, even though it is not explicitly mentioned,"[7(p. 47)] so I will "ditto" that.

The association between anxiety and dizziness

Many different theoretical models have been presented to explain the association of anxiety with dizziness and decreased balance control, which speaks to the fact that there are numerous vestibular connections throughout the central nervous system that could provide a plausible explanation. Balaban[56] described three different vestibular-limbic neural circuits, which involve different brainstem nuclei that form part of the reticular activating system (RAS). The RAS is responsible for regulating state of arousal, as well as the thalamic and cortical areas they project to. The circuits are briefly summarized below:

- **Vestibulo-parabrachial network.** Cells within the *parabrachial nucleus (PBN)*, which is located in the dorsolateral pons of the brainstem, communicate information regarding whole body rotation and body position relative to gravity (linear acceleration) to neural circuits involved in anxiety responses. These neural circuits include the *amygdala*, the *hypothalamus*, and a region in the *ventromedial prefrontal cortex* that is responsible for the inhibition of emotional responses such as fear. In Chapter 4, we identified these structures as being among the brain structures most implicated in PTSD, so it is no surprise that so many trauma survivors have vestibular symptoms, nor that the PBN is considered a neural substrate for anxiety and panic disorders.[57] Balaban[56] theorized that the processing of body motion is likely to be context dependent since the connections between the vestibular nuclei and these higher-level structures along the PBN pathway are reciprocal.
- **Ceruleo-vestibular network.** Noradrenergic (norepinephrine-releasing) neurons in the *locus ceruleus* of the pons project to the vestibular nuclei, motor pathways, and PBN networks, which are thought to influence vestibular-related motor actions in relation to changes in alertness, vigilance, and arousal.[56]
- **Serotonergic network.** Serotonin-releasing (and other) neurons project from certain *raphe nuclei* in the brainstem to vestibular nuclei, limbic forebrain regions, and/or the spinal cord, suggesting they may help to coordinate vestibular, autonomic, and emotional responses.[56]

Balaban et al.[57] hypothesized that the locus cerulus and raphe nuclei/serotonergic network interact closely together to influence the vestibular nuclei, amygdala, and cerebral cortex including with regard

171

to "the sensorimotor, interoceptive and cognitive components of comorbid balance, migraine and anxiety signs and symptoms."[57(p. 7)]

Vestibulo-sympathetic reflexes and baroreceptors

There is also considerable research evidence showing that bodily movements in space adjust blood distribution throughout the body and that these effects are controlled by the sympathetic nervous system. These reactions are called **vestibulo-sympathetic reflexes**.[58] When blood pressure is low, the vestibulo-sympathetic responses are intensified and when blood pressure is high they are significantly diminished. The vestibulo-sympathetic reflex results from hair cell firing from either or both of the otolithic organs, which modulate muscle sympathetic nerve activity (MSNA).[59] The contributions of the vestibular system to blood pressure control are higher in an upright position.[60] The vestibulo-sympathetic reflexes are thought to interact with the baroreceptors in a complementary way to maintain homeostasis of the cardiovascular system.[58]

Baroreceptors are mechanoreceptors located in the carotid sinus and the aortic arch that respond to changes in tension in the walls of the arteries. If the blood pressure increases suddenly (such as when doing Legs Up the Wall in a yoga practice), the baroreceptors are stretched, sending impulses to the solitary nucleus in the brainstem and on to the vasomotor center in the brainstem, which inhibits sympathetic tone and increases vagal tone on the SA node of the heart. Heart rate is then slowed to reduce the pressure. Yates et al.[58] reported that vestibulo-sympathetic reflexes can be activated as soon as movements are initiated that affect blood distribution, prior to actual blood pressure changes, whereas the baroreceptors react to changes in blood pressure as soon as they occur but not prior. Arterial baroreflex control over muscle sympathetic nerve activity is continuous and dynamic throughout movement, changing to meet the intensity of exercise.[61] Except indirectly through the baroreceptors, the parasympathetic nervous system itself does not have a "reflexive" relationship with the vestibular system, as does the SNS, though regular dynamic exercise c1an increase vagal tone.[62] Notably, slow breathing (six breaths/min) was found to improve baroreceptor sensitivity and reduce blood pressure in people who have hypertension.[63]

The link between rocking and relaxation

It has been intuitively understood across thousands of years and different world cultures that rocking movements can produce a relaxation response and even lull people of all ages to sleep, from infants in the cradle to elderly folks in rocking chairs; yet, surprisingly, there remains a lack of high quality empirical evidence to establish rhythmic input as relaxing.[64,65] There are also so many different variables that can be manipulated with regard to vestibular stimulation that it is impossible to make a blanket statement that "linear" or "rotary" stimulation is calming or excitatory to the nervous system. We will begin to try to tease out some of the issues here, but to do so we first need to identify the types of movement input we are talking about:

- There are *three pure planes of linear (aka translational) movement*: **heave** (up and down), **sway** (side to side), and **surge** (forward and backwards), but the otoliths are also stimulated by any combination of these movements.

- There are *three pure planes of rotary movement*: **pitch** (i.e. rotating about the lateral horizontal axis, such as occurs when shaking the head "yes"); **yaw** (i.e. rotating about the vertical axis, such as occurs when shaking the head "no"); and **roll** (i.e. rotating about the longitudinal horizontal axis, such as occurs with ear down tilt). Again, there are numerous combinations of these movements that would stimulate the semicircular canals as well.

There are many movement combinations in which the otoliths and/or semicircular canals can

Guideline 3
Yoga can promote effective sensory, motor, and cognitive processing of traumatic experiences and thus aid healing

be activated. For example, slow rocking in a rocking chair or over a therapy ball is usually considered to be a linear form of movement (which is believed to inhibit the SNS and activate the PNS); however, they are also examples of pitch rotation and thus provide semicircular canal stimulation as well, which has traditionally been considered stimulating as a generic category of movements. In fact, pitch movements of the head that are produced from a natural upright posture are known to stimulate both the semicircular canals and the otoliths in a coordinated fashion.[66] This is good to know since several of the slow, rhythmic movement patterns presented in this book involve a combination of pitch rotations with surge linear movements, such as the Down Dog to Up Dog and Modified Hare to Knee-Down Up Dog flows. Also, any rotational movement of the head stimulates all of the semicircular canals to one degree or another.[66] Thus, a simplified explanation of the effects of pitch, roll, yaw, heave, surge, and sway movements is likely impossible.

Some have, though, tried to pin it down. Winter and colleagues[67] were the first to study the effects of each of these movements when passively applied using a motion simulator (hexapod) and found:

> *Yaw rotation was associated with feeling more comfortable, pitch rotation with feeling more alert and energetic, and roll rotation with feeling less comfortable. Heave translation was associated with feeling more alert, less relaxed, and less comfortable and surge translation with feeling more alert. Biomarkers were not affected. In conclusion, we provide first experimental evidence that passive rotational and translational movements may influence mood states on a short-term basis and that the quality of these psychotropic effects may depend on the plane and axis of the respective movements.*[67] *(abstract)*

First, I would like to say that due to my own training, experience, and clinical observations as an occupational therapist, there are some results I am happy with in this study and some that I am not. The comfortable feelings elicited by *yaw* rotation (horizontal rotation) support my decision to include certain rhythmic moves used in the Sensory-Enhanced Yoga program, such as the Dynamic Sidelying Twist – Upper Body Variation and Dynamic Thread the Needle. But the *pitch* results conflict with the training I received from Sensory Integration International many years ago, as well as my own experiences as an occupational therapist in which I witnessed many of my clients quickly calm in response to slow rocking in a forward-backward direction over a therapy ball.

Let's take a closer look at the study. The 23 healthy volunteers were secured in a four-point safety harness in a chair with a headrest that was mounted to the platform and the stimulations occurred in "complete darkness" (p. 2) so there could be no interference from the visual system on the effects of the vestibular input. They were rotated at .25 Hz, so it took four seconds to complete a cycle, and for the pitch rotations, they were tilted 12 degrees backwards from vertical and 12 degrees forwards from vertical, that is, 24 degrees from "peak" to "peak". Normally, rocking chairs do not displace a person forward from a vertical position, and usually, the feet are positioned on a stable, horizontal surface (i.e. the floor), not a tilting surface, while the rocking is occurring. Tilting floors and forward-tipping chairs are not typically encountered in daily life and thus I am not that surprised that the movements triggered alertness and an increased feeling of energy (both suggestive of SNS activation). As Balaban[56] noted, context likely plays a big role in how we experience vestibular input and I wonder if context may have played a big role with regard to the findings of this study.

Chapter 13

Many highly influential occupational therapists have emphasized that the most important variables to consider when presenting therapeutic vestibular stimulation are the speed, intensity, rhythmicity, and duration of the input.[7,16,68] Linear movements, usually with a rotational component, such as swings and therapy balls, have been more frequently emphasized for the purposes of calming, possibly because rhythm is more easily presented within the context of linear movements, and because movements directly over the axis of rotation have more easily produced symptoms of hypersensitivity in clients. There are exceptions, such as Rood's slow rolling technique,[68] which is simulated with dynamic Sidelying Twist – Upper Body Variation (see Chapter 17).

There are many parameters to consider when using vestibular stimulation therapeutically (see box on the right). I suspect that the parameter of vestibular input that most affects its impact on the nervous system is whether it is perceived as enjoyable or not by the person experiencing it, which depends on the context. I also suspect that Rood was right all along in thinking that the speed, intensity, and rhythm of a stimulus are among the most important variables, but we need to do more empirical testing to find out, and these should occur within the context of yoga if we want to apply the findings to yoga.

Considerations for vestibular stimulation

When designing studies or interventions utilizing vestibular stimulation, it is recommended that you consider:

- speed, amplitude, rhythm, and plane/axis
- whether the movement is actively or passively generated
- the specific muscles that are producing the movements (if active)
- whether the head is rotating directly over the axis of movement or is orbiting at some distance from the axis
- the orientation of the head during the movement
- the orientation of the arc of movement in relation to the center of gravity
- whether the motion device (if any) is stabilized from below vs suspended from above, which affects the quality of motion
- stability of the feet or other supporting body parts and their angle in relation to the surface of the earth
- most important of all, *context*.
- Among the context variables are one's sense of safety and groundedness and the expectation of either a pleasurable or an unpleasant experience.

The effects of movement on respiration

The effects of vestibular input on PTSD-associated health conditions

Hypertension and cardiovascular disease

Higher rates of hypertension and cardiovascular disease have been found in PTSD populations.[69–71] Also, a recent study by Morris and colleagues[71] found a significant association between increased heart rate in the early aftermath of trauma and subsequent PTSD symptoms, suggesting that a high heart rate poses a risk factor for the condition. Since yoga[72] and vestibular stimulation[73] have separately been found to benefit the cardiovascular system, it would be highly worthwhile to conduct research to determine if therapeutic vestibular stimulation imbedded *within* yoga accentuates these effects and whether that, in turn, affects PTSD symptomology. Lending support for this hypothesis is the fact that brainstem areas that regulate cardiovascular functions receive both direct and

Guideline 3
Yoga can promote effective sensory, motor, and cognitive processing of traumatic experiences and thus aid healing

indirect inputs from the vestibular nuclei,[58] which in turn project to higher brain centers that are implicated in PTSD,[56] as mentioned earlier.

Insomnia

The medial vestibular nucleus is connected to brain areas associated with sleep, arousal, and homeostasis.[74] Reciprocal projections between the medial vestibular nucleus and hypocretin neuropeptides (formed in the hypothalamus) have been found, strongly suggesting a relationship with the sleep–wake cycle.[64,74] Indeed, Krystal and colleagues[48] found that vestibular stimulation via TENS-type electrodes placed over the mastoid processes shortened the amount of time it took to fall asleep in those who had an average sleep onset latency of ≥ 14 minutes.

A natural vestibular stimulation study conducted by Bayer and colleagues[75] also supports a connection with the sleep–wake cycle. They assigned 12 adult males two 45-minute midday naps on a rocking bed, once while it produced slow lateral rocking motions and once while it was stationary, and found that the vestibular stimulation facilitated transition from wake to sleep and also increased the duration of stage N2 sleep. The stimulation also resulted in a sustained increase of slow brain wave oscillations and spindle activity. Bayer and colleagues[75] believe their results are most likely due to somatosensory and vestibular inputs to the thalamic nuclei, which could affect neuronal synchronization within thalamo-cortical networks.

A modified replication of Bayer et al.'s study by Omlin and colleagues[76] did not show similar improvements in sleep onset; however, they believe this was because their participants were already good sleepers and the study was conducted at night. In contrast, many of the military personnel enrolled in the Iraq Yoga Study were sleep deprived and demonstrated significant sleep improvements following participation in the yoga protocol, which included slow, active rhythmic movements as one of several therapeutic sensory modalities. Additional research is needed to identify the contribution of vestibular input to the positive effects experienced by the participants.

Chronic subjective dizziness

Indovina and colleagues found that sound-evoked short-tone burst vestibular input resulted in significantly less activation of the hippocampus, ACC, and anterior insula in patients with chronic subjective dizziness (CSD) as compared to healthy controls, which these researchers pointed out are the same areas shown to be hypoactivated during trauma-related re-experiencing symptoms in those who have chronic PTSD.[77-80] As the hippocampus, ACC, and anterior insula are richly innervated by vestibular nerve fibers, and are hypoactivated in both chronic PTSD and CSD, this raises the question as to whether a similar form of therapeutic vestibular stimulation may benefit both conditions. If the above brain areas are hypoactive in PTSD (and possibly CSD) ***due to hyperactivation of the amygdala*** (according to the neurocircuitry model of PTSD; see Chapter 4), then theoretically inhibitory rather than facilitatory vestibular techniques should be used to inhibit the amygdala, which may in turn help to rebalance the relationship between the amygdala and these higher brain structures. However, this is 100% conjecture and studies are needed.

Substance abuse

A study was recently conducted by Cross et al.[81] to determine how adding vestibular stimulation via use of a rocking chair compared with treatment as usual for homeless veterans undergoing treatment for substance use disorder. The results showed that veterans who scored highest on the Expectancy Scale of the Alcohol Craving Questionnaire (ACQ) rocked more, presumably to self soothe, and also found that greater time rocking was associated with fewer urges and desires connected with the intent and plan to drink, as revealed by results on the Purposefulness Scale of the ACQ. They conclude that rocking in a rocking chair may improve the ability to self-regulate mood and cravings for alcohol and thus potentially reduce the risk of relapse and chronic homelessness.

The effects of natural, active vestibular input on stress reduction

While a mountain of basic research has been conducted on the effects of vestibular stimulation on the nervous and cardiovascular systems, mostly with animals, there are far fewer published studies to my knowledge that have investigated the use of natural vestibular stimulation for stress reduction in humans, and it is very rare to find a study that investigated the effects of *active* vestibular stimulation on stress reduction. Many of these studies were conducted quite recently at the Little Flower Institute in India. At this Institute, K. S. Sailesh and his colleagues have performed over a dozen studies investigating the effects of natural vestibular stimulation, i.e. active swinging on a standard playground-type swing, on various physiological functions and conditions, including stress and cardiovascular parameters,[73] insomnia,[82] hypothyroidism,[83] psychoneuroimmuno modulation,[84] and depression in underweight women.[85]

All of these studies produced positive findings, but to highlight just one,[73] 240 healthy college students were randomized to four groups: 60 males/stimulation group; 60 females/stimulation group; 60 males/control group, and 60 females/control group. The participants consented to swing on a swing in a back to front direction, according to their level of comfort, following standardized methods. A comparison of pre- and post-tests found that cortisol, stress score, pulse rate, systolic, diastolic, and mean blood pressure were significantly lowered in the male and female vestibular intervention groups following vestibular stimulation and remained within normal limits. The researchers reported that their findings are consistent with prior study results suggesting that the vestibular system causes the release of GABA from the substantia nigra and also activates hippocampal neurons, thereby inhibiting the HPA axis.[73,86,87]

A word on vestibular remediation

Exercise-based approaches have also long been used successfully to enable the central nervous system to compensate for vestibular deficits.[88,89] Some of these exercises resemble common yoga movements, including a few of the famous Cawthorne-Cooksey exercises which were first published over 70 years ago and are still popular today.[90] Examples include performing head movements (independent of eye movements), performing shoulder shrugs and shoulder circles, forward bending activities, and performing movement transitions from sitting to standing and vice versa. While these exercises start out slow and are perhaps relaxing, they are gradually increased in speed in an effort to stimulate a habituation effect in the central nervous system. In contrast, the slow, dynamic yoga movements provided in this chapter are expressly designed to rebalance the ANS toward increased parasympathetic activation and thus remain slow and rhythmical. In this book, we provide a few suggestions to compensate for vestibular hypersensitivity, but do not address remediation.

Other considerations for practice

Below I share some information learned from the courses completed for the **Sensory Integration and Praxis Tests** certification (Boston, 1995), which included a course on sensory integration intervention, and suggest how this information may be applied within yoga.

- **Slow, rhythmical movements** such as rocking in a rocking chair or hammock tend to be very calming due especially to the influence of the otoliths on the reticular activating system (RAS).

Guideline 3
Yoga can promote effective sensory, motor, and cognitive processing of traumatic experiences and thus aid healing

The movements presented in the sample slow and rhythmic flows section (p. 178) are designed to simulate these activities to bias the ANS toward parasympathetic activation; however, watch for individual reactions, especially vestibular sensitivity.

- The otoliths can influence the RAS in either direction. For example, jumping on a trampoline or bouncing on a therapy ball can be very arousing to the nervous system. In yoga, this movement can be simulated by jumping from one asana to another as is common in a power yoga class. We avoid jumping in Sensory-Enhanced Yoga classes due to its arousing effects.
- The very calming effects of slow *passive* rhythmical movement may last from two to six hours.[91,92] The duration of effects from active rhythmical yoga movements is not yet known.
- Prone rocking on a therapy ball is often used in neurorehabilitation to decrease ANS arousal. Supine rocking on a therapy ball often produces the opposite reaction and is to be avoided with individuals who have PTSD. It stimulates protective extension responses and stimulates the ANS (i.e. is arousing). For these same reasons, backbends in yoga tend to be very alerting (so we only use gentle ones with the head upright), while dynamic forward folds tend to be calming.
- Forward inversions tend to be calming (e.g. Standing Forward Fold, Downward-Facing Dog). Down Dog is less apt to elicit dizziness than a Standing Forward Fold due to the grounding of both hands and feet (proprioceptive input helps to modulate vestibular input).
- The traditional treatment for vestibular hypersensitivity in the sensory integration field is to combine proprioceptive activities, that is, heavy muscle work, with linear (especially forward/backward) movement activities. Combining active, heavy muscle work with movement through space helps the nervous system modulate vestibular sensations, whereas passive movement (such as being swung or spun) is much more apt to cause dizziness or nausea

Rotary stimulation

- Do not attempt to treat trauma survivors with rotary stimulation. This means even being cautious with standing rotations from side to side (e.g. "empty coat sleeves", with arms loosely swinging), which can stimulate dizziness, anxiety, and disorientation. Rotary stimulation has been shown to induce a vestibular-evoked stress response expressed by increased ACTH, noradrenaline, and adrenaline while caloric stimulation of the semicircular canals (which simulates rotary stimulation) has been shown to increase cortisol levels and reduce serum levels of GABA, glutamate, and glycine (Saman, Bamiou, Gleeson, and Dutia, 2012, citing Kohl, 1985 and Dagilas et al., 2005, respectively).[93-95]
- Using EEG, Gale et al.[96] found that both transient and constant-velocity passive whole body yaw rotations were associated with a significant suppression of alpha power (8–13 Hz) bilaterally localized over the temporo-parietal scalp regions, which they suggested reflects cortical vestibular processing. Chapter 4 mentioned that alpha power has been associated with neural inhibitory mechanisms (Clancy et al.'s Sensory Hypothesis of PTSD). Findings from studies cited by Benedek and colleagues as well as their own study have shown that alpha power increases in the right parietal cortex when bottom-up processing of environmental stimuli is inhibited, in order to enable focused attention on internal thought processes.[97] Thus, it is not surprising that horizontal rotation **decreases** alpha power in this region due to the intensity of sensory input that is being processed. One can surmise that not a lot of concentrated thinking is going on when a person

Chapter 13

is spinning in circles. These EEG studies together may partially explain why rotary vestibular stimulation has been observed to be an excitatory rather than calming therapeutic technique.

Sample slow and rhythmic flows

The key is to make sure the flow is in fact *slow* and *rhythmical*. It is important not to pause at the end ranges but instead to smoothly "swing" back and forth. A suggested pace is 7–10 times per minute (inhaling in one direction and exhaling in the other), depending upon the amount of exertion the activity demands. For example, Down Dog to Up Dog flow is much more physically demanding than the dynamic Sidelying Twist – Upper Body Variation and thus requires a greater rate of respiration to support cardiovascular requirements. This pace is somewhat faster than the *ideal resting* rate of 5–6 breaths per minute proposed by Brown and Gerbarg,[98] yet is still slower than the *average resting* breathing rate of 12–20 breaths per minute (according to the Cleveland Clinic), and is within the guidelines (6–10 breaths per minute) suggested by Russo and colleagues to produce the PNS effects, as discussed in this chapter.

At the suggested pace of 7–10 breaths/movement cycles per minute, the movement is hypothesized to:

- provide sufficient input to the vestibular receptors to be adequately registered and produce a calming response
- increase tidal volume/depth of breathing to compensate for the decreased respiratory rate which will enhance the PNS effects as well as improve ventilation.

Cautions:

- Do not concern yourself with breath rate until after you have mastered diaphragmatic breathing.
- Once diaphragmatic breathing is mastered, start at the breathing rate that comes most naturally to you when you perform the movements and very gradually reduce the rate with practice.
- Only perform these movements at the 7–10 breath per minute rate if it comes easily for you without causing stress or discomfort.
- My suggestion is not to go below 7 breaths per minute with moderate movement or 10 breaths with intense movement (e.g. Down Dog to Up Dog).
- The reader is advised that these claims have yet to be empirically studied within the context of slow rhythmic yoga movements and are based on analyzing relevant studies and on personal experimentation and observations of students.

Try combining two or more flows together in the same plane of movement to achieve an optimal duration of approximately three consecutive minutes. Following are examples (see Chapter 17 for descriptions).

Performed sitting in a chair

- Cat-Cow (chair version)
- Setting Sun (Sun Breath to Forward Fold; place hands on thighs during forward fold to protect lower back, lifting tailbone as you fold)
- Dynamic Knee to Chest to Extended Leg
- Dynamic Cat-Cobra (chair version)
- Dynamic Thread the Needle in Chair
- Sun Breath Twists

Performed on a mat

- Cat-Cow
- Tiger Flow
- Hare (*crown of head close to floor*) to Knee-Down Up Dog
- Down Dog to Up Dog
- Dynamic Sidelying Twist – Upper Body Variation
- Dynamic Vajrasana (Extended Kneeling to Child)

Guideline 3
Yoga can promote effective sensory, motor, and cognitive processing of traumatic experiences and thus aid healing

- Sitting Dynamic Head to Knee
- Dynamic Pyramid (Standing) (*not shown in this book*)
- Dynamic Warrior I

Neutral warmth

Neutral warmth is a technique that works by affecting the temperature receptors in the hypothalamus and parasympathetic nervous system. It refers to maintaining body heat by wrapping the body (or body part to be relaxed) with a cotton flannel or fleece blanket or a down comforter. In therapeutic settings, it is used for 10–20 minutes. Neutral heat is heat no greater than body temperature so as to avoid a rebound effect in 2–3 hours.[99-101] Dougherty explained the connection between warmth and the parasympathetic nervous system:[102]

> *Activation of warm-sensitive neurons results in an activation of neurons in the paraventricular nucleus (PVN) and lateral hypothalamus that result in heightened parasympathetic outflow to promote the dissipation of heat.*

Placing a Mexican blanket on yoga participants during final relaxation is an example of using neutral warmth to calm, but there are other times during yoga practice when draping a blanket over one's body may be therapeutically beneficial, such as when performing seated warm-ups or reclined yoga forms. As mentioned in Chapter 12, a blanket can also help to reduce a sense of vulnerability during certain yoga forms for individuals who have experienced sexual trauma.

Some general effects of posture families are listed in the box on the right. You may also find Appendix B, Sensory qualities of selected yoga forms and rhythmic flows, helpful in applying the information learned in Guideline 3.

Some general effects of posture families

1. **Forward bends.** Tend to be calming to the nervous system and are traditionally recommended for anxiety or stress relief, but be careful how you present them to reduce the risk of eliciting dizziness in those trauma survivors who exhibit vestibular hypersensitivity. A standing *half*-forward fold with hands on a chair seat or on the thighs and head kept above hip level is better tolerated for some people than a full forward fold. Supporting the crown of the head on a tall block during a forward fold also helps to modulate vestibular sensations.

2. **Backward bends.** Tend to be energizing and are often recommended to treat depression. However, they can stimulate ANS arousal and should be presented in a carefully thought-out manner with those who have PTSD. Positioning the head behind the center of gravity (such as in Camel) is likely to increase hyperarousal so it is best to choose backbends that maintain the head in a more vertical position, such as Cobra or Upward-Facing Dog. Also, when heart-opening (chest-expanding) yoga forms are presented, they should ideally be well grounded; thus, Cobra is an ideal choice due to the increased contact with the earth.

3. **Twists.** Are very calming in general. They help to release stress in the gut, which is considered to be the "2nd brain" as it is controlled by the vagus nerve. Eighty percent of the vagal nerve fibers are afferent and are considered to have a significant influence on emotional well-being. The closer to the ground and the more supportive the twist form is, the more calming the effects are. Conversely, the more balance or effort that is required in a twist, the less they will produce a calming effect; in fact, a revolved standing twist will likely increase hyperarousal.

Chapter 13

4. **Lateral bends.** Due to their asymmetry, lateral bends may be more difficult for those who have decreased body awareness and motor planning ability. Therefore, you may need to assist (preferably verbally unless trust has been developed). Also, some lateral bends (such as Triangle) position the head in extreme positions away from the center of gravity, which may elicit dizziness in those susceptible to this symptom. This effect can be mitigated by providing strong muscle input and/or by reducing the balance demands, for example, by coming into Triangle via Extended Side Angle (when ready for Triangle).

5. **Balance forms.** Promote sensory integration on many levels and are especially powerful for helping to improve focus, bringing the mind back to the present moment. However, relatively gentle balance forms with the head upright and in midline (such as Tree or Eagle), or which are low to the ground and carry a minimal risk of injury (such as Spinal Balance), are more therapeutic for PTSD than forms that would more strongly stimulate the sympathetic/fight–flight nervous system, such as Crow.

6. **Proceed with caution.** Wide-legged yoga forms can make some individuals with PTSD feel very vulnerable, especially those who have suffered from sexual abuse. Consider who is in your yoga session before you present these forms. Standing wide-legged forms tend to be perceived as less threatening than reclined wide-legged forms. If you choose to present Bound Angle, for example, it is best to also present an alternative yoga form ("or you can choose to do this …") (see Chapter 12 for full discussion).

Guideline 4
New beliefs and attitudes more easily take hold when we first prepare the body to receive and accept them

Without this awareness of bodily feeling and attitude, a person becomes split into a disembodied spirit and a disenchanted body. — Alexander Lowen[1(p. 2)]

We intuitively gauge a person's emotions not only from their words and facial expressions, but also from their posture and movements. Thus, on some level we all know that emotions are registered and held throughout the **body**mind, not just the mind. For example, depressed people tend to walk slower, with a more slumped posture, and demonstrate less arm swing and more lateral swaying movements of the upper body.[2] However, posture does not just *reflect* emotion, it *induces* emotion. Nair et al.[3] found that assuming an upright sitting posture can reduce fear, increase self-esteem, and cause a person to feel more enthusiastic, excited, and/or strong, whereas a slumped posture can cause a person to feel more fearful, hostile, nervous, dull, passive, quiet, sleepy, and/or sluggish. Furthermore, a set of experiments conducted by Veenstra and colleagues[4] found that **posture can also play an important role in helping a person recover from a negative mood that has already been activated**. Thus, one may logically argue that yoga—an activity that stretches people in all sorts of ways in which typical activities do not—is well-suited to be a natural mood lifter, which in turn tends to inspire more positive attitudes and beliefs.

If linking posture to one's personal beliefs feels like a stretch, just imagine a counselor trying to help someone take a more optimistic or calmer perspective of a situation while their body is sending strong alarm signals that conflict with that. Dychtwald[5(pp. 11-12)] described in detail the many ways that emotions can become blocked and expressed in the body structure, affecting one's attitudes and beliefs. Though I personally believe he overstated the case in certain body structure presentations that have a genetic basis, there is enough deep wisdom in his book to highly recommend it for anyone doing this work, particularly yoga therapists. Dychtwald[5 (pp. 11-12)] used a quote by Ida Rolf which I will re-quote here since it perfectly underscores this fourth guideline of Sensory-Enhanced Yoga:

An individual experiencing temporary fear, grief, or anger, all too often carries his body in an attitude which the world recognizes as the outward manifestation of that particular emotion. If he persists in this dramatization or consistently re-establishes it, thus forming what is ordinarily referred to as a "habit pattern", the muscular arrangement becomes set ... Since it is not possible to establish a free flow through the physical flesh, the subjective emotional tone becomes progressively more limited and tends to remain in a restricted, closely defined area. Now what the individual feels is no longer an emotion, a response to an immediate situation, henceforth he lives, moves, and has his being in an attitude.[6 (pp. 9-10)]

Through a carefully designed yoga practice delivered within the context of a "safe container" we can help trauma survivors safely release trauma-based muscular tensions and protective holding patterns. As the bodymind comes to feel safer and freer, spaces

Chapter 14

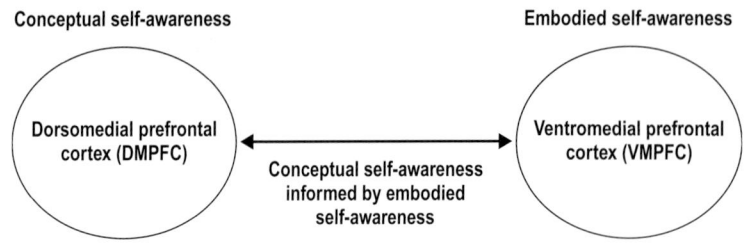

Figure 14.1

The power of language in the context of yoga (adapted with permission from Alan Fogel[7])

will open in the body in which new beliefs can begin to take hold. Alan Fogel[7] conceptualizes this beautifully from a neural standpoint in a portion of a figure in his own book, ***Body Sense*** (depicted in Figure 14.1). Of course, brain structures do not operate in isolation but rather as a component of larger systems of neuronal activation, as discussed in Part 1; however, we will limit the discussion here to these two brain structures for the sake of simplicity.

To summarize Fogel, the dorsomedial prefrontal cortex (DMPFC) is continuously active during our waking hours and is involved in our ongoing stream of thought. Among other things, it is concerned with language-based self-judgments, that is, our ***conceptual self-awareness***. In contrast, the ventromedial prefrontal cortex (VMPFC) has direct links to the body through the interoceptive and body scheme networks (including the insula) and is concerned with ***embodied self-awareness***, that is, judgments based on what we feel in our bodies. ***Conceptual self-awareness is informed by embodied self-awareness***. If we are exhibiting an anxious, tense posture or a slumped, depressed posture, the VMPFC will communicate that to the DMPFC, which then forms a conceptual thought such as "I can't handle this job" or "I will never amount to anything." Conversely, if we free up the constrictions in the body and facilitate a freer and more relaxed, grounded, and receptive body posture, the VMPFC will inform the DMPFC of the change, leading it to adjust its thoughts to align with this new felt-experience ("I've got this!" or "I am okay just as I am").[7]

Interestingly, Roy and co-workers[8] found that the vmPFC is more associated with positive emotions while the dmPFC is more associated with negative emotions, further supporting the idea that embodied self-awareness is the better place to "be." Mindfulness-based practices have also been shown to successfully address a related issue: ***ruminations and intrusive thoughts***. The pregenual anterior cingulate cortex (pgACC) has been associated with ruminative thinking in depressed individuals, who have also been shown to demonstrate increased functional connectivity between the pgACC and posterior cingulate cortex (PCC), the latter of which, like the dmPFC, is involved in self-reflection and emotional regulation.[9] Therefore, this may represent the neural correlates of excessive ruminative thinking related to self-reflection seen in people who are depressed. However, findings from a recent study by Yang et al.[9] in which 13 novices received 40 days of training in mindfulness-based stress reduction (MBSR) revealed decreased functional connectivity of the pgACC (presumably less rumination) with both the PCC and the dmPFC following the training, showing one possible neural pathway as to how mindfulness-based practices may reduce intrusive thoughts in individuals who have PTSD.

And really, this is what Guideline 4 is speaking to: clearing out the negative ruminations, worries, and intrusive thoughts from the ***entire body***mind via the practices presented in Guidelines 1, 2, and 3, and then using the art of language to encourage more positive thoughts and attitudes to flourish after the body has

Guideline 4
New beliefs and attitudes more easily take hold when we first prepare the body to receive and accept them

been prepared to receive and accept them. This same exact process is embedded in the kosha model of the ancient yogis as one progresses from feeling *safe* (in the annamaya kosha), *calm* (in the pranamaya kosha), *clear* (in the manomaya kosha, *uplifted* (our current topic, here in the vijnanamaya kosha), and *empowered* (in the anandamaya kosha). Progress at the level of the vijnanamaya level/Guideline 4 is also measured by the ability to assume a "*witness mentality,*" that is, the ability to emotionally detach from emotive and sensory events in a conscious and mindful way and simply notice them with equanimity and without getting engulfed by them, such as when attending to the breath, following a body scan, or holding a yoga form. The concept of a "witness mentality" is explicitly taught in Sensory-Enhanced Yoga classes. Other practices are discussed below.

Positive suggestions and affirmations

The **Sensory-Enhanced Yoga** method advocates the use of posture-inspired positive suggestions and self-chosen affirmations to enhance the healing power of yoga. These techniques help to counteract negative thought patterns that can result from traumatic experiences, and open the mind-body to more positive beliefs, attitudes, and emotions. They tend to be much more powerful when presented within the context of yoga, since, as we have just learned, how we feel in our bodies has a huge influence on how we conceptualize who we are.

Positive suggestions include statements made by the yoga instructor to draw the student's awareness to the emotional effects that tend to be naturally elicited by a particular yoga form or movement. For example, many yoga forms may naturally encourage a sense of emotional "grounding" due to the enhanced physical grounding they provide. These include forms where the energy moves downward into the earth (e.g. Downward-Facing Dog), the feet are encouraged to root solidly into the floor (e.g. Mountain and other standing forms), and/or there is heavy activation of the leg muscles and a lowering of the center of gravity such as in the squatting postures (e.g. Chair form, Victory Squat, Knee-Down or Standard Lunge).

Other forms tend to psychologically open the heart center, particularly those that expand the chest (e.g. Triangle, Cow Face Stretch, Cobra, Warrior I variations). Some forms have a self-nurturing quality, such as when hugging the knees into the chest, or a quality of feeling supported, such as lying in Child form. Yoga forms that provide a balance challenge foster emotional steadiness, while forms that position the head off-kilter change the view, quite literally inviting the person to open their minds to a different perspective on the world. The teacher or therapist can point these things out during the yoga session, as mindfulness to these qualities may accentuate these effects.

However, not everyone will feel the effects, especially if they are experiencing mental distress. So we try to word the suggestions not by implying that they feel these qualities (which may backfire) but rather as an invitation to draw the quality into their bodymind. Alternatively, asking students to *inhale* a quality is an innocuous way to invite it into the bodymind as you are not suggesting it is already present in the person but rather something outside of them being invited in, and better yet, being invited in on the power of the breath. Inviting the quality in on the thread of the breath may possibly enhance integration of sensation and emotion, since all three—sensation, emotion, and breath—are integrated in the insula.

A few examples of positive suggestions are listed below; typically a few are presented per class.

Knee(s) to Chest (hugging knees)

For the beginning of class: "This tends to be a self-nurturing yoga form. Can you invite some self-compassion into your practice today?"

Chapter 14

This is a good segue to remind students to listen to the messages of their bodies and minds during practice and make any adjustments as necessary, or even to get out of a yoga form or breathing practice if it is uncomfortable, and also to remind students that the goal of yoga is to enhance their own health and well-being and not to compete with others in the room.

For the end of class: "If you like, you might draw your knee(s) into your chest and give yourself a hug, thanking your body for everything it has done for you today." — *Thanks to Sadie Crane.*

Dynamic Cat to Cobra (in chair): "As you exhale into Cat, you might invite tension to roll off your back, and as you inhale into Cobra, invite self-compassion to flow into the increased spaciousness around the heart center." — *Thanks to Meaghan Tweedie.*

Spinal Balance: "Inhale steadiness and confidence into the very core of your being."

Thread the Needle (Table Twist): "Welcome the different point of view and notice how this affects your bodymind." — *Double meaning.*

Downward-Facing Dog: "Sense your connection to the earth through the palms of your hands and the soles of your feet." — *Simply drawing awareness to the literal contact with the earth may promote a psychological sense of grounding.*

Down Dog to Up Dog Flow (or Hare to Knee-Down Up Dog Flow): "What happens when you release the effort and resistance and just "go with the flow?" — *Double meaning.*

Child: "Rest in the center of your being, releasing all tension and effort."

"Breathe in, rest your eyes, and allow yourself to sink downward into the support of the earth." — *Thanks to Kate O'Donnell.*

Mountain: "Can you stand strong while keeping your heart soft, using the breath?" — *Discriminating two positive yet somewhat opposite qualities in the bodymind.*

Or simply: "Strong spine, soft heart." — *Short and sweet suggestions work, too.*

Victory Squat: "Sense the strength of your legs firmly planting you on the earth." — *This yoga form requires strong engagement of the leg muscles which can help a person to better sense their legs and, in turn, their contact with the ground.*

Chair: "From a grounded base, invite your heart to soar toward the sky. Feel your energy flow up from your strong connection to the earth."

Cow Face, Triangle, Warrior I — bent arm variation or with Vajrapradama Mudra, or another chest expander: "With the expansion of the ribcage, you may sense increased spaciousness around the heart center. If it feels right for you, you might focus your breath right into the heart space, and with each exhalation, imagine it radiating in all directions."

Warrior I or Lunge with Arms Extended: "Warrior I [or Lunge] tends to elicit different qualities in different people … you may notice a sense of grounding … or balance … or perhaps a sense of receptivity as you reach up toward the sky … connect with sensation … what quality or feeling does this yoga form most draw out for you?"

"This yoga form tends to elicit a sense of receptivity … You might consider if there a personal quality you would like to receive and, if you like, invite it into your being with each breath."

Warrior II: "Warrior II can be very helpful for drawing a sense of strength and power into the mind and body. Is there a place in your own body where you feel strong in this yoga form? Even if only in a single

Guideline 4
New beliefs and attitudes more easily take hold when we first prepare the body to receive and accept them

muscle, you might try directing your breath to that area and notice how that affects your experience."

"The more we claim our power, the easier it is to move beyond our perceived limitations."

"Sense your connection to the Earth through the strength of your legs and know that in whatever direction you head, you always have the solid earth beneath your feet to support you every step of the way."

"If you like, you may choose to repeat to yourself: 'I choose today to take a few moments to be a Warrior ... I feel_____' and fill in the blank" — *Thanks to Tracey Champagne, who uses it with survivors of domestic violence.*

Dynamic Standing Side Angle to Reverse Warrior: "Notice how the strength of your legs supports the flexibility and movement of your upper body to change your point of view." — *Thanks to Nicole Cipriani.*

Standing Forward Fold: "Imagine releasing all tension, worries, and burdens to the floor."

Coming up from Wide-Legged Forward Fold into Five-Pointed Star: "Coming into your Star, you might choose to shine your heart forward, opening it to new opportunities and possibilities from the universe." — *Thanks to Sadie Crane, who uses it with the recovery population.*

Tree: "Welcome the sway—it is an essential part of the process of moving into balance, both in mind and body."

Seated or Reclined Twist: "You might imagine squeezing out all tension and worries."

"When you meet resistance, pause and breathe ... soon you will find space to continue your movement forward, even if just a tiny bit ... As on the mat, so in life ... when you find resistance, pause and breathe ..."

Legs up the Wall (or other inversion): "Invite deep healing to flow into your heart."

Generic (for any yoga form):

"Notice sensation."

"Can you step back to witness the sensations without getting engulfed by them?"

"Find a balance between effort and ease" — *Thanks to Lindsay Thelin Wagner.*

"Can you find the ease in the flow?"

"You may find it helpful to focus on the thread of your breath."

"You might try sending your breath into the knots of tension, inviting them to soften and release with each exhalation."

"If you like, try breathing into [the space between your shoulder blades, your left ribcage, your right hip joint, your lower back, etc.] and notice the effects." — *The breath actually reaches most of the areas listed here, but even when it doesn't, imagining it can sometimes produce a strong visceral sensation of it happening, likely via the insula.*

"Let your own experience be your guide." — *Learning self-trust.*

"You are free to make your own choices and decisions in your practice."

"Notice the tone of your emotional self as you assume this yoga form. If you feel you could benefit from feeling a bit more _____ [uplifted, grounded, balanced, etc.], you might try ____ [suggest a modification]."

"If you like, you might _____. How does that feel?"

Chapter 14

Self-chosen positive affirmations are commonly used in cognitive therapy, and consist of repeating positive statements, either to oneself or out loud, to counteract negative thinking patterns and drive one toward more positive thoughts and experiences. Pairing affirmations with specific asanas that embody their essence brings the power of the thought not only into the mind but also into the body, where trauma (and often negativity) is stored. If you decide to incorporate affirmations into a therapeutic yoga practice, it is recommended that a student-directed approach be used. One particularly effective method for using affirmations in the context of yoga is to ask the student (or group) what quality a particular asana suggests to them in their felt body sense and invite them to create an affirmation that incorporates this quality. Several possible qualities could be suggested to help with the process, such as described in the Warrior I example in the above list. Encourage the student(s) to focus on sensation during the yoga form so the affirmation will arise naturally from their "feeling" state rather than "thinking" mind. Inviting the person to create their own personalized affirmation based on a positive "felt experience" that a yoga form is already drawing into consciousness is quite possibly the safest and most effective way to introduce an affirmation.

In contrast, a recent study found that positive affirmations that are imposed upon people may backfire for individuals who have low self-esteem, causing the person who recites them to feel worse.[10] However, they only tested one affirmation, "I am a lovable person," which is a sweeping, emotionally loaded statement, and was imposed on the test subjects. To explain their findings, the study authors surmised that the subconscious mind might argue with the conscious mind, which is directing the affirmation, creating internal conflict. They also speculated that the "backfiring" would be more likely to happen with global statements such as "I am a generous person," versus moderately positive statements that are more specific, such as "I give generous gifts," to use their own example.

Wood and colleagues found that allowing or even encouraging the person to experience disconfirming thoughts along with the affirmative thoughts, rather than fighting the contradicting thoughts, diminished the potentially harmful effect of the positive affirmations for those with low self-esteem. This finding occurred when they suggested the participants focus on ways the statement was true of them and/or was not true of them, which may have communicated to them that such thoughts were to be expected. This draws to mind certain yoga nidra practices, such as iRest®, which work with the concept of opposite emotions and opposite beliefs as a therapeutic strategy with documented success.[11] However, with iRest, the student chooses the emotion or thought they wish to work with (giving them the locus of control) and the "opposites" are experienced using a body sensing rather than an analytical approach, which helps to re-link bodily sensation and emotion to support a healthy mind–body connection.

The Sensory-Enhanced Yoga program is careful to avoid sweeping statements when presenting positive suggestions or affirmations. For instance, you will notice the positive suggestion for Knees to Chest is presented as a gentle invitation to connect with a "feeling state" just for the present moment and within the context of a specific activity: "This tends to be a self-nurturing yoga form. Can you invite some self-compassion into your practice today?" This is a far cry from asking the person to globally state "I am filled with self-compassion," to which declaration disconfirming examples may leap to mind. Similarly, emotionally laden statements such as "I forgive myself," which have actually been used in some veteran yoga classes, are not appropriate in any group yoga practice. Only a qualified mental health counselor should handle such emotionally charged issues.

In my own private yoga therapy practice, I typically invite clients to generate a personal affirmation at the end of a yoga therapy session (as taught to me in

Guideline 4
New beliefs and attitudes more easily take hold when we first prepare the body to receive and accept them

the Integrative Yoga Therapy program), and every one of them thus far has welcomed the opportunity and has experienced no difficulty generating one. By the end of a yoga therapy session, they have gone through the steps of body sensing, identifying their feeling and emotional states, and articulating the issues and goals to be addressed during the session. They have also hopefully moved closer toward achieving their stated intention for practice during the yoga therapy session itself. In many cases the affirmation that bubbles up in their bodymind is closely aligned with their intention for practice, though this is certainly not always the case.

I do steer clients away from global, emotionally charged statements that are opposite to their current felt sense. For example, if someone with depression suggests an affirmation such as "I feel happy and upbeat every moment of my life"—which is bound to backfire right out of the gate—I will often suggest one of the many excellent affirmations from ***Mudras for Healing and Transformation***,[12] which are often *process-oriented* rather than statements of an achieved "end state." For example, one suggested affirmation for depression is, "As I nourish my inner being, I experience greater enthusiasm and vitality" (permission granted by the authors), which includes an attainable plan to reach the stated goal. Worded in this manner, the affirmation is much more likely to resonate for someone at any stage of healing for depression, and be received as a very hopeful, self-empowering message by the bodymind.

Tips on creating effective positive affirmations

1. A single sentence in simple language tends to be most effective (and easy to remember!).
2. The affirmation should be stated in the first person: "*I am …*", "*I feel …*", "*I have …*" "*As I …*"
3. Use positive language, e.g. "*I open my heart to happiness*" vs "*I am no longer depressed.*"
4. Structure the affirmation in the present tense, as the subconscious mind is operating in the present moment.
5. When creating affirmations for challenging or emotionally charged issues, consider choosing "**process-oriented**" affirmations, e.g. "*Listening to my heart, I am wisely guided on my life's journey*" rather than global "**end-state**" affirmations such as "*I always take the right course of action in every situation,*" to avoid generating disconfirming messages from the mind.
6. When repeating the affirmation, draw it into your entire being using all of your senses, including the sensory input from the muscles holding the posture that embodies the essence of the statement.

Note: If you find that your "gut" disagrees with your self-chosen affirmation, allow yourself to feel as you do without trying to suppress or judge it. You might try using the sensations of the yoga form as your "inner resource" to help guide you toward a more positive viewpoint. However, if the affirmation is disturbing to you, release the affirmation and simply allow the bodily sensations of the form or movement to speak to you. Later, you may want to reframe the language, using the above tips.

Guided meditations

Guided meditations are another "top-down" approach that can be effectively used to promote healing from trauma and to promote self-regulation. They can be easily embedded into a yoga class but need to be presented within the parameters of the therapist's training and in a manner that fosters the "safe container" for the student(s). An example of a particularly effective form of guided meditation is yoga nidra, otherwise known as "yogic sleep." Yoga nidra produces a deep state of relaxation in which the physical body is asleep while the mind is awake yet at rest and more readily capable of accessing the subconscious. The iRest program, in particular, has been formally studied to

Chapter 14

document its effects on the symptoms of PTSD, with positive results.[11] Certain components of that program are commonly integrated within veteran yoga classes by instructors who have received formal training in iRest practices, particularly the body sensing, breath awareness, inner resource, heart-felt desire, and intention for practice scripts, which can be easily incorporated into a primarily asana-focused class. Please refer to the iRest website (https://www.irest.us/) for further information regarding this program.

When working with traumatized populations, it is usually best to present meditations that help to keep the person grounded in their bodies (such as through focusing on sensation and breath) rather than take them on a "trip" somewhere, such as to a beach or some other specific type of place. For one thing, the therapist does not really know if the student(s) really would enjoy a trip to that particular place. A beach scene may seem innocuous but maybe not so much to someone who fought on a beach in Vietnam, or to someone who didn't have such a good experience behind the sand dunes. Also, mental trips encourage dissociation from the body, when what we really want is to encourage re-connection with the body.

Zeidman and Maguire recently presented study findings to suggest that the anterior hippocampus constructs internal representations of environments based on incoming sensory information and/or prior experience, which is essential in order to "vividly re-experience past events, simulate future events and imagine fictitious scenarios, in addition to experiencing the environment we currently inhabit."[13 (p. 3)] As the anterior hippocampus is particularly implicated in PTSD, it is conceivable that the ability to construct internal scenes may be affected in some individuals with the condition, which should also be taken into consideration when choosing mindfulness-based strategies. That is, it may be best to avoid visual meditation scripts unless they are self-generated and within the person's ability to access.

One self-generated script that has been found to be helpful for many (though not all) traumatized individuals is the **Inner Resource** (discussed in Chapter 11). In this case, the person has full control of the scene, and it is a "go-to" place in those instances where it may not feel safe in that moment to be in the body in the present setting (such as inside an MRI machine, to use a personal example!). So it is actually a condoned form of short-term dissociation used for an adaptive purpose and in a mindful way.

Gratitude meditations are another form of meditation that has been found to be helpful among traumatized populations. Vieselmeyer and colleagues[14] conducted a self-report questionnaire study of 359 students, faculty, and staff who were present during a campus shooting and found that both "resilience and gratitude can be conceptualized as protective mechanisms, with resilience operating to prevent adverse outcomes while gratitude may promote positive outcomes following trauma" (abstract). They concluded that interventions for trauma survivors should cultivate gratitude as a way to decrease post-traumatic stress and increase post-traumatic growth. Gratitude practices have also been helpful following earthquakes[15] and substance misuse,[16] among other situations.

A gratitude meditation while in Mountain

contributed by Sadie Crane

I invite you to join me in a gratitude meditation here [in Mountain], or you may choose to focus on your own experience of Mountain ... If you are joining me, begin by sensing the strength in your legs as they carry you along this Earth, and send them your gratitude ... Then bring awareness to the area around the abdomen and send gratitude to this area as it takes in nutrients, assimilates, and lets go of what is no longer serving us ... Then draw your awareness to your heart center, where

Guideline 4
New beliefs and attitudes more easily take hold when we first prepare the body to receive and accept them

we cultivate gratitude, joy, and compassion for ourselves and others ... If you like, you may bring someone or something into that area that you are grateful for ... Next, invite in a sense of gratitude for your arms, for they allow us to hug our loved ones ... Then draw awareness to your head ... Inviting a sense of gratitude for your mouth, as it allows us to speak our truth ... For your ears, as they allow us to hear the harmony of life ... For your eyes, as they allow us to see the beauty of the world ... And finally, for your mind, which allows you to endeavor creativity.

Sadie writes, "This meditation works well with the recovery population because most still struggle with low self esteem and are uncomfortable with their changing bodies, but it may not be suitable for all populations, especially those with disabled body parts or senses."

Mudras

Mudras are amazing tools that can take a meditation practice to a whole new level. According to Joseph and Lilian Le Page, mudras are "gestures of the hands, face and body that promote physical health, psychological balance, and spiritual awakening."[12 (p. 7)] Who is not familiar with the image of a yogi sitting in Lotus meditating, using a hand mudra? Yet very few Americans understand what a mudra is for or how it may impact the bodymind.

Mudras have been used in India for approximately 2000 years as well as in other countries and religious traditions, including Christianity.[12] As I know from personal experience and from my training in the Integrative Yoga Therapy (IYT) program, mudras can have a very powerful effect on a person's breath, energy level, state of alertness, level of relaxation, mood, clarity of mind, and can facilitate higher states of meditation and well-being. However, when I was told on the first day of IYT training that we were going to learn mudras, I had a sinking feeling that I signed up for the wrong program. After all, we move our hands all the time in our daily lives, so how could simple hand gestures affect so many core qualities? I wasn't the only one in the room who was skeptical, so we experimented with several mudras without being told what effects we should feel. Sure enough the majority of the students (including me) experienced very similar and powerful effects from these mudras, particularly with regard to how they affected our breath and the breath-related movement of energy in the body.

When we position our arms, hands, and fingers in certain ways, it produces subtle shifts in posture and muscle contractions around the ribcage and other parts of the body. For example, when the tips of the **index fingers** are gently pressed together in front of the solar plexus, with the remaining fingers relaxed inward toward the body, while assuming an upright posture with shoulders relaxed and elbows held slightly away from the body, in *Tarjani* mudra, the chest expands and the breath naturally rises upward into that greater expansiveness, promoting an uplifting quality. Yet when the **little fingers** are pressed together, with all other fingers relaxed inward, in *Kanishtha* mudra, it produces a subtle postural and energetic shift which draws the breath and energy down toward the base of the body, extending the exhale and promoting a sense of grounding and calming.[12] Biomechanical postural shifts are not the only explanation or even the primary explanation for the effects of mudras, as there is a lot we still do not know about the energy systems of our bodies. The rich nerve endings of our palms and fingers, which are highly represented in the sensory homunculus of the brain, certainly play an important role.[12]

The best resource for mudras to promote self-regulation and trauma healing is ***Mudras for Healing and Transformation***. The mudras in Table 14.1 and Table 14.2 are examples taken from it. They do not

Chapter 14

constitute an exhaustive list. They have been found especially beneficial for my students and the students of other SEYI faculty who have struggled with issues of anxiety and trauma. Each mudra has different effects, which are explained in the book, so you will want to read the descriptions carefully and choose accordingly. Each person will experience the effects of some mudras more powerfully than others, and in slightly different ways, so allow your students to experience several of them to see which ones seem to work best for them.

Table 14.1 Recommended mudras for PTSD and related disorders*

	Guideline	I am:	Mudra(s)	Rationale	Affirmation
Annamaya	1. A sense of safety is essential for healing	SAFE	Adhi (11) Bhu (40) Prithivi (15)	Promotes embodiment, grounding, and sense of safety. Directs breath to the pelvic floor	"As I become more safely present in my body, I develop greater trust in myself and the world around me"
Pranamaya	2. The most direct and powerful way to self-regulate is through control of the breath	CALM	Pala (36) Dvimukham (70) Adhi (11)	Cultivates the diaphragmatic breath; relieves anxiety	"As I follow the rhythmic rise and fall of my breath, I experience a greater sense of calm and tranquility"
Pranamaya			Purna Svara (10)	Cultivates full yogic breathing; integrative on all levels	"As the wave of breath flows through my being, I sense my inherent wholeness"
Manomaya	3. Yoga can promote effective sensory, motor, and cognitive processing of traumatic experiences and thus aid healing	CLEAR	Ishvara (86) Dvimukham (70) Ushas (73) Adhi (11)	Draws the senses inward, instilling an inner silence; subtly digests accumulated thoughts and feelings	"As my senses turn inward, my mind moves toward stillness and greater clarity"
Vijnanomaya	4. New beliefs and attitudes more easily take hold when we first prepare the body to receive and accept them	UPLIFTED	Ushas (73) Chaturmukham** (80) Vajrapradama** (35) **use with grounded yoga forms; avoid if experiencing anxiety	Promotes confidence, vitality, and enthusiasm; supports the treatment of depression	"As my mind becomes more calm and clear, I more easily recognize life's infinite possibilities"
Anandamaya	5. Self-empowerment is born on the wings of the spirit rising from the mind-body connection	EMPOW-ERED	Hakini (6) Chaturmukham**(80) Purna Svara (10) **use with grounded yoga forms; avoid if experiencing anxiety	Optimizes health and healing at all levels of our being. Brings equilibrium to the L and R sides of the body	"As all facets of my being move into harmony, I step forward into life more confidently to manifest my life vision"

Mudras that are bolded are shown and described in Table 14.2. Unbolded mudras (and fuller descriptions of the bolded mudras) can be found in the source book (see footnote*)

*Columns 3 and 4 are from the second edition of Mudras for Healing and Transformation, by Joseph and Lilian Le Page © 2014. Reprinted with permission. The numbers refer to numbers in the book. The affirmations were also inspired by it.

Guideline 4
New beliefs and attitudes more easily take hold when we first prepare the body to receive and accept them

Table 14.2 A sampling of mudras for self-regulation and trauma healing*
The mudras are most effective when performed in a sitting or well-grounded standing position. With all of the mudras, it is important to state as the final step: "relax the shoulders down and away from the ears, keeping the spine naturally aligned."

ADHI (11)	BHU (40)	CHATURMUKHAM (80)
1. Curl the fingers loosely around the thumbs, forming soft fists. 2. Rest the hands face down on the thighs or knees.	1. Fully extend the middle and index fingers into a "V" position (peace sign); tuck the ring and little fingers into the palm; and place the thumbs over the tucked fingers 2. Plant the tips of the middle and index fingers firmly to the earth, out to the sides of the body, forming your upper body into a triangular mountain shape	1. Assume Hakini mudra, except: 2. Extend the thumbs straight up *This mudra is uplifting and supports the treatment of depression. Do not use if experiencing acute anxiety, as this mudra is more energizing than the others presented here*
DVIMUKHAM (70)	**HAKINI (6)**	**ISHVARA (86)**
1. Hold the hands facing upward below the navel 2. Touch the tips of the little and ring fingers to the same fingers on the opposite hand 3. Rest the hands below the navel, with the forearms against the belly or onto the lap	1. Gently touch the tips of all the fingers and thumbs to the same fingers on the opposite hand, in front of the solar plexus 2. Hold the hands open and rounded as if holding a globe 3. Keep the forearms parallel to the earth	1. Interlace the fingers to the outside with the base of the palms touching 2. Extend the little and index fingers 3. Place the thumbs alongside each other, resting them onto the index fingers 4. Rest the forearms onto the abdomen, with the extended fingers facing forward

— continued —

Chapter 14

Table 14.2 continued

PALA (36)	PRITHIVI (15)	USHAS (73)
1. Cup the hands and place the left hand with the palm upward four finger-widths below the navel 2. Place the right hand with the pam downward at the level of the navel, just above the left hand, with the hands gently touching the abdomen 3. Hold the elbows slightly away from the body	1. Touch the tips of the thumbs to the tips of the ring fingers of each hand while extending the other fingers straight out 2. Rest the backs of the hands on the thighs or knees	1. Interlace the fingers loosely and rest the hands on the lap, with the palms upward 2. The tips of the thumbs may lightly touch each other

*These mudras are from *Mudras for Healing and Transformation*, by Joseph and Lilian Le Page (2014) which provides two full pages of information for each (including a guided meditation) plus 98 additional mudras. This brief version of the mudras is presented here with the authors' permission, but advanced training is highly recommended. Learn more at https://www.iytyogatherapy.com/

**The numbers refer to the numbered mudras in the book, *Mudras for Healing and Transformation*.

***The mudras are meant to be performed by both hands, but can be done with one in the case of mobility issues.

Guideline 5
Self-empowerment is born on the wings of the spirit rising from the mind-body connection

To lose our connection with the body is to become spiritually homeless. Without an anchor we float aimlessly, battered by the winds and waves of life. — Anodea Judith[1(p. 54)]

You will know how to act when you know who you are. — Stephen Cope[2(p. 208)]

Oftentimes people walk out of a yoga class with a freer body, a clearer mind, and in higher spirits. Whereas before class they may have been debating whether to go to yoga class or fix themselves a bowl of Ben and Jerry's and sit in front of the TV, after class they are making a beeline to the Whole Foods store for a spinach salad. They feel healthy and want to keep that good feeling going. And most importantly, they have more trust in themselves that they can. They feel empowered. This "yoga effect" can be particularly therapeutic for those who have been traumatized and lost their sense of agency in the world. As explained by Ritu Sharma, "When people experience trauma, they may experience not only a sense of emotional disregulation, but also a feeling of being physically immobilized. Body-oriented techniques such as yoga help them increase awareness of sensations in the body, stay more focused on the present moment and hopefully empower them to take effective actions."[3]

David Emerson uses the term "empowerment" in the context of yoga to describe "giving our clients the space to have their own experiences without anything being imposed from the outside—namely, your experience or your ideas about what an experience within a yoga form might or should be."[4(p. 21)] So this brings us squarely back to Guideline 1, the importance of providing a sense of safety for our students by, among other considerations, giving them choices and thus a sense of control over their own process of yoga. When we place the locus of control on our students for their own experiences, they literally operate on their own power on the mat. For true healing transformation to occur, however, it is necessary to help the student take their power off the mat and into the world and their daily lives, and this is what Guideline 5 is all about.

In this book we have focused on states of trauma, i.e. **distress**, but there is a positive type of stress, referred to as **eustress**, that is essential in fostering a sense of empowerment. Though the concept of eustress as introduced by Hans Selye[5] is familiar to most people who have studied psychology, Kupriyanov and Zhdanov[6] recently pointed out that it has been insufficiently explored, which they attributed to a lack of defining criteria to distinguish it from other forms of stress. After a careful review of the topic, they proposed that, "Distress is a type of stress that leads to deterioration of the adaptive capabilities of the organism and eustress is a stress that initiates an increase in adaptive capabilities."[6(p. 181)] They further explained: [6(p. 181)]

Chapter 15

Adaptation and stress phenomena have a causal relationship wherein the onset of stress initiates adaptation. The evolutionary history of all life forms may be treated as a history of organisms combating stressors, thus bringing about destruction (distress) and gains (eustress). When using the term "eustress", we want to emphasize the positive, constructive value of the stress response. The initial purpose of the body's reaction to stress and stressors is to overcome the adverse impact of the external environment. Nature created a mechanism that allows the body to activate all of its resources to survive in adverse conditions. Therefore, most anti-stress programs aimed at decreasing stress levels are misguided; they intend to reduce stress levels rather than to control the stress response by converting the response to a eustress reaction.

This concept of healing being necessarily an active versus passive endeavor is not new to the field of trauma. Indeed, van der Kolk[7] has discussed the importance of action for the successful resolution of the stress response and the deleterious effects of immobilization following trauma, using as an example the "ongoing fear, depression, rage, and physical disease"[7(p. 54)] caused by elevated stress hormones in men who were strapped down during their evacuation from Hurricane Katrina rather than allowed to help with the recovery efforts. Similarly, Peter Levine's Somatosensory Experiencing program and Pat Ogden's Sensorimotor Psychotherapy programs are both founded on the premise that trauma healing requires a physiological release of stress energy through some form of mobile action.

Empowerment itself requires energy, and our energy levels are controlled by the ANS. When the ANS is seriously out of balance and affecting a person's emotional stability and/or ability to function, the person is said to be operating outside the window of tolerance. Ogden speaks of working at the **edge** of the window of tolerance rather than trying to keep the person smack in the middle of that window, totally within their safety zone and devoid of challenge. In order to move forward in life one must literally move forward, and that requires energy, which in turn requires activation of the SNS. The thing is, the person must be able to rise to meet life's challenges **and also** calm the nervous system once a challenge has passed. So we place our treatment emphasis at the lower koshas (i.e. first guidelines) at the beginning, and then carefully open Babette Rothschild's soda bottle (see Chapter 12) just a little bit at a time, providing the "just right challenge" that will activate the nervous system in an adaptive way as well as allow it to return to a calm resting state afterwards. Another of Rothschild's analogies[8(p. 79)] is that of teaching someone to drive. She explains:

Only when my student (and I) were secure in her ability to find the brake pedal and stop the car reflexively did I deem it safe for her to use the gas pedal and learn to (slowly) accelerate, while periodically returning to the brake pedal—stop and go.

Empowerment through occupation

In one important way, we can think of Guideline 5 as somewhat of the reverse of Guideline 1. Whereas Guideline 1 is about creating a safe environment to influence the healing process, Guideline 5 is about the healing process empowering the person to influence their environment, i.e. engage in the world. Working through the koshas over the course of time, a person develops clarity of mind and purpose as well as the intrinsic motivation to live in a manner consistent with their values, goals, and interests. Thus, empowerment is born of well "being" but is expressed in the "doing" of life, which involves living and working in the world around us, not spending the complete entirety of our lives sitting in meditation. Meditation is a means of discovering our true nature, our deepest heartfelt desires, and purpose, not the end goal.

Guideline 5
Self-empowerment is born on the wings of the spirit rising from the mind-body connection

But neither is **achievement** the end goal, for yoga teaches us the importance of non-attachment. Stephen Cope does an amazing job explaining this concept in the context of the Bhagavad Gita:[2(pp. 127-8)]

In this third lesson, Krishan is transmitting to Arjuna one of the most brilliant discoveries of the ancient yoga tradition: the power of nonattachment. Give yourself entirely to your work, yes. But let go of the outcome. Be alike in success and defeat. Krishna is emphatic on this point: You cannot devote yourself fully and passionately to your dharma without engaging this principle.

Why? Over the course of hundreds of years of practice, yogis had discovered that clinging to outcome has a pernicious effect on performance. Clinging (or grasping) of any kind disturbs the mind. And this disturbed mind, then, is not really fully present to the task at hand. It is forever leaning forward into the next moment—grabbing. And, not being present for the moment, it cannot fully devote its powers to the job at hand.

Thus, it is the *process* of unfolding one's potential that is the important thing, not an achieved end state, which is how I conceive the term "self-actualizing" in Figure 15.1B. A person's potential unfolds when their actions align with their most deeply held values and goals, and when they are fully engaged in that process in present moment awareness. In other words, "self-actualizing" is a process in which one's being and doing are in sync. To better explain this relationship, I conceptualized a **Model of Well-Being and Well-Doing**. It is presented in three parts simply to fit in all of the text information.

The process of **Well-Being** (Figure 15.1A) was described on pp. 120–122; it is simply another way to depict the **Transdisciplinary Model of Post-Traumatic Growth**. As explained previously, it is proposed that through this process, a person can come to feel **safe** (annamaya kosha), **calm** (pranamaya kosha),

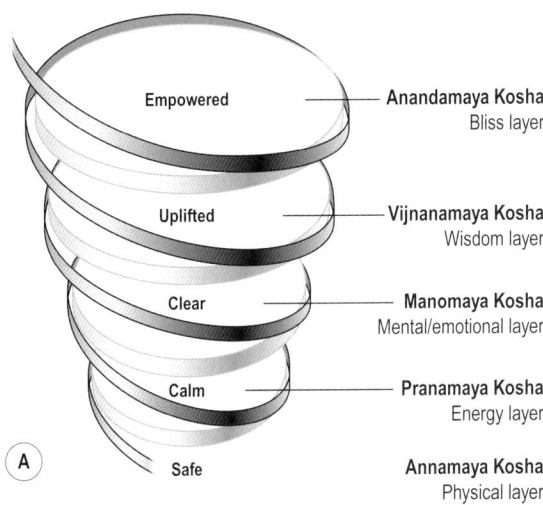

Figure 15.1A
A Model of Well-Being

clear (manomaya kosha), **uplifted** (vijnanamaya kosha), and **empowered** (anandamaya kosha).

Figure 15.1B depicts a **Model of Well-Doing**. I didn't quickly whip this up: the text on the side of the spiral actually came from my old master's thesis, which I literally dusted off the shelf after 34 years, titled *"Toward a unified theory of occupational therapy: an analysis and synthesis of developmental and systems theories."* This time, as with the **Model of Well-Being**, I displayed on the spiral itself the core quality of each stage of the process, almost like an affirmation.

The process goes as follows: when we learn to "do," we first acquire skills, and at that point we can only say we are **capable** of performing the skill. We then integrate these skills together into cohesive occupational behaviors as we engage with the world, at which point we can say we are showing **competence**. We then need to learn to balance and adjust our activities and actions within the context of time and circumstances; hence, we become **adaptable**. Over the course of time,

Chapter 15

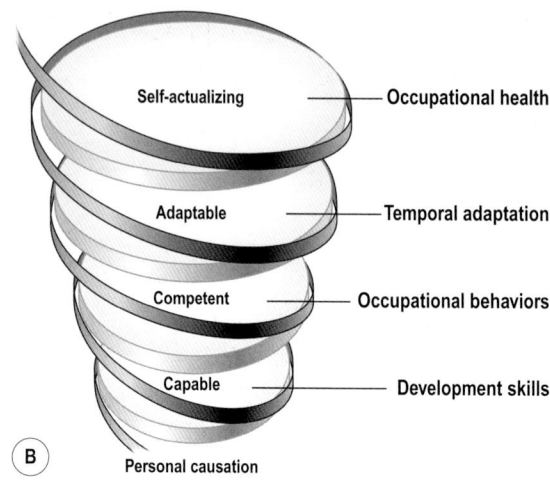

Figure 15.1B
A Model of Well-Doing

as we engage in occupations, we connect more deeply with our felt purpose in life, which causes us to spend more time doing the things that matter most to us. This leads us to unfold our potential, and thus we become *self-actualizing*.

The *Model of Well-Being and Well-Doing* (see Figure 15.1C) is—as you will have guessed—the relationship between being and doing. Each of the spirals closely influences the other; in fact, they are only separable for the purposes of explaining their togetherness! If we are not feeling safe, if we are anxious, if our head is not clear, if we have negative attitudes or beliefs floating around in our head, then we are not going to be present and fully engaged in the activities we need and want to do. Conversely, if we are particularly challenged in learning a skill, or putting skills together into occupational behaviors, or balancing or adjusting our activities to meet both our own needs and the demands of the environment, then our head will likely be filled with negative self-talk—it most certainly won't be clear; we will likely feel anxiety, and depending upon the circumstances, we may even feel unsafe.

Readers who are occupational therapists will recognize that the **Model of Well-Being and Well-Doing** was inspired by the **Person-Environment-Occupation-Performance (PEOP) Model**, which well conceptualizes the relationship between the healing process and environment.[9] The **Model of Well-Being and Well-Doing** actually fits inside the PEOP model and adds an additional layer of complexity to it by describing the ever-evolving processes of being and doing. The PEOP model—developed by Drs Carolyn Baum, Charles Christiansen, and Julie Bass—is intended as a model of practice for occupational therapists. The model describes how the characteristics of the person and environment interact to influence the performance of everyday occupations including daily living tasks as well as activities performed during leisure, at work or in school.

The first part of the treatment process using the PEOP model, as in yoga therapy, is to gather information about the **roles, activities, and goals** of a client. So both professions (occupational therapy and yoga therapy) are concerned with health and well-being and utilize information on roles, activities, and goals to achieve it. Where they most diverge is with regard to the tools of their trade. Whereas yoga therapists use primarily *yoga forms, breath work, and meditation practices* to support health and well-being at every level of the koshas (**physical, energy, emotional/mental, wisdom, bliss**), occupational therapists use *direct engagement in purposeful activities* (usually the functional activities of everyday life) to support the **physiological, neurobehavioral, psychological, cognitive, and spirituality** aspects of being (reordered from the PEOP model to show the resemblance to the kosha model). Yoga is one of those purposeful activities: the American Occupational Therapy Association suggests that occupational therapists "consider helping clients integrate wellness practices such as yoga and progressive muscle relaxation into their daily routines."[10(p. 2)]

Guideline 5
Self-empowerment is born on the wings of the spirit rising from the mind-body connection

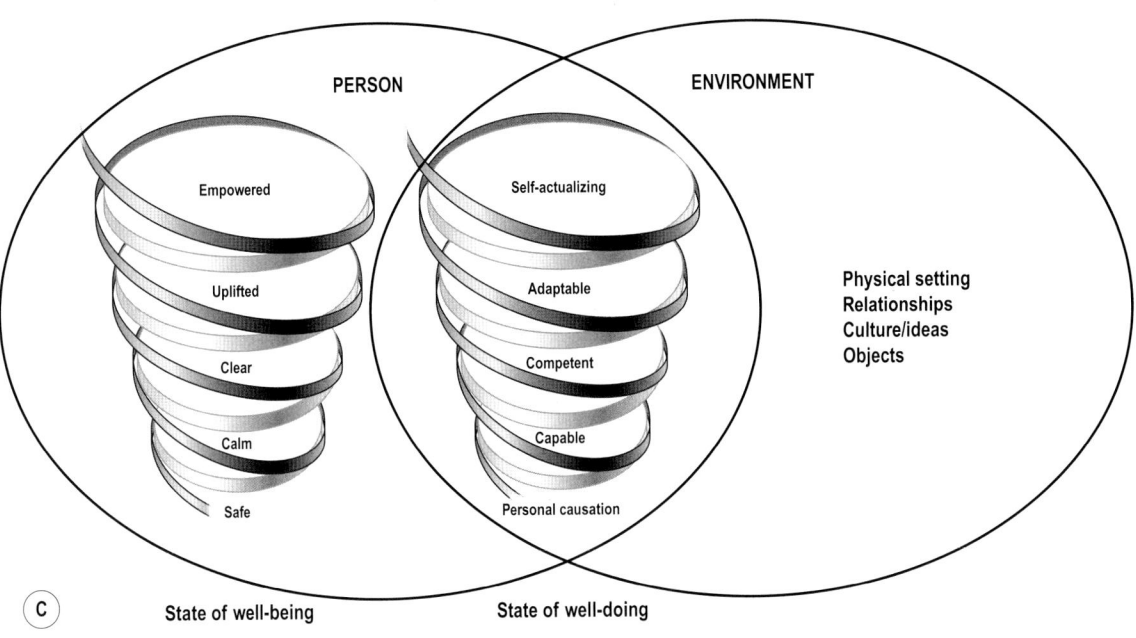

Figure 15.1C
A Model of Well-Being and Well-Doing

In the overarching occupational therapy models for practice, including the PEOP, the different aspects of being are frequently kept in separate boxes or bullets with no identified process that relates one to the other. While these overarching, practice-wide models do leave room for other theoretical models to be incorporated into them (such as the sensory integration model which does identify a relationship between different aspects of being), to my knowledge there is no model used in occupational therapy that explains this relationship as it applies to mental health practice. However, the kosha model does explain this relationship, and it is a relationship that applies across the board, regardless of age, health condition, or level of well-being. The ***Transdisciplinary Model of Post-Traumatic Growth*** is based on the kosha model and extends it by addressing the interaction between the individual and the environment, through occupational engagement and by recognizing the effect the environment can have on the well-being of the individual.

Yoga therapists may have cornered the market with regard to the **relationship between** the intrinsic factors (aka layers) of a person, but when it comes to the actual "doing" of things, occupational therapists certainly have the edge. After all, the yoga therapist does not typically walk off the yoga mat with their client and into their world to watch them engage in activities and analyze what specific factors are impeding their occupational performance (nor are they trained to do so). Thus, we can confidently say that yoga is especially concerned with an internal concept of well-being, or we might even say, the health of the **default mode network** ("off-task" state; see Chapter 4), while occupational therapists are especially concerned with the externalization of well-being, that is, well-doing, or one might say, the health of the **central executive network** ("on-task" state).

Chapter 15

However, due to the ultimately inseparable nature of being and doing, both professions necessarily overlap to some degree, but working together, they could potentially create a powerful "functionally connected network" for healing trauma (pun intended). An ultimate goal would be for these various professionals (and professions) to form collaborative relationships with one another not just within institutional settings such as schools, shelters, or hospitals, but also in community settings and across settings, thereby creating networks of referral systems to support the recovery and empowerment of traumatized individuals whatever their circumstances may be.

A few suggestions for promoting self-empowerment both on and off the mat

1. We can help our students identify the state of their own valued goals and interests by using a structured approach such as the **Wellness Survey for Post-Traumatic Growth** (see Table 15.1).
2. Through the practice of yoga nidra (such as iRest®; www.irest.us), we can guide our students to find their "sankalpa" (resolve), which can take two forms: one is the "heartfelt desire" and the other is a specific intention or goal. In the "heartfelt desire" exercise, students are guided into a deep state of meditative relaxation and then asked to become aware of their heart's deepest desire, something they wish for more than anything else. The answer emerges from the depths of the self and informs the mind of the direction that needs to be taken. There is an art and science to teaching this practice, and professional training is suggested. The following article provides a good introduction: https://yogainternational.com/article/view/how-to-create-a-sankalpa. You can learn more at www.irest.us.
3. During a yoga session, we can suggest specific ways to incorporate yoga tools into everyday life, such as chair yoga, breath work, mudras and/or meditations, to help the students learn how to self-regulate off the mat as well as on the mat. This is the yogic version of helping a person develop a "sensory diet", a term coined by occupational therapists. The more we can stay self-regulated, the more empowered we will be to set goals and meet them.
4. As emphasized earlier, it is crucial that we give our students choices and thus a sense of control over their own experience of yoga, to allow them to operate on their own "power" on the mat.
5. Most importantly, we can listen to ourselves and our students. As Joseph Le Page points out, "listening already contains within it the answer to our questions" (IYT training manual). He adds:

As we learn to listen to ourselves, we also learn to listen to others. As we listen, we also teach the art of listening. Teaching the art of listening is synonymous with teaching yoga, as both help us open the door to who we really are.

The Wellness Survey for Post-Traumatic Growth

I will close this chapter on empowerment by presenting the **Wellness Survey for Post-Traumatic Growth**, which you may find helpful for organizing your intake interview with new clients who have experienced trauma (Table 15.1). As mentioned on the form, many of the items were inspired by or found on materials developed by Joseph Le Page and were chosen (with Joseph's permission) based on their relevance for trauma healing. They were also reorganized into the kosha model format to align with the **Transdisciplinary Model for Post-Traumatic Growth**. The scoring is not standardized and is not terribly meaningful beyond helping to grossly identify the aspects of one's being (physical, energetic, emotional/psychological, wisdom, or bliss) that appear to be most in need of support. The overall pattern might suggest where along the healing process a person falls, as outlined by the model.

Guideline 5
Self-empowerment is born on the wings of the spirit rising from the mind–body connection

The final section was made more "bliss-sensitive" by renaming it Integration/Resources (not the Bliss Body) and by asking (for example) if there are *moments* in which they feel at peace, etc. The intention of the questions in this section in particular is to help identify resources that may facilitate the healing process through *follow-up questioning*. For example, one might inquire "Can you give an example of when you feel more at peace?" and then determine how frequently the person engages in that activity. I would like to collect some data on this form, so if you would like to contribute towards that effort (by administering the forms with a cover sheet and sending copies to SEYI), please contact me at lynn@sensoryenhancedyoga.org.

See page 200 for Table 15.1 Wellness Survey for Post-Traumatic Growth*
By Lynn Stoller, M.S., OTR/L, C-IAYT, RYT 500/E-RYT © Sensory-Enhanced Yoga Institute, 2018. All rights reserved.

Chapter 15

Wellness Survey for Post-Traumatic Growth, page 1
How true do these statements feel to you?

| 0 Never | 1 Rarely | 2 Sometimes | 3 Often | 4 Always |

PHYSICAL BODY	ENERGY BODY
I feel fully connected to my body and am receptive to its sensory messages	I feel connected to my breath
I feel firm, solid, and stable	My belly naturally expands with each inhalation
My body feels comfortable and free from chronic muscle tension	I enjoy full, easeful breathing
I assume an upright and relaxed posture	I am generally calm and tranquil
I like how my body feels when I move through my available range of motion	I naturally smile as I approach and greet people
I easily tolerate bodily sensations without becoming engulfed by them	I live life without fear
I feel completely at home in my body	My digestive system runs smoothly
I maintain healthy physical boundaries with others	I get sufficient sleep
I am attentive to my body's needs (e.g. for healthy nourishment, sufficient sleep, medical care)	I maintain calm under stress
I feel firmly connected to the Earth	I return to my point of balance easily after stressful situations
I feel safe and secure	I have all the energy I need to carry out my daily activities
I am comfortable with heights and moving platforms (e.g. escalators)	I "go with the flow" in my daily life
I feel comfortable in novel environments	I easily adjust my energy level to the situation at hand
I feel comfortable around people, including standing close to them	I balance rest and activity
TOTAL SCORE	**TOTAL SCORE**

Guideline 5
Self-empowerment is born on the wings of the spirit rising from the mind-body connection

Wellness Survey for Post-Traumatic Growth, page 2
How true do these statements feel to you?

| 0 Never | 1 Rarely | 2 Sometimes | 3 Often | 4 Always |

EMOTIONAL/MENTAL BODY
- I am aware of and welcome my feelings and thoughts
- I express my feelings freely yet thoughtfully
- I enjoy a variety of sensory experiences (e.g. music, touch, visual/art, nature, lively settings, smells)
- I feel completely present in this moment
- My mind feels clear and free from intrusive or ruminative thoughts of the future or the past
- I feel connected to the world around me
- I can focus and concentrate well on the task at hand despite mild distractions
- I am fully engaged in my daily activities
- I feel compassion towards myself and others
- I experience difficult emotions without identifying with them
- I meet life's challenges with equanimity
- I am warm and friendly
- I enjoy positive self-esteem
- I am upbeat

TOTAL SCORE

WISDOM BODY
- I view situations with objectivity
- I am able to stand back and be a witness to my thoughts and emotions
- I observe my limiting beliefs without identifying with them so completely
- I always look at the bigger picture
- I trust in the guidance of my inner being
- I listen to my heart with sensitivity
- I am practical in relation to my goals and plans
- I readily let go of that which no longer serves me
- I am open to life's infinite possibilities.
- I embrace difficult situations as opportunities for learning
- I am hopeful
- I am open-minded to different perspectives
- I sense my inherent wholeness
- I am open to change and transformation

TOTAL SCORE

Chapter 15

Wellness Survey for Post-Traumatic Growth, page 3
How true do these statements feel to you?

| 0 Never | 1 Rarely | 2 Sometimes | 3 Often | 4 Always |

Note: "Suffering" is said by the ancient yogis to be the most common condition of human beings, so if you are not "feeling the bliss", you have plenty of company. In this section, we are looking for potential resources that can help us guide you during difficult times to find your own unique doorway to a sense of well-being and renewal.

INTEGRATION/RESOURCES
I experience moments of peace and tranquility
I have moments where I forget my troubles and experience pleasure in whatever it is that I am doing
I accept life as a gift and a blessing, despite its hardships
I like to get out into nature and "smell the roses"
I retain a sense of my inherent wholeness and "true self" even during times when it feels like life is trying to pull me apart
I have personal connections with others that are meaningful to me and that I can draw on during difficult times
I can still laugh at things that are funny in spite of it all
I am able to use my mind to generate positive memories, images, or other sensory impressions (e.g. sounds, smells) that draw in a sense of safety, peace or even joy
What I feel, think, say, and do are congruent with each other
I have moments when I connect to a clear sense of direction and purpose in life
I find meaning in the work I do for a living
I have hobbies and/or other interests that bring me comfort or joy
I make time in my schedule to do activities that nurture me
I feel a sense of personal empowerment in the areas of life that are most important to me
TOTAL SCORE

*Many of the items used in this form were inspired or taken from materials developed by Joseph Le Page and were chosen based on their relevance to trauma healing and reorganized into the kosha model format, with his permission.
By Lynn Stoller, M.S., OTR/L, C-IAYT, RYT 500/E-RYT
© Sensory-Enhanced Yoga Institute, 2018. All rights reserved.

PART 4

Putting the practice together

Structuring the practice 16

In crafting and teaching sequences to others, it calls on us to more fully assess, anticipate, and honor the realities of students in our classes, thereby offering them a pathway that makes yoga work for them. — Mark Stephens[1(p. 15)]

This chapter discusses how to structure a Sensory-Enhanced Yoga class for trauma survivors or those who have related conditions such as anxiety, attention deficit hyperactivity disorder (ADHD), bipolar disorder, or mixed anxiety/depression. Though the book is heavily focused on trauma, the information is very useful for these other folks as well.

The most important suggestion I can give you is to start where the person is at the moment. Someone who has ADHD may be quite fidgety; one such student (a young adult) began the school year in my yoga class by repetitively rolling up and unrolling the edge of his mat, and taking his socks off and putting them on, and didn't stop fidgeting for the first several yoga sessions. The transformation was remarkable as he learned to come to complete stillness quite easily within a couple of months of starting the program. The key for him was to start the class at a fast enough pace so his mind wouldn't wander off to other thoughts and actions, and then gradually slow him down during the course of the yoga session. He also benefitted from intense proprioceptive feedback through weight-bearing forms and using the yoga strap. Yoga was the one thing he was adamant should stay in his Individualized Education Plan to help him stay alert and focused and able to better access his school curriculum.

Another student, who was very obese, depressed, and had low energy, needed to start at a much slower pace and very gradually have the pace picked up during the session to move him in a more energetic and upbeat direction. The problem was, both students were in the same class. We had the obese student sit in a chair much of the time, perform modified moves, and take rests when he needed to. In this class, I had the benefit of an assistant who could also provide him with some suggestions. In some classes, a physical or occupational therapist would work one-on-one with a student who had severe physical challenges, physically helping the student perform many of the moves, and would also address other motor goals during times when the rest of the class was doing something that couldn't be approximated by the student.

Students who use wheelchairs have usually been taken out of the wheelchair and positioned with props on the floor or a mat table for yoga class but this is not always the case. I once had a very anxious student with very limited mobility who routinely spent each yoga class fully reclined in his power chair with a weighted bag on his lap. He listened to his special music on his headphones during asana instruction and took off the headphones during the initial centering and final relaxation/meditation sections of class so he could benefit from them.

Chapter 16

Another challenging scenario is working with people who have mixed anxiety and depression. The protocol for treating anxiety involves moving the energy downward to help ground the individual, while people in depressed states need to be uplifted. In a mixed case, chest-expanding (heart opening) yoga forms, which are ideal for depression, should be well grounded, such as with the Warrior I series and some of the arm stretches with a strap, so as not to induce anxiety.

Unfortunately, in a group class all of the students will likely not have the same needs; however, I have found that it somehow all works out by planning in advance how you might modify yoga forms and movements for those in your class who are likely to struggle with them—*before* the yoga class starts. Also, when planning the class, a general rule of thumb is to repeat large chunks of it from week to week and maintain a consistent structure, as people tend to like repetition and can relax more into a class when they feel it is somewhat predictable. (For students with special needs, this is crucial.) But at the same time, it is good to also include two or three novel moves to keep the class fresh. Themed classes work well especially in community settings, such as a focus on the breath, grounding, resiliency, and so on.

When designing a yoga therapy session, it is important to carefully consider every element for maximum therapeutic effect: the initial centering, choice of breath work, yoga form selections, flow components, the final relaxation segment, all meditative elements (including any mudras) and thoughtful sequencing of all of the above. This chapter presents a few sample scripts as a starting point. Since the focus of this book is to help people heal from trauma, high anxiety, and/or related autonomic nervous system disorders, it is very helpful to use any opportunity you can to help students move out of their minds and safely back into their bodies. "Body sensing" language and body scans are very useful in this regard. You will notice these elements in the initial centering script, tension/relaxation exercise, and the two scripts for Savasana (the final relaxation portion of class). Since the breath is so important for self-regulation, it is drawn into virtually every element of a class (as discussed in Guideline 2.)

Table 16.1 shows a sample class sequence that includes chair options for those who need or prefer to use one. Oftentimes, students who use chairs are able to perform some standing yoga forms, too. With the older adults, the difficulty with mat work is usually the transition up and down from the mat. Some will choose to get down on the mat for final relaxation, but not for the earlier yoga forms, as one trip down to the floor is enough for them. Some of my students who remain in the chair during final relaxation find it helpful to have another chair positioned in front of them with a blanket folded over the backrest to rest their heads on (see Crocodile in the Chair, Figure 13.18). Or, you can turn the second chair to face the person and place a bolster on it for Restorative Child (Figure 13.6). You might also offer to add a weight on their back to provide enhanced deep touch pressure.

When working with a group of individuals with mixed mobility levels, it is ideal to have present an assistant who is also a registered yoga teacher or an allied health professional who can assist with the demonstrations and be an extra set of eyes to be sure everyone's needs are taken care of. Whether teaching solo or with an assistant, I mostly provide oral instructions for the mat forms while my assistant or I model the chair version, which the chair yogis follow Simon Says style. I say *some* things specifically to the people in the chair, but generally speaking, the chair moves are much more easy

Structuring the practice

Table 16.1 Sample Sensory-Enhanced Yoga® class

	Segments	On a mat	Using a chair
1	Segment A: Breath work prep	Reclining Symmetrical Stretch Reclined Half-Moon Stretch — *Breathe into stretched ribcage* Knees to Chest	Sitting Sun Breaths Sitting Half-Moon Stretch — *Breathe into stretched ribcage* Dynamic Knee to Chest to Extended Leg
2	Segment B: Centering/body sensing/breath	Initial Centering Script	Initial Centering Script
3	Segment C: Supine forms	Leg Stretches With Strap — *Also ankle circles/flex/extend without strap* Supine Twist — *Knees to chest – counterform*	Sitting Leg Stretches (optional: with strap) — *Can support leg on another chair when using strap, if desired* — *Also ankle circles/flex/extend without strap* Sun Breath Twists in Chair — *Then hold twist; repeat on opposite side*
4	Segment D: Table forms	Cat/Cow Rhythmic Flow: — *Down Dog to Up Dog* *and/or* — *Modified Hare to Knee-Down Up Dog* Spinal Balance	Cat/Cow in Chair Rhythmic Flow: — *Setting Sun* (*Sun breath into forward fold with palms on thighs to protect back.*) Sitting Spinal Balance – raise arm overhead and opposite leg
5	Segment E: Standing Stretches with strap	Mountain Mountain *(with Strap)* Standing Side Bend *(with Strap)* Standing Twist *(with Strap)* Cow form *(Arm Version with Strap)* Standing Yoga Mudra *(with Strap)* -OR- *Sensory-Enhanced Moon Salute*	Sitting Mountain *Sitting Extended Mountain (with Strap)* *Sitting Side Bend* *(with Strap)* *Sitting Twist (with Strap)* *Cow form (Arm Version with Strap)* *Sitting Yoga Mudra (with Strap)* -OR- *Sensory-Enhanced Moon Salute*
6	Segment F: Standing forms	Warrior I and/or II Standing Forward Bend Tree	Warrior I and/or II in chair — *Front thigh over corner or parallel to front of chair if possible* Sitting Forward Bend (two-stage) Modified Tree Using Chair or Wall (*if capable*)

— continued —

Chapter 16

Table 16.1 continued

7	*Segment G:* Prone forms	Crocodile Baby Cobra or Cobra — Then Knee to Chest as counterform	Sitting Crocodile Dynamic Cat to Cobra — Hands on thighs with elbows out for Cat — Arms hold lower back of chair in Cobra
8	*Segment H:* Savasana	Savasana (and Restorative)	Savasana (and Restorative)
9	*Segment I:* Advanced Breathing Practices and Mudra Meditations	Alternate Nostril Breathing or Sitkari Breath Client-Centered Mudra Meditation	Alternate Nostril Breathing or Sitkari Breath Client-Centered Mudra Meditation

to follow as there are fewer critical alignment cues and I can effectively communicate some of them with a gesture, such as an upward move of my hand along the midline of my body to remind the group to lengthen up through the spine while I exaggerate the move. If I tried to verbally communicate every detail to both groups of students, the class would hardly be relaxing at all as then people have to figure out who I am talking to and there would be twice as much chatter from the teacher. When I don't have an assistant in class, I still spend a good part of my time in the chair as there are enough experienced students in class who can serve as visual models on the mat for any newbies. But I do some demos on the mat, too.

The duration of a class can vary depending upon the endurance and needs of the people within it. In a school environment, 15–20 minutes each morning in the classroom can get the day off to a really great start. Even a minute or two can be very helpful during transition times, to get up and do a few stretches in coordination with the breath. Done in this manner, the yoga techniques are used as "sensory diet" tools to help students stay self-regulated during the school day. Weekly yoga groups in school settings are generally the same length as a class period, but for a classroom of students with short attention spans or low endurance, the class period may be broken up into two activities or yoga and a break time. Community classes for adults, on the other hand, are often scheduled for 70–75 minutes. This allows time for a proper final relaxation period. One-hour classes work well when there are a lot of chair users since an hour is a long enough time to sit in a chair; however, most of the people in my classes can stand for portions of time which allows a 70-minute class time to work. My own natural teaching style best lends itself to a 90-minute class, which allows me to fit in everything I would like to include, from soup to nuts, but alas, for many of the students I teach this would be too long of a time frame.

When sequencing the class, you can start in any position. I prefer to start a class either in sitting position (to do some neck, shoulder, and trunk warm-ups) or in a reclined position with the Breath

Structuring the practice

Prep stretches as shown in the sample class plan. Also as shown in Table 16.1, the Breath Prep stretches have a chair version for those who have mobility limitations. I move into Table fairly early in the practice to really warm up the spine prior to moving into the standing forms. There is always at least one Downward-Facing Dog (in fact, usually at least a couple) in my classes as they are so therapeutic on many levels (see Appendix B). Downward-Facing Dog can be done on the mat, up to a wall, or using the back or seat of a chair. I usually transition people from the table forms to the standing forms by going through Downward-Facing Dog. I often save Cobra and Bridge to the end, after the standing forms, when the body has been well stretched. (I learned that this is the classic way of sequencing these yoga forms, which is reflected in many yoga books.) After every backbend, it is always important to present a forward fold as a counterform, such as Knees to Chest, Child, or a Standing Wide-Legged Forward Fold. Windshield-wiping the legs also helps to loosen up tension in the lower back area following a backbend performed from the prone position. Offering a restorative form (see Chapter 13) is often well received at the end of class, before final relaxation.

During final relaxation, I often suggest placing a bolster or rolled blanket under the thighs (or a block under each thigh, at the lowest height), and placing a folded blanket under the head, if they are reclined on a mat (see Supported Savasana). Raising the thighs reduces the potential for strain in the lower back. Some people need a lot more support under their heads, especially if they have kyphosis, in which case I build up the supports, as the chin should ideally be lower than the forehead. Some people may choose to remain in another restorative yoga form during the guided relaxation, while others may choose to sit in a chair, in a restorative form or not. I use several different scripts for final relaxation, but every one of them includes some sort of body sensing and breath awareness element. As mentioned earlier, I stay away from sending people on "trips" to places in guided meditations when working with traumatized individuals unless they create the trip themselves (to access their Inner Resource).

Being trained in iRest® Level 2, I occasionally venture further than the body sensing and breath awareness elements into exploring opposites of feeling, emotions, or thoughts, but am more apt to do this in a one-to-one yoga therapy session rather than within the limited time frame of a group asana-based yoga class. This process helps to reconnect bodily sensation with emotion, thus restoring the body representation maps that Damasio described (Chapter 3). However, staying in the body sensing and breath awareness levels is generally recommended during the early stages of healing with this population. I should mention here that iRest is a practice of personal exploration, not a relaxation technique per se, though oftentimes relaxation occurs during the process. It is very important to have advanced training in this technique as well as the prerequisite skills and knowledge for doing the work if you choose to incorporate it into a yoga class.

The following pages present a few basic scripts for the initial centering and final relaxation portions of class to help get you started. The Integrative Yoga Therapy and iRest programs offer a wide variety of therapeutic scripts for yoga and meditation and are highly recommended sources for further learning.

Chapter 16

Initial centering script for a yoga session

Positioning

I invite you to lie down on your mat, arranging your body so that you feel completely supported by the surface on which it rests.

You may wish to place a rolled blanket or a bolster under your knees.

And you may want a knee pad or blanket under your head.

Allow your legs to drop to the floor, and your arms to drop away from your body, palms turning upwards.

Make whatever adjustments you need to bring a deeper sense of ease into your body and mind … (*pause*)

Listening to the body and mind

Please always listen to your own body and mind during the practice. If you experience any discomfort at any time, please re-adjust your body, or even get out of a yoga form. You can then join back in when you are ready.

It is also possible for emotions to arise in any mind-body practice. If you can welcome them, instead of fighting them, it will often help them move through the mind and body towards resolution. I am here for you if you need me, and if you feel the need to stop, I just ask that you remain in the room, perhaps sit along the wall, until the practice is over as it is important to feel grounded before you leave and I'll want to be sure you're okay.

Sensing surroundings

Now begin to sense your surroundings … the room around you … the sounds … without resisting them or grasping them … Notice the surface that is supporting the weight of your body … the points of contact between your body and the floor … the tactile sensation of your entire body … simply allowing sensations and perceptions to arise naturally …

Body sensing

And then turn your awareness inward, and begin to scan the body, beginning with the feet and slowly working your way upwards, just noticing what sensations are present … in your feet … soles and tops of the feet … legs … both the lower legs and thighs … inside and outside … hips and buttocks … lower, mid, and upper back area … simply noticing sensation … abdomen … sensing the internal organs … moving up to the heart center and the area inside the ribcage … Now scanning the arms, noticing sensation in the palms … scanning from the hands and all the way through and into the shoulders … and then moving over to the neck and throat area … just noticing what is present there … and into the face … jaw … eyes … forehead and scalp … and even the thoughts inside your head … what messages are you receiving from your body and mind today?

Intention for practice

Perhaps using this information, develop an intention for your practice today … Maybe you would like to feel more calm, a sense of peace … become more flexible or strong … eliminate an area of physical tension … achieve mental clarity … or perhaps some other physical or mental benefit of practice … Take a few moments to experience your intention for today's practice.

Breath awareness

And notice the body breathing itself … without controlling it in any way, simply be aware of the movement of air in and out of the body … Notice the quality of your breath today … is it slow, deep, and relaxed ... short, shallow, or constricted ... just notice the quality of your breath in this moment.

Inner Resource

This is a natural spot for the Inner Resource to be inserted (see Chapter 10).

Preparing the body for breath work

We'll begin to prepare for our breath work by performing a few stretches first.

(*Perform the three Supine Stretches:* **Symmetrical Stretch, Half-Moon Stretch, and Knees to Chest**.)

Diaphragmatic breath

(*From Knees to Chest position*) And now stretch the legs back out on the floor as we prepare to move into the diaphragmatic breath, breathing all the way down into the lower lungs. This results in a slower, deeper breath that helps to relax the mind and body.

You may wish to place a weight [sandbag] or a hand on your belly, which can help invite the muscles of your belly to soften, and also encourages a longer exhale, which is calming to the nervous system.

Release the muscles of your throat ... and invite the belly to soften.

Inhale deeply through your nose ... feeling your belly gently expand against your hands or the weight. As you exhale through the nose, feel your belly sink back toward the spine ...

Continue inhaling and exhaling through the nose ... slowly ... smoothly ... letting your breath flow naturally ... belly expanding on the inhale ... belly sinking on the exhale ...

After 3–5 min Try removing the weight now and continue with the breath ...

Complete yogic breath

When the diaphragmatic breath is well-established, you might begin to expand the breath into the complete yogic breath ... First the belly expands as you draw the air into the lower lungs, and when the lower lungs are full, continue to inhale more air filling up the entire lungs, fully expanding the ribcage in all directions.

Then slowly exhale the air completely out of the lungs. You may wish to slightly contract the abdomen at the end of the exhale to release the last remnants of air. (*Perform about six complete breaths.*)

And now return to a more gentle, relaxed, diaphragmatic breath. (*Proceed to asana session.*)

Chapter 16

Tension/relaxation exercise (body sensing)

A tension/relaxation exercise can be presented at the beginning of an asana practice for the body-sensing component. The works of several individuals influenced this version. I would especially like to acknowledge the influence of Richard Miller and Emily Hain.

Introduction

I invite you to participate in a body sensing exercise. First, I will ask you to squeeze a body part, hold it, and then release it. As you squeeze, think of hugging, rather than clenching. Afterwards, I will invite you to notice the sensations in your body. You may notice some sensation or you may notice very little sensation. There's no need to try and change your experience. Please breathe at your own pace so that it remains easy and comfortable. If you choose not to participate, feel free to move however it feels good for you or simply rest.

Mouth and face

If you would like to try this exercise, first draw your attention to your mouth. If you like, open your jaw, and stick out your tongue ... then close the mouth, purse the lips together, and scrunch the face toward the tip of your nose, squeezing your eyelids tightly shut ... and then when you are ready, let go of all the muscles of the face, letting the face completely soften ... and notice sensation.

Neck and shoulders

Now, you might try scrunching your shoulders off the floor and towards your ears ... drawing tension into the shoulders ... shoulder blades ... and neck ... this whole area ... while letting your hands, mouth, and eyes remain completely at rest. Neck and shoulders full of tension ... mouth and eyes at rest ... and when you are ready, completely release your shoulders to the floor, and notice sensations that are present.

Left hand

Now, if you wish, slowly make a fist with the left hand, lifting the arm slightly from the floor. Tighten the fist ... forearm ... elbow ... upper arm ... building tension all the way up the left arm ... the right arm remains completely at rest ... mouth and eyes are soft ... but the left arm is full of tension. Then completely release the arm to the floor, and notice sensation.

Right hand

Now you might slowly make a fist with your right hand, lifting the arm slightly from the floor. Tighten the fist ... and bring the tension into the forearm ... elbow ... upper arm ... building tension all the way up the right arm ... but the left arm and muscles of the face remain at rest ... Then completely release the arm, allowing the arm to feel completely supported by the floor, releasing all control of the muscles, and notice sensation.

Hips and buttocks (omit if you suspect sexual trauma)

Next, you might feel down into your hips and buttocks ... if you like, you could tighten the buttocks, lifting the hips off the ground ... Mouth completely at rest ... eyes at rest ... the hips and buttocks completely tense ... and then allow the hips and buttocks to completely release back to the floor, noticing sensations that are present.

Left leg

Now, if you like, begin to hug the muscles of your left leg into the bones ... Maybe raise it off the floor a little bit ... and slowly bring tension into the foot ... ankle ... calf ... knee ... and thigh ... tense the toes toward you ... and then tense them away from you ... holding the entire foot, leg, and hip in full tension ... while the right leg, arms, and face remain at rest ... and when you are ready, slowly release the leg ... let it completely rest on the ground ... and notice sensation.

Right leg

Now you might try hugging the muscles of your right leg into the bones ... Perhaps raise it a tiny bit and begin to tense the foot ... the ankle ... calf ... knee ... thigh ... tense the toes toward you ... and then tense them away from you ... holding the tension ... both arms and left leg remain completely at rest on the floor ... mouth and eyes remain soft ... but the right leg is completely full of tension ... and then when you are ready ... let go of the leg ... and let it completely rest on the ground ... noticing all sensations.

Noticing sensation with body at rest (softer, slower voice)

Notice sensation in the face ... the jaw ... tongue resting at the back of your throat ... the entire inside of the mouth ... lips ... corners of the eyes ... forehead ... and scalp.

Sense the neck and throat ... inviting the throat to completely soften.

Sense the arms ... all the way to the hands and fingers ... left and right ... Arms full of sensation ... and completely at rest on the floor ...

Sense the upper back ... middle back ... simply noticing what is there ... and follow sensation around the body into the abdomen ...

Sense the belly ... inside and outside ... noticing the belly gently rise and fall with the breath.

Follow sensation down through to the lower back ... and into the hips ... inviting any remaining muscle tension you find there to completely release ...

And then sense your way down through the thighs ... lower legs ... and feet ... both feet and legs simultaneously ... full of sensation and completely resting on the floor.

Now draw your awareness to the entire body ... feeling all of the sensations simultaneously ... front and back ... right and left sides ... inside and outside ... and welcoming every experience that is now present in awareness ... (*Allow several minutes of rest.*)

I now invite you to begin wiggling your fingers and toes ... or make any movements you'd like to make to help you become more alert ... yet rested ... grateful for taking this time for yourself ... and when you are ready, slowly open your eyes and come fully back to your wide-awake and alert state of being.

Chapter 16

Sample script for Savasana

Roll your head from side to side, then let it rest in a comfortable position back in the center. Allow your jaw to drop open if it wants, and the tongue to fall to the back of the throat. Soften the eyes, and invite the worry lines to melt right off the face …

And notice the tactile sensations of the ears … cheeks … nose … both eyes … forehead … the whole face and scalp.

And we will continue to focus attention to points throughout the body … with no need to do anything, just notice and feel …

… the back of the head and neck … shoulders … and follow sensation down through the shoulders and into the arms …

Be aware of your right arm … right shoulder … upper arm … lower arm … and hand … becoming aware of sensation throughout entire right arm.

Then shift awareness to your left arm … left shoulder … upper arm … lower arm … and hand … becoming aware of sensation throughout the entire left arm.

And bring your attention into your throat and allow it to soften …

Draw your awareness from the throat down to the chest and heart center … into your ribcage and around to your upper back … down to your lower back … and around to your belly … noticing sensation inside and around the belly area …

Draw attention to the right hip … upper right leg … lower right leg … right foot … entire leg from the hip to the foot.

Then shift your awareness over to the left leg … left hip … left upper leg … left lower leg … left foot … entire left leg …

Feel both feet and legs simultaneously … simply noticing sensation …

Allow all of the sensations throughout the entire body blend together … so the entire body is perceived simultaneously … front side and back side … right side and left side … inside and outside … feeling the entire physical body as pure sensation … and welcoming every experience that is now present in awareness … (*pause for several minutes*)

You may begin to wiggle your fingers and toes, taking your time as you now transition into your waking life … stretching however you wish … You may wish to lie on one side for a few additional moments before coming up to a sitting position … and when you are ready, slowly open your eyes and come fully back to your wide-awake and alert state of being.

A short grounding Savasana

Roll your head from side to side, and then let it rest in a comfortable position back in the center ... Allow the jaw to fall open if it wants, and the tongue to fall to the back of the throat. Soften the eyes, and the muscles of the forehead ...

Soften the throat ... soften the belly ... and become aware of your breath, the natural spontaneous breath with no need to change it ...

And become aware of the meeting points of the body and the floor, inviting the muscles of your body to completely soften downward into those points of contact ...

The back of the head ... shoulder blades and back of the torso ... back of the arms and hands ... the calves ... and the heels ...

The sensation of all points simultaneously ... inviting your whole body to feel completely supported and at rest ...

Total awareness of your body lying in complete stillness ...

Breathing in and breathing out ...

And welcoming every experience that is now present in awareness ... (*Pause for several minutes, then invite back to a state of alertness as with the previous script.*)

Savasana with 41 points

(Adapted from the traditional 61 Point Meditation)

Roll your head from side to side, and then let it rest in a comfortable position back in the center ... Allow the jaw to fall open if it wants, and the tongue to fall to the back of the throat. Soften the eyes, and the muscles of the forehead ...

Sense all of the points of contact between your body and the floor, and invite your body to soften downward into those points of contact.

Soften the throat ... soften the belly ... and become aware of your breath, the natural spontaneous breath with no need to change it ...

And now we will focus our attention to different points throughout the body, like a butterfly landing for a split second before flitting off to the next spot. There is no need to do anything but simply notice ...

(Stay just long enough on each point for the students to register it, but not long enough for the mind to wander, i.e. about six seconds, including the time it takes to state the body part.)

1. The point between the eyebrows
2. Hollow of the throat
3. Right shoulder joint
4. Right elbow joint
5. The bend of the right wrist
6. Center of the right palm
7. The bend of the right wrist
8. Right elbow joint
9. Right shoulder joint
10. Hollow of the throat
11. Left shoulder joint
12. Left elbow joint
13. The bend of the left wrist
14. Center of the left palm
15. The bend of the left wrist
16. Left elbow joint
17. Left shoulder joint
18. Hollow of the throat
19. Heart center
20. Solar plexus (just below the bottom of the breast bone)
21. Navel center (two inches below the physical navel
22. Right hip joint
23. Right knee joint
24. Right ankle joint
25. Center of the sole of the right foot
26. Right ankle joint
27. Right knee joint
28. Right hip joint
29. Navel center (two inches below the physical navel)
30. Left hip joint
31. Left knee joint
32. Left ankle joint
33. Center of the sole of the left foot
34. Left ankle joint
35. Left knee joint
36. Left hip joint
37. Navel center (two inches below the physical navel)
38. Solar plexus
39. Heart center
40. Hollow of the throat
41. Center between the eyebrows (repeat this last one three times)

Description of therapeutic yoga forms 17

There is more to practicing asanas correctly than merely the physical aligning of the body. The classic poses, when practiced with discrimination and awareness, bring the body, mind, intelligence, nerves, consciousness, and the self together into a single, harmonious whole. — B. K. S. Iyengar[1,2(p. 62)]

The yoga forms in this chapter are presented in the order listed in Table 16.1, Sample Sensory-Enhanced Yoga class, with a few additional yoga forms sprinkled in between them. The chair versions are listed at the end of the chapter, but as mentioned earlier, many people who mostly use a chair are able to perform the standing yoga forms on the mat. Also, the chair versions of yoga forms are ideal for small spaces, such as counselor offices, even if the person is capable of doing yoga on a mat. So feel free to mix and match according to ability and interest level. Since some of the people who will use this material will likely not be registered yoga instructors, I did not include yoga forms that I was concerned might be presented in an unsafe manner. However, there are key cues included in the descriptions below that are important to state to the student in order to maintain the integrity of the musculoskeletal system. The reader is encouraged to generously sprinkle invitational language (e.g. "if you like", "you might", "if it feels right") to these descriptions according to what phrases feel most natural to the reader. There are also numerous additional cues that could have been added to these descriptions, but that would have been overwhelming for new learners and are also not essential for the purpose of healing psychological conditions. Nonetheless, it is recommended that readers who are not registered yoga instructors or certified yoga therapists be mentored by one when learning how to present these forms to their therapy clients.

Supine forms

Supine Symmetrical Stretch (Figure 17.1)

- Reach your arms above your head to the floor behind you.

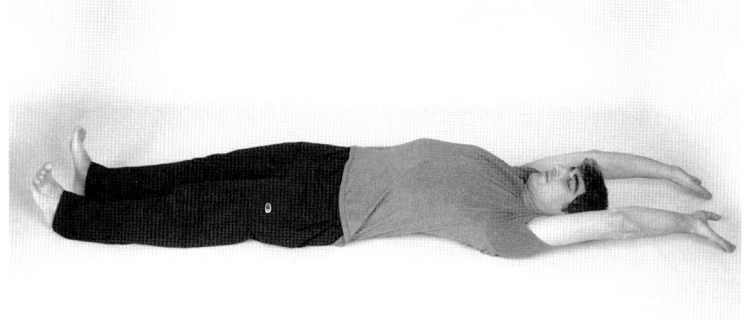

Figure 17.1

Supine Symmetrical Stretch

Chapter 17

- Stretch your hands and feet away from each other.
- Hold the stretch, feeling the entire body lengthen from your fingertips through the arms, torso, legs, and through the heels.
- Take several nice slow deep breaths in and out.
- Release, and rest.

Supine Half-Moon Stretch (Figure 17.2)

- *(From Supine Symmetrical Stretch position)* Walk your heels to the left and at the same time, bring your left arm back down to your side while continuing to stretch your right arm overhead.
- With your body curved in this "C" position, stretch out the entire right side of the body, from the heel, through the leg, right side of the torso, right arm, and all the way through to the fingertips of the right hand.
- *Direct the breath into the right ribcage*, feeling the small muscles between the ribs expand with each inhalation and release more and more with each exhalation.
- Repeat steps on the other side.

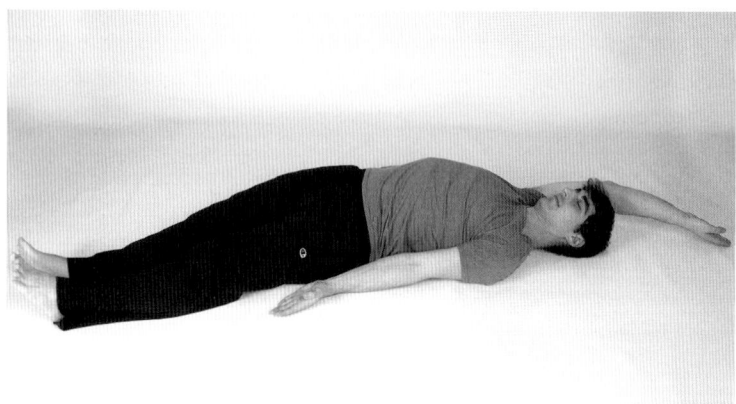

Figure 17.2
Supine Half-Moon Stretch

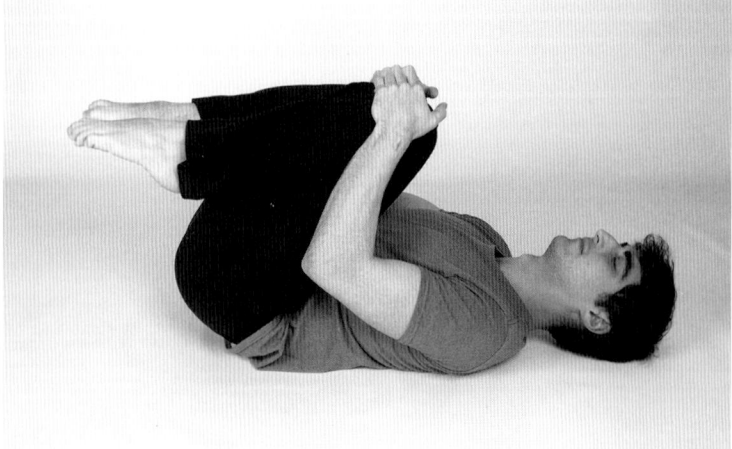

Figure 17.3
Knees to Chest

Description of therapeutic yoga forms

Knees to Chest (Figure 17.3)

- (*From supine*) Draw your knees into your chest, clasping your hands around the knees or placing each palm on a knee. Simply let the weight of your arms slowly release the thighs toward your body.
- Take several nice slow breaths through the nose, noticing where you feel the movement in your body as you breathe. You may feel it around the abdomen, or mostly in the chest area, perhaps in both areas, or you may not notice much bodily movement at all. You may even notice your knees moving slightly away from your body as you inhale, and move closer to your body as you exhale, as your belly rises and falls with the breath. Simply observe where the movement occurs with your own breath, with no need to change anything.
- Now you might slowly move your knees side to side, to begin to loosen up any tension in the lower spine, or maybe place a palm on each knee and move the knees together in a circular direction, as though drawing circles on the ceiling (or sky), first one way … and then the other way … or even in opposite directions.
- Feel free to explore, rolling over any spots on the lower back where you feel tension.
- You may notice that when your knees are held further away from your body, you roll lower down on the spine, and when your knees are held closer to your body, you roll higher up on the spine. This may help you locate the spots that you need to release.

NOTE: It is suggested that the above three stretches are presented before introducing the diaphragmatic breath in a treatment session. These simple stretches use movement to stretch the ribcage, creating more space for the breath, and/or bring awareness to the breath as it is.

Leg stretches with a yoga strap (Figures 17.4–17.6)

IMPORTANT NOTE: *These leg stretches are not recommended for people who have experienced sexual trauma.*

Leg Stretch 1 (Figure 17.4)

Prepare the strap for the leg stretches by forming a small loop with the buckle.

- Start in supine position, with both knees bent and feet flat on the floor. Bend your left knee toward your chest, and position the loop of the strap over the sole of your foot.

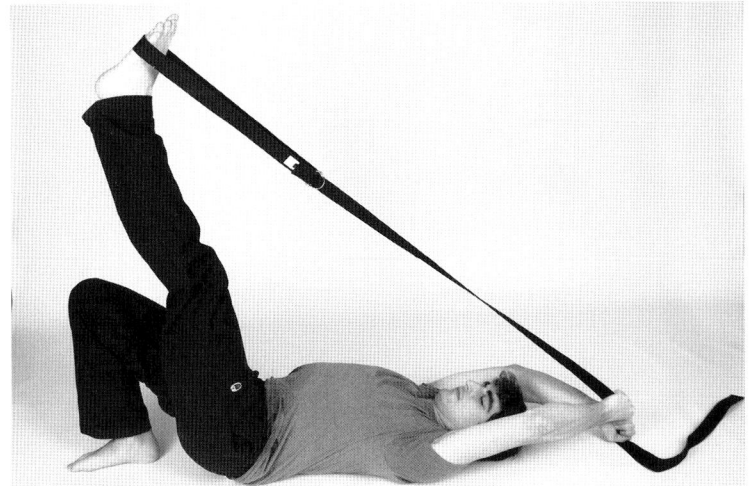

Figure 17.4

Leg Stretch 1

Chapter 17

- As you slowly raise your leg upward, slide both hands down the strap until your arms are stretched over and behind your head.
- Only raise your leg to the point where you just begin to feel the stretch without bending your knee. Then back off slightly, to allow the muscles to release in the stretch and avoid eliciting the stretch reflex.
- As you feel the muscles release, you may pull slightly on the strap to invite your leg to slowly stretch a bit further into the space created by the release—it may be just a half inch.

Leg Stretch 2 (Figure 17.5)

- To prepare for the next stretch, extend your opposite leg on the floor.
- Bring your left hand down to hold the strap halfway between your left foot and right hand.
- Allow your leg to lower to the left side, until it is about a foot off the ground, keeping the sacrum pressed into the floor and the abdominal muscles engaged.
- Take the far end of the strap with your right hand, pulling the strap behind your head. Allow your

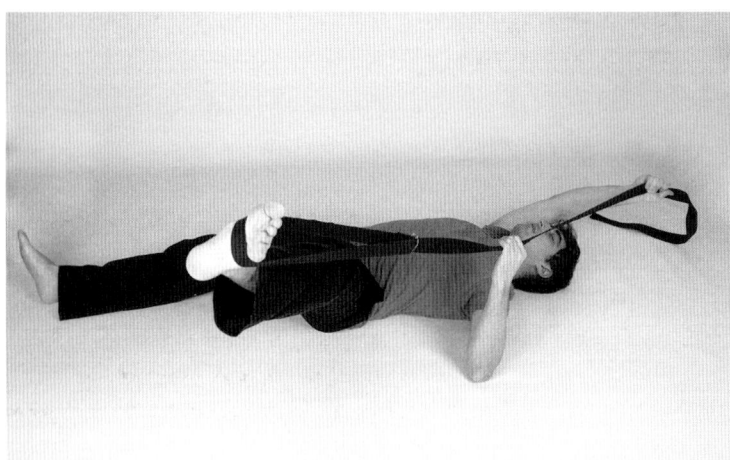

Figure 17.5
Leg Stretch 2

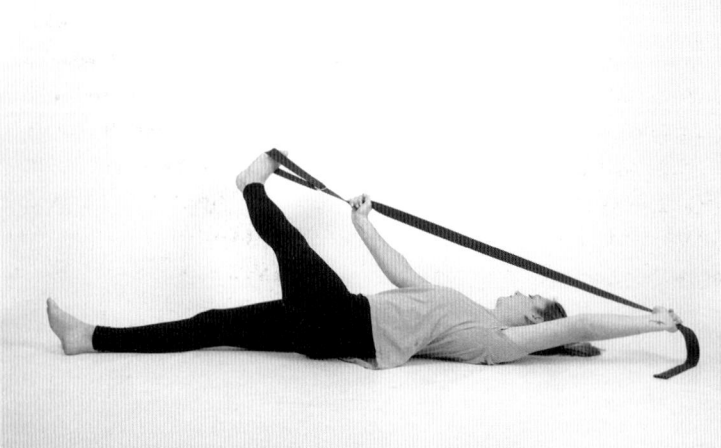

Figure 17.6
Leg Stretch 3

Description of therapeutic yoga forms

left elbow to rest on the ground to provide better leverage with the strap.
- Hold for several long breaths, then slowly raise the leg back overhead.

Leg Stretch 3 (Figure 17.6)

- Switch hand positions (now your right hand is halfway between your right foot and right arm, and your left arm is stretched over/behind head).
- Lower the left leg over toward the right side, coming over only as far as you can while keeping your sacrum grounded on the floor (your left hip will rise a bit). Hold for several long breaths.
- Slowly return to center, hold the strap ends with both hands, draw the knee to the chest, and release the strap from your foot.

NOTE: After performing the three leg stretches with one leg, rest for several breaths, and then repeat the stretches with the opposite leg.

Supine Twist (Figure 17.7)

- Draw the knees to the chest, then release the hands from the knees and position your arms out to the sides in a "T" position, with palms facing up.
- Draw in a nice slow breath, and as you exhale, slowly lower your legs partway down to the floor on the L side, then as you inhale, draw them back to center.
- Then, as you exhale, lower them part of the way to the right side, and inhale the legs back to center.
- Repeat slowly, exhaling to one side, inhaling to center, and exhaling to the opposite side, while keeping the back and shoulders on the floor and legs together.
- Then lower your legs all the way to the floor on the left side allowing them to completely rest on the floor.
- Invite your right shoulder to also release down to the floor, and invite any other muscles that you don't need right now to soften and release.
- You may wish to turn your head to face opposite your knees or keep your head in the center.
- Focus on your breath ... you might imagine your spine as a spiral staircase in the twist, sensing the breath climb up the staircase as you inhale and lengthen the spine, then sensing it sink back down to the base of your spine as you exhale.
- Repeat steps on the opposite side.

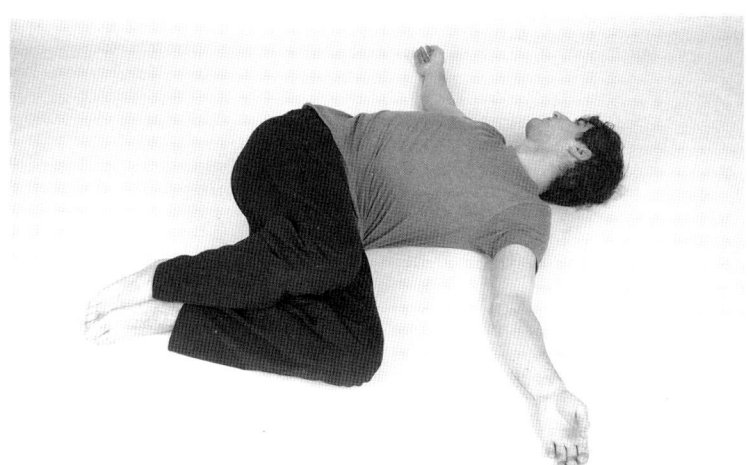

Figure 17.7
Supine Twist

Chapter 17

NOTES:

1. If your knees do not come all the way down to the floor, rest them on a bolster or folded blanket. You can also place a folded blanket between your legs. It is important that you feel completely supported to help you release unnecessary muscle tension.
2. The abdominal area has a very strong connection with the brain via the vagus nerve. Eighty percent of the vagal nerve fibers are afferent, and contribute to our emotional states (e.g. butterflies in the stomach). Twists are wonderful for releasing stress in the abdominal area. They also work like a sponge, squeezing out the stagnant body fluids and toxins while in the twist so that fresh, oxygenated blood will flow into the area as you release the twist.

Dynamic Sidelying Twist – Upper Body Variation

This is an adaptation of the *Slow Rolling Inhibitory Technique,* which has been used for decades by physical and occupational therapists to reduce hyperarousal of the autonomic nervous system (ANS). To perform this technique in the traditional manner, the therapist holds the client's hip and shoulder while

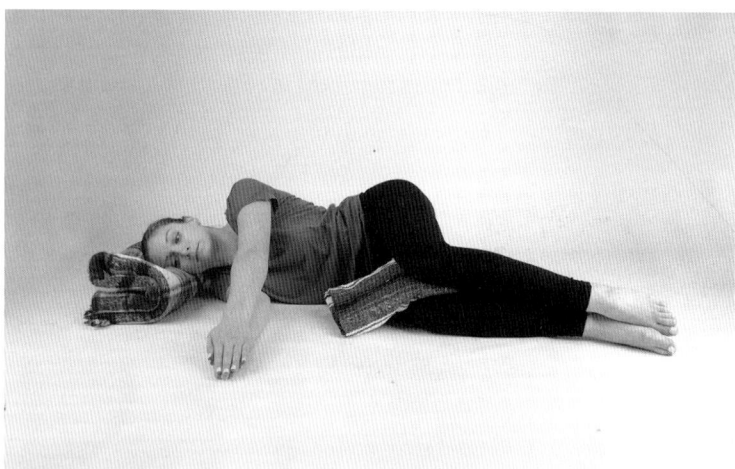

Figure 17.8

Dynamic Sidelying Twist – Upper Body Variation 1

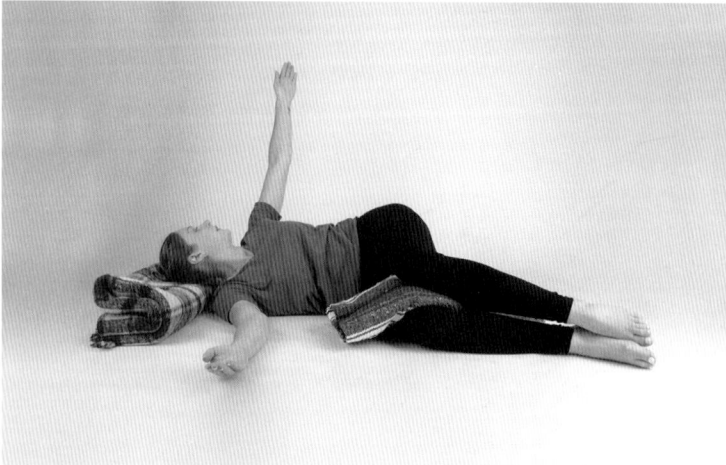

Figure 17.9

Dynamic Sidelying Twist – Upper Body Variation 2

Description of therapeutic yoga forms

rolling them slowly and rhythmically from supine to sidelying.[3(p. 77)] Follow these steps to perform the active yoga version:

- Start in sidelying, with your arms stretched straight out and your palms together. Align your hips and knees at 90 degrees (Figure 17.8).
- On an inhalation, slowly raise your top arm up and overhead (Figure 17.9), continuing until it rests on the floor on the opposite side of the body. As you do this, follow the moving hand with your head and eyes. Once the arm is placed on floor, invite both shoulder blades to rest on the floor (Figure 17.10).
- As you exhale, slowly lift your arm back up and over to its original position, so your palms are together once again. Again, head and eyes follow the hand.
- Repeat approximately six times on one side, then rest in the "twist" on that side, with both arms in a T-position, with your head facing opposite the legs.
- Repeat steps on the opposite side.

Yoga forms from Table

"Table" is the term yogis use for the basic hands and knees position. The purpose of the position is to

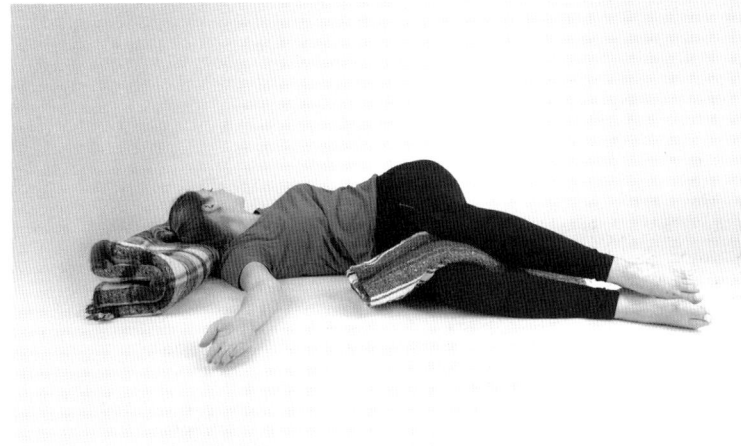

Figure 17.10

Dynamic Sidelying Twist – Upper Body Variation 3

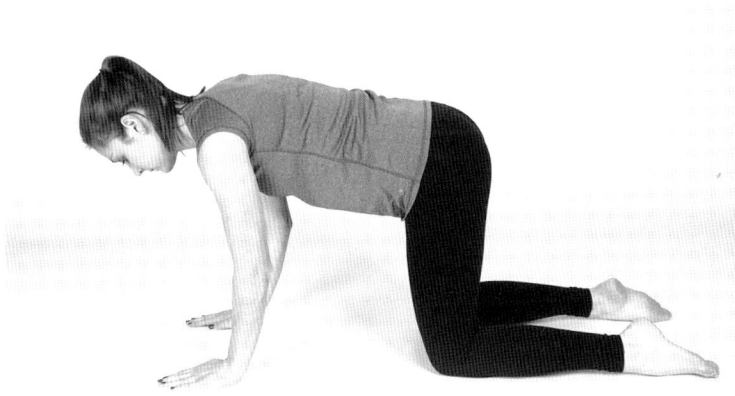

Figure 17.11

Table

Chapter 17

facilitate good alignment in yoga forms that originate from this position. It is a good idea to offer Child as a resting form between other Table forms that require heavy muscle work or balancing effort, such as Spinal Balance or Downward-Facing Dog.

Table (Figure 17.11)

- Come onto the hands and knees.
- Place the knees directly under the hips, hip distance apart.
- Position the creases of the wrists directly under the shoulders, shoulder width apart.
- Gaze downward, keeping the neck long and in line with the rest of the spine.

Cat/Cow (Figures 17.12 and 17.13)

- Come into Table (see above).
- As you inhale, lift the tailbone, allowing your belly to release downward, forming a small hollow in the lower back (similar to a cow), as you lift your head to look straight ahead.
- As you exhale, tuck your tailbone under and round your back up toward the ceiling (like an angry cat), pulling your navel up toward your spine, and allow your head to drop between your arms.

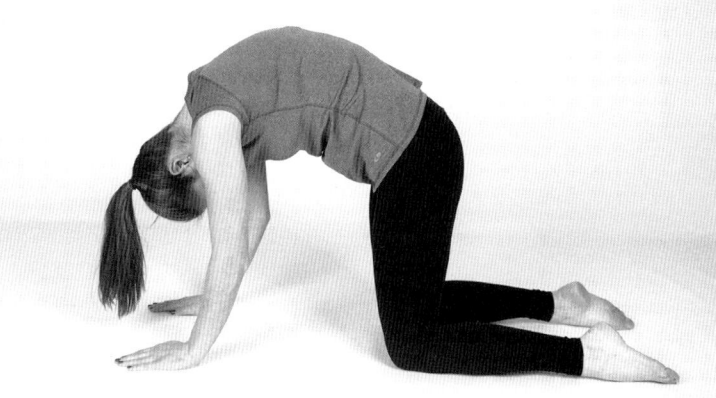

Figure 17.12
Cat

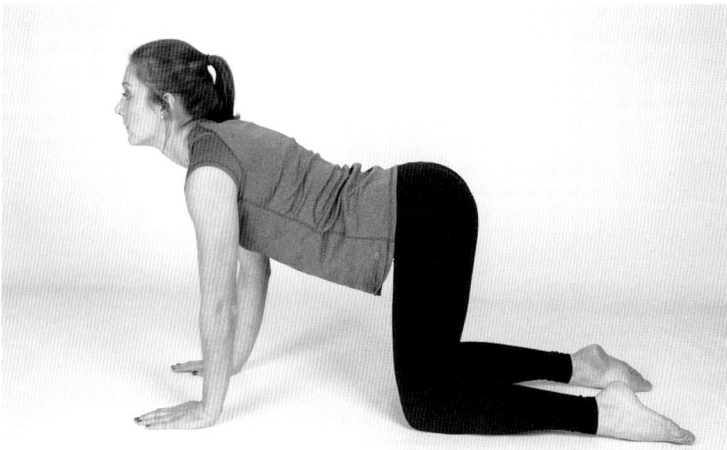

Figure 17.13
Cow

Description of therapeutic yoga forms

- Alternate between cat and cow several times, inhaling as you move into cow, and exhaling as you move into cat.
- Keep the arms straight but don't lock the elbows.

Alternative flow (Chakravakasana): Inhale into Table and exhale into Child.

Tiger Flow to Spinal Balance (Figures 17.14–17.16)

- (While in Cat/Cow flow …) If you choose, on your next exhale, you could pull your left knee in toward your forehead (Figure 17.14), and as you inhale, extend your left leg so it is parallel to the floor (Figure 17.15). (Repeat three more times.)
- The next time you raise your left leg parallel to the floor, hold it here as you continue to breathe. You can either press through the heel or point the toes. Focus your gaze downward to keep your neck long.
- You can decide to stay right where you are or challenge your balance more by hovering your left palm an inch or so off the mat, or by raising your left arm parallel to the floor, stretching through the fingertips (Figure 17.16).

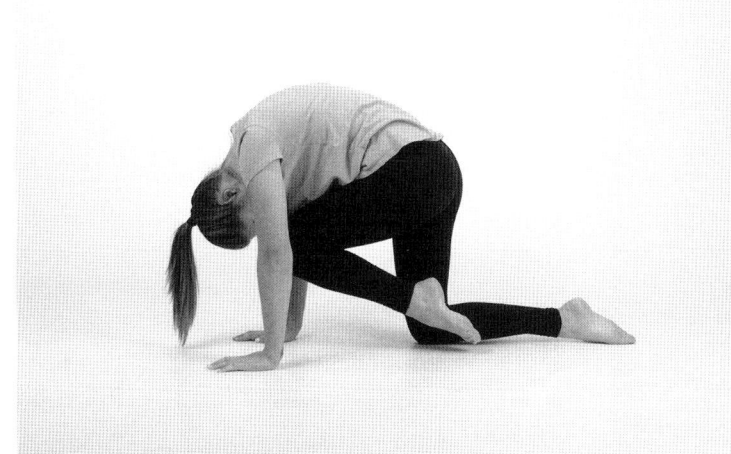

Figure 17.14
Tiger Flow to Spinal Balance 1

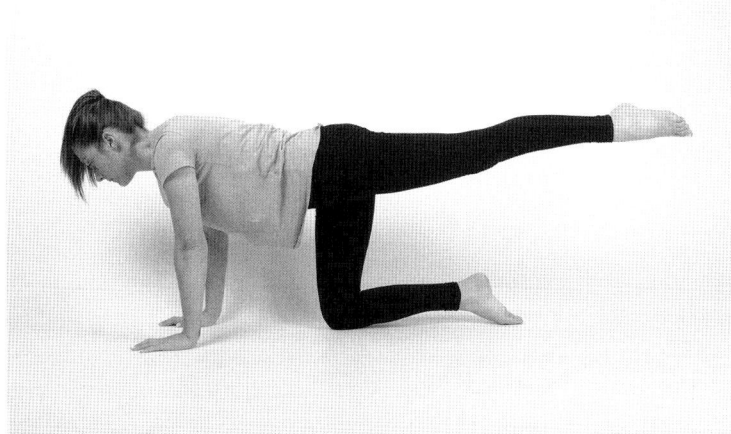

Figure 17.15
Tiger Flow to Spinal Balance 2

Figure 17.20) or Child as you sweep your right arm down to return the back of your hand against your sacrum. The crown of your head (Modified Hare) or forehead (Child) should barely hover over or lightly rest on your mat.

- Repeat these steps on your left side.
- Continue with this flow, slowly and smoothly with your breath, alternating sides with each inhale.
- Complete four rounds per side.

NOTE: Modified Hare is friendlier on the knees than coming all the way down into Child. The trunk and arm portion of this flow can also be done while sitting on the edge of a chair.

Modified Hare to Knee-Down Up Dog (Figure 17.21 and 17.22)

- From Table, lower your forearms to the floor to *position the crown of your head close to but not touching the mat*. (Your hips will shift backward but stay lifted off your legs.)
- Then slide your hands forward to fully extend your arms, and plant your hands slightly wider than shoulder-width apart. This is Modified Hare (Figure 17.21).

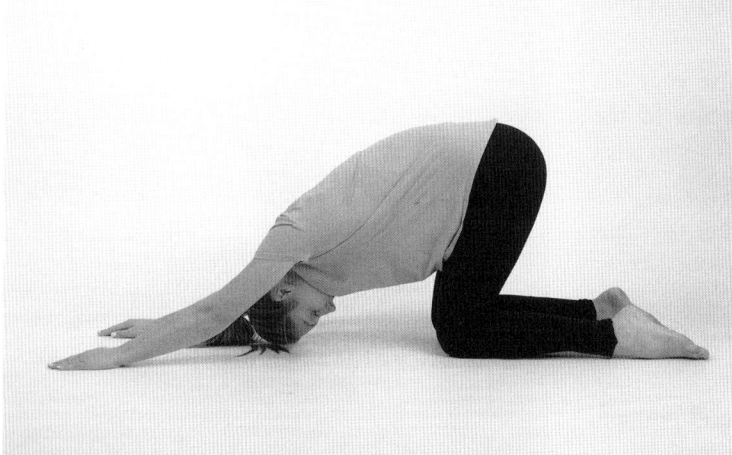

Figure 17.21
Modified Hare to Knee-Down Up Dog 1

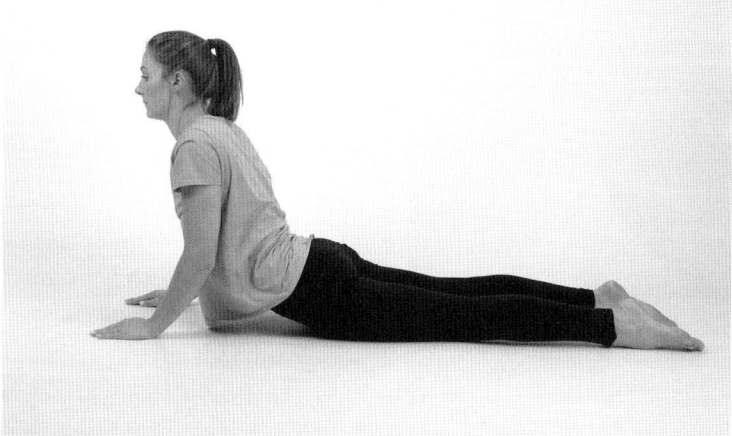

Figure 17.22
Modified Hare to Knee-Down Up Dog 2

Description of therapeutic yoga forms

- As you inhale, rise up through Table and continue to swing your hips forward and down as you lift your chest up through your arms, drawing your shoulder blades down and toward your spine (Figure 17.22). Keep your elbows slightly bent and your arms engaged, pushing the arms downward. Gaze straight ahead.
- As you exhale, return to Modified Hare.
- Continue to alternate between the forms, slowly and rhythmically, with the breath, inhaling into Knee-Down Up Dog and exhaling into Modified Hare.
- Perform 6–10 rounds.

Downward-Facing Dog (Figures 17.23 and 17.24)

- From Table, move your hands one "hands-length" forward.
- As you inhale, curl your toes under, and as you exhale, raise your hips into the air, lifting your knees off the ground.
- Keeping your knees bent, press the floor forward and away from you with your arms, to lengthen the spine.
- *Lift your tail and drop your chest.*
- Keep your head in line with your arms.
- Distribute the weight throughout your palm and fingers, especially the web space.

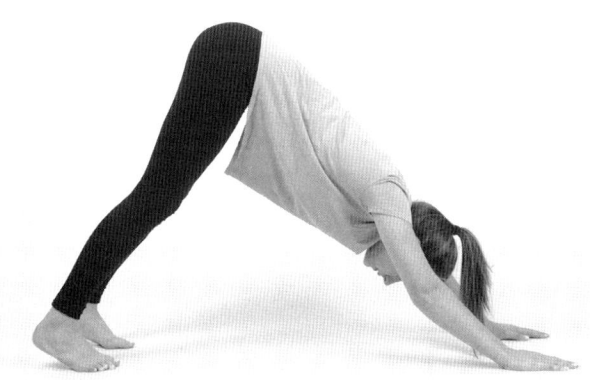

Figure 17.23
Downward Facing Dog – *Correct*

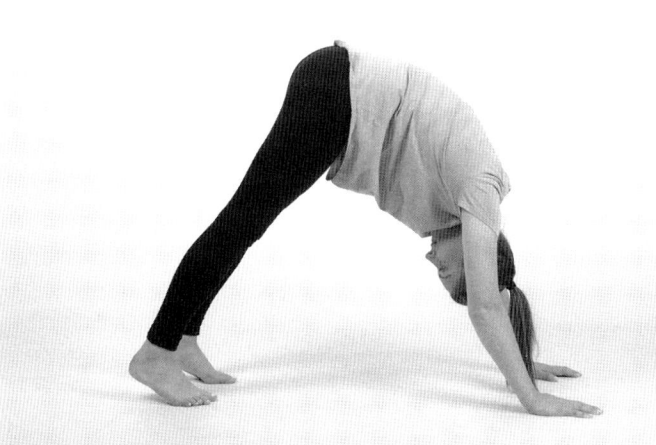

Figure 17.24
Downward-Facing Dog – *Incorrect*
(Note rounded back; to correct, *bend the knees and push the floor forward and away from you as you lift your "tail" and drop the chest.*)

Chapter 17

- You might like to "walk your dog" by alternately pressing one heel lower to the floor while bending the opposite knee, to loosen the hamstrings.
- As you are ready, rise up on the balls of your feet and then slowly press both heels downward toward the floor to straighten the legs only as far as is comfortable, but not at the expense of losing the length in the spine and straining the back (Figure 17.23).
- *Teachers*: If you see something like this (Figure 17.24), determine whether the hands are too close to the feet (as they are here), and again coach your student to bend the knees (to help release the hamstrings), lift the tail (without over-arching the back), and push the floor forward with the arms to lengthen the spine.

Down Dog to Up Dog Flow (Figures 17.25 and 17.26)

- Assume Down Dog (Figure 17.25), but position your hands slightly wider than shoulder distance apart.
- On your next inhalation, swing your hips down as you lift your chest up through your arms, staying

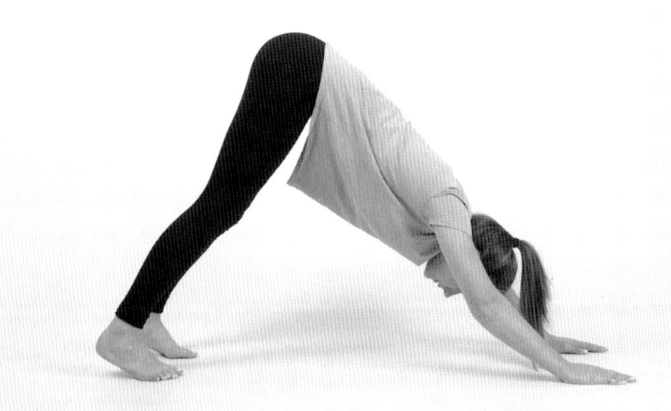

Figure 17.25
Down Dog to Up Dog Flow 1

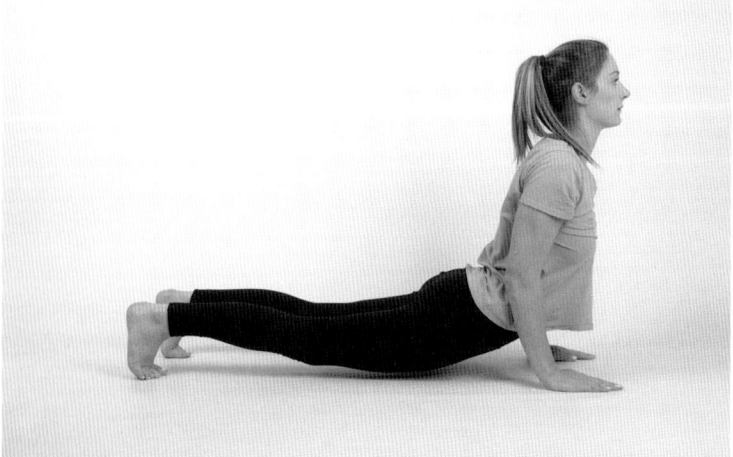

Figure 17.26
Down Dog to Up Dog Flow 2

Description of therapeutic yoga forms

on the toes of your feet (Figure 17.26). As you lift your chest up through the arms, draw the shoulder blades down and toward the spine, keeping your elbows slightly bent and close to your sides. Gaze straight ahead or slightly downward.

- As you exhale, push yourself back into Down Dog, pressing the floor forward and away with your arms as you lift your hips back up in the air, bending your knees as necessary to achieve a lengthened spine.
- Continue to alternate between the two forms, very slowly and rhythmically, with the breath, inhaling into Up Dog and exhaling into Down Dog.

Caution: Do not attempt this powerful flow unless you can safely assume each of the two yoga forms and have sufficient strength and endurance to perform the flow. This is not a move for beginners, but is a wonderful flow for those who are fit enough for it as it combines powerful therapeutic deep touch pressure (through the palms), proprioceptive input (through heavy muscle work), and slow, rhythmic movement.

Alternative option: Flow between Down Dog and Plank.

When doing rhythmic flows, do not pause at the end ranges, but instead move similar to a slow swing or rocking chair, theoretically to obtain the optimal inhibitory effect on the autonomic nervous system.

Child (Figure 17.27)

- From Table, separate your knees further apart, then lower your hips to your heels and drape your body over your legs.
- You may rest your arms alongside your body (Figure 17.27), or for an active stretch, feel free to extend them out on the floor over your head for Extended Child.
- Rest your forehead on the floor. If your forehead doesn't reach, you can support your head on a block or on your fists stacked on top of each other.
- Rest in the center of your being, releasing all tension and effort.

NOTE: If this is hard on your knees, you can place a cushion between your hips and your heels and may also want to place a folded blanket over your mat prior to assuming Child. Also see **Restorative Child**, in Chapter 13.

Standing forms

In yoga, all standing forms start from **Mountain**, which is a straight upright posture with the feet hip distance

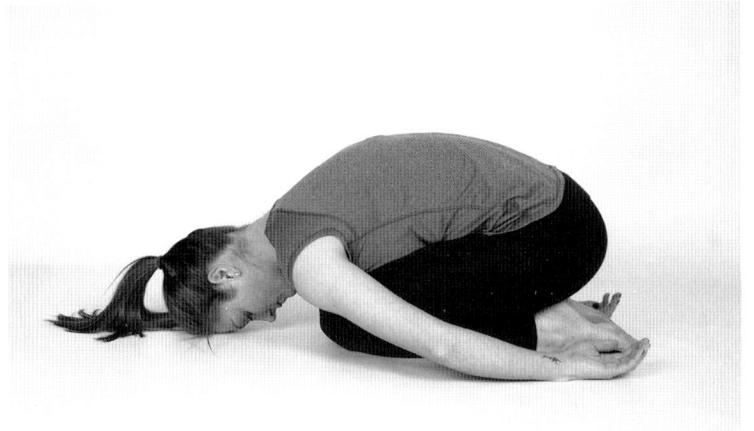

Figure 17.27
Child

Chapter 17

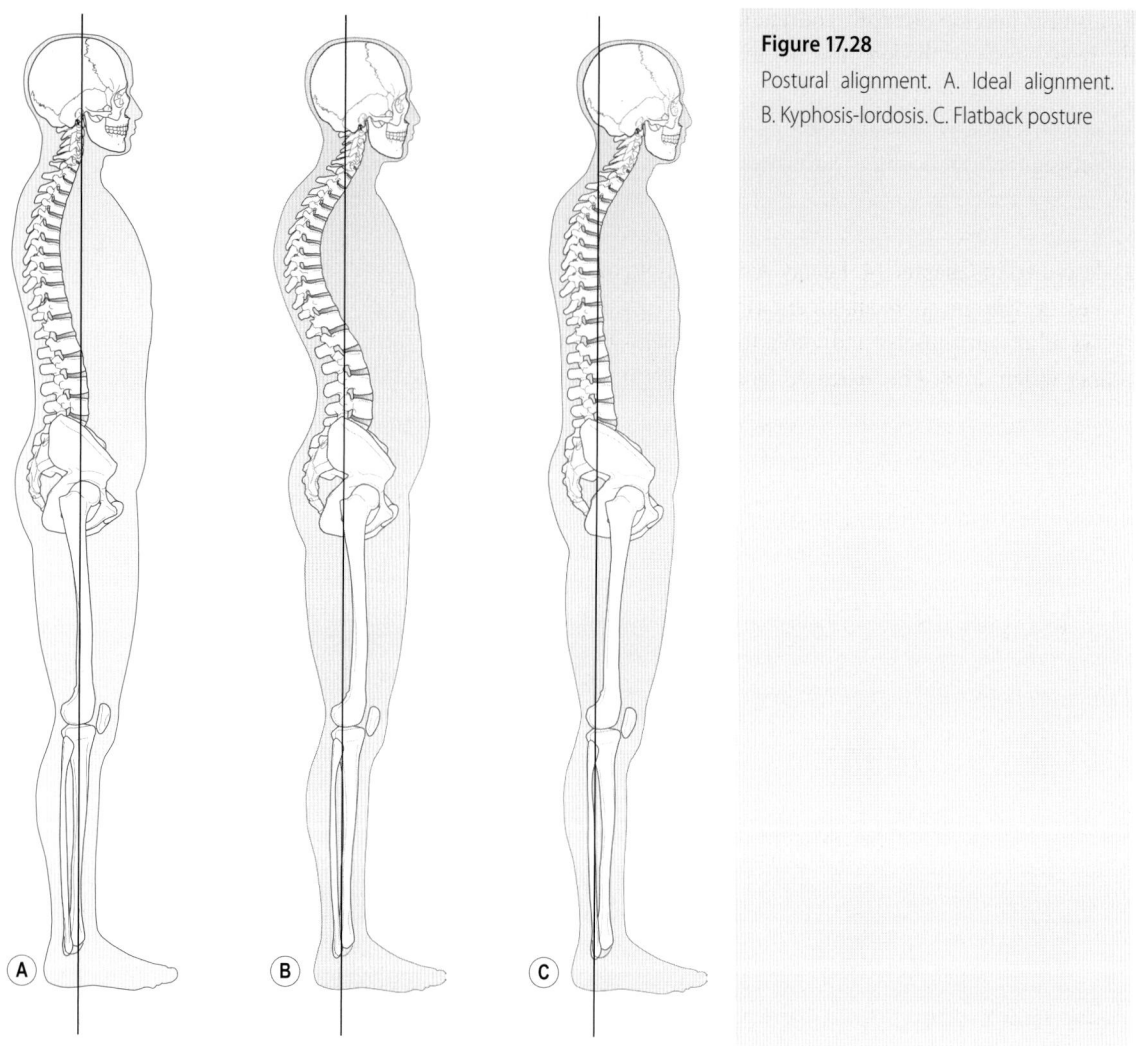

Figure 17.28
Postural alignment. A. Ideal alignment. B. Kyphosis-lordosis. C. Flatback posture

apart and the body well aligned over the center of gravity. **Mountain** helps us to become better aware of and improve our postural alignment both on and off the mat. Yet it goes deeper than that, as our postural alignment defines our very relationship to gravity. Many idioms in our culture acknowledge the relationship of gravity to our sense of well-being. When we are experiencing a lot of stress in our lives, and especially when undergoing major life or relationship changes, we talk of feeling "knocked off-balance" or "off-kilter." As you learned earlier (Chapter 13), this is not simply a figure of speech, as our level of stress can actually influence the functioning of the labyrinth of the inner ear, which is responsible for our sense of head movement through space, i.e. our vestibular sense.

Virtually all standing forms provide a balance challenge, and thus stimulate and strengthen the functioning of the labyrinth. Even forms that challenge balance more subtly, such as **Mountain**, serve this purpose by drawing our attention to the subtle details of our head and body position in space. Most standing

Description of therapeutic yoga forms

forms also develop strength and endurance, through the heavy work of the legs and the effort required to position the arms in space. Enhanced physical strength and endurance contributes to a sense of mental strength and endurance, and "grounding." This is an example of the power of the body to influence the mind. We can accentuate this effect by providing positive suggestions, as described in Chapter 14. Finally, when we hold our bodies upright in good alignment (Figure 17.28), it allows all of our muscles and joints to work with the proper weight load. The increased length in the spine frees up space in the abdominal cavity for the organs to function more efficiently. The lungs can expand more freely, improving respiratory function, which in turn supports all of the cells of the body.

Spine neutralizers for standing yoga forms

In yoga school, we learn the importance of offering a spine neutralizer following yoga forms that strongly pull the spine out of its natural shape. The best counterform for most standing yoga forms is a **Standing Forward Fold** (or **Wide-Legged Forward Fold**). The appropriate counterform for forward folds is a mild backbend, such as Baby Cobra, Crocodile, or if standing, placing the palms on the lower back, and on an inhalation, lengthening the spine upward while slightly leaning back, drawing the shoulder blades together to expand the chest. It can be okay to string two or three yoga forms together that stretch the spine in a similar way (e.g. twists or backbends) before offering the counterform, but this depends on the amount of stress the yoga form puts on the spine as well as one's level of endurance holding the form.

Mountain

Mountain is built from the ground-up, starting with the feet. **Position the feet hip distance apart** means the distance between the centers of each hip joint, which is far closer to midline than the fleshy parts of our hips (Figure 17.29). When the feet are positioned correctly, typically you can place a fist or two at most between the feet.

You might next make the suggestion to **position the toes straight forward**, though keep in mind that each body is different, and for some, pointing the toes is a long term goal to strive for (or even contraindicated if it causes the hips and knees to turn inward or outward).

Next, you might suggest to **rock slightly forward and backward ... and left to right ... to feel all four sides of the feet ... and then plant the entire surface of both feet (except for the arches) into the floor, aligning the body so the center of gravity is directly over the arches of the feet**. Not only does this help with alignment, but it draws the client's attention to their connection with the earth, which can help to foster a sense of security for those who are anxious and feeling like they are floating in space.

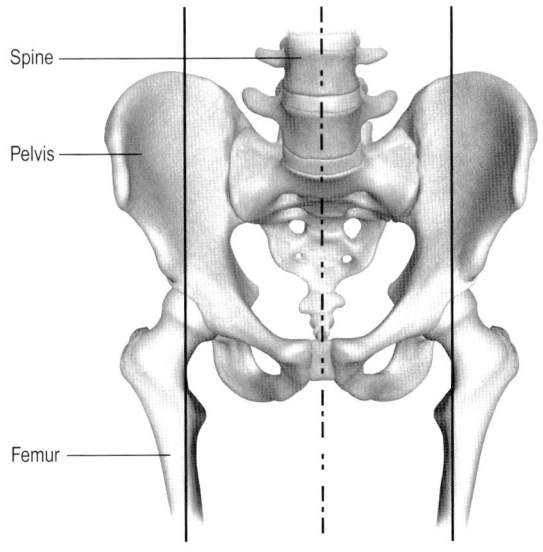

Figure 17.29

Center of hip joints

Chapter 17

Next, ask your client to **engage the muscles of the legs**. However, since this can be too "abstract" for those who have lost the connection to their bodies, I find it helpful to add, **and lift the knee caps to engage the quadriceps muscles**. Lifting the knee caps can be a more accessible feat to accomplish.

To level the pelvis and align the lower spine, you might suggest your client **engage the core by gently moving the navel toward the spine**. A suggestion to **slightly tuck the tail** also works well for many people to level the pelvis. However, individuals who have a flat lower back (reduced lumbar curve) or who rest their torso on their pelvis will benefit from the opposite suggestion to **slightly lift the tail**.

Next, for seasoned yogis, it is usually enough to say "lengthen the spine all the way up through the crown of the head"; however, people starting out in yoga often have little awareness of how to make that happen. So, it is helpful to say, **imagine there is a string coming down from the ceiling, attached to the crown of your head, gently pulling the crown of the head upward, stretching the spine nice and long ...**

Or, alternatively, you might suggest the following: *lift the waist out of the pelvis ... and then lift the ribcage out of the waist.*

Then, **while maintaining the length in the spine, allow the shoulders to release downward away from the ears, allowing gravity and the weight of your arms to do all the work, without effort.**

Next, we have an opportunity to enhance self-awareness of the amount of effort they are expending in the form: **notice the muscles of your face ... whether they are relaxed or tense, and invite them to soften and release.**

And finally, and always, reconnecting to the breath: **sense the increased spaciousness within the abdominal cavity ... and how this affects the breath ... just notice the breath, without any need to change it ...**

Standing stretches with strap

One way to provide enhanced muscle and joint input in standing is by using a yoga strap. Here are some suggested stretches:

Extended Mountain (Figure 17.30)

- Fold the strap in half and hold it with both hands, positioning your hands slightly more than shoulder width apart.

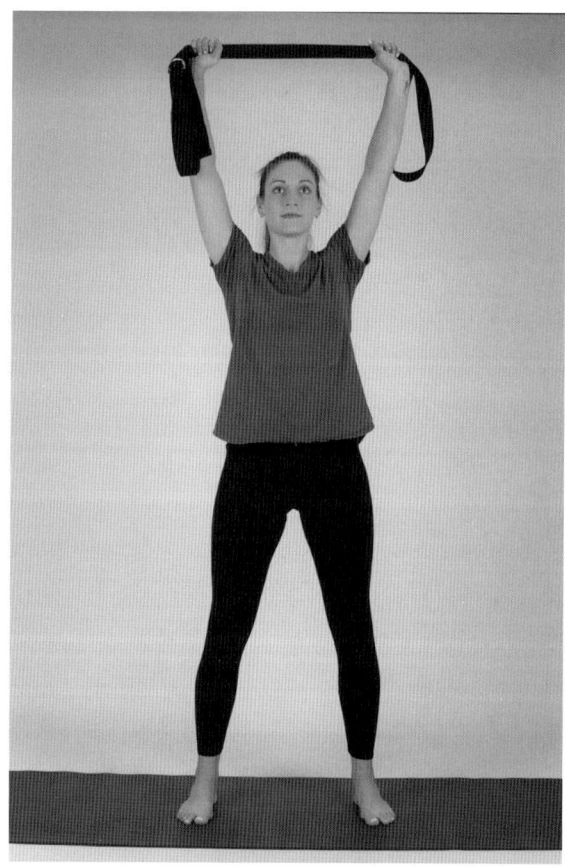

Figure 17.30
Extended Mountain

Description of therapeutic yoga forms

- Then assume Mountain, taking several breaths in this position.
- On your next inhalation, raise your arms overhead. Release your shoulders down away from your ears.
- Pull your arms out against the strap in this position to increase muscle activation in the arms. Hold in Extended Mountain for 3–4 breaths.

Side Stretch (Figure 17.31)

- Fold the strap in half and hold it with both hands, positioning your hands slightly more than shoulder width apart.

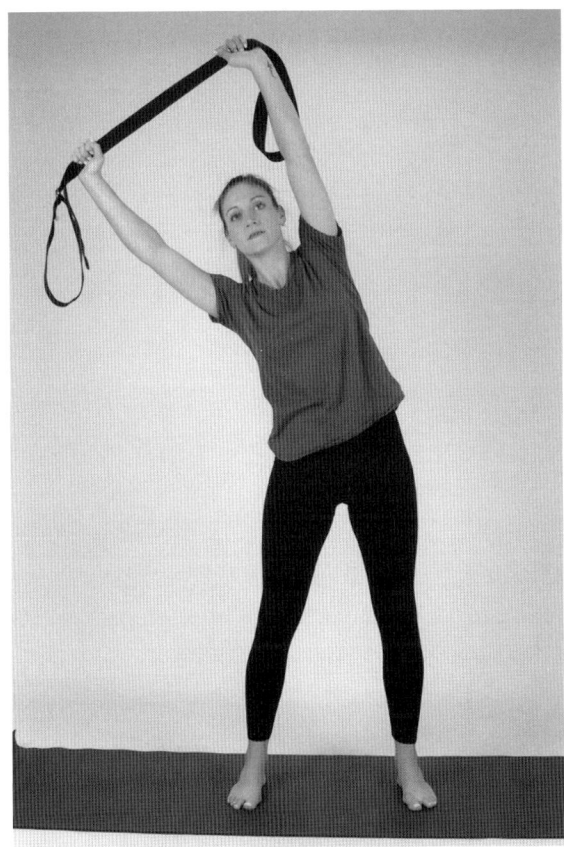

Figure 17.31
Side Stretch

- As you inhale, raise your arms overhead. Release your shoulders down away from your ears while pulling your arms out against the strap to increase muscle activation in the arms.
- As you exhale, bend toward one side, while lengthening upward.
- Be sure not to collapse the underside—stretch that side, too.
- Take a few breaths into the side of the ribcage that is being stretched.
- Inhale back to center and exhale to the opposite side, repeating the steps on that side.

Standing Twist with Strap (Figures 17.32 and 17.33)

- Stand with feet slightly further than hip distance apart, with toes pointing slightly outward.
- Hold the strap in your fists, so that your fists are just a bit more than shoulder distance apart, with arms in front of you at the level of the shoulders, elbows straight.
- Bend the knees, keeping the torso vertical.
- Keep the hips facing forward throughout the twist (this is key to avoid torqueing the knees, and to ensure that the twist is actually happening in the spine).
- Inhale, and as you exhale, twist the torso so the arms swing toward the left, keeping shoulder blades drawn back and down, and your gaze following your left hand.
- Inhale back toward the center, and exhale to the opposite side.
- Repeat until you have completed about three twists per side, moving smoothly with your breath.

CAUTION: The twist is not intended to be held, but is a movement flow with the breath.

Chapter 17

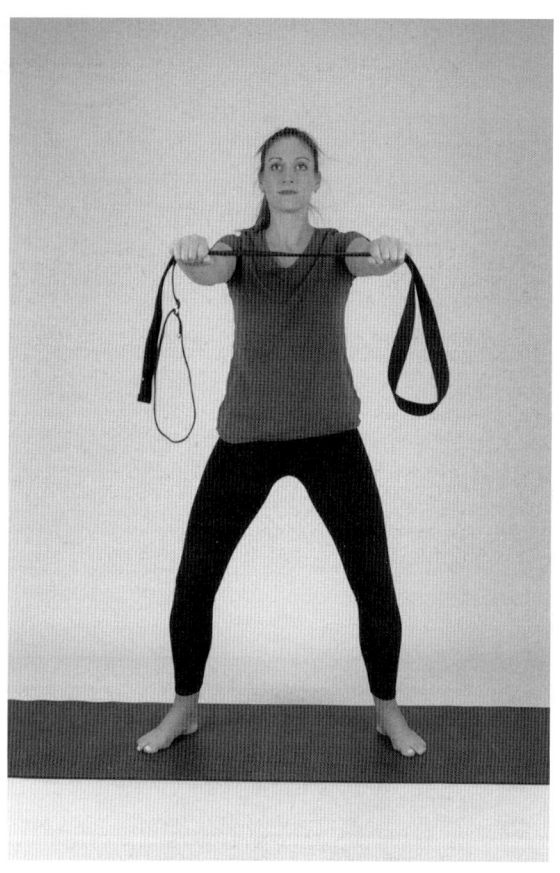

Figure 17.32
Standing Twist with Strap 1

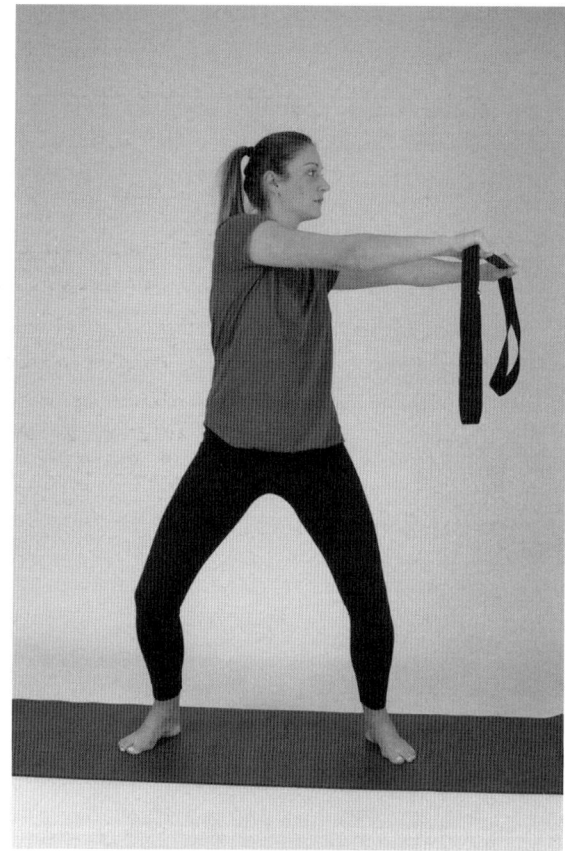

Figure 17.33
Standing Twist with Strap 2

Cow Face (Arm Version) (Figure 17.41)

First comes the Warm-Up Stretch (Figures 17.34 to 17.40).

Start with a few **Modified Sun Breaths** as a warm-up exercise, as follows:

- Place your palms together at the heart center (Figure 17.34).
- As you inhale, swing your arms out to the sides (Figure 17.35) and overhead, and re-connect your palms overhead (Figure 17.36).
- Exhale as you bend your elbows so your connected palms point down behind your neck (Figure 17.37). Try to keep your upper arms close to your head.
- Inhale your palms back overhead (Figure 17.38).
- Exhale as you swing your arms out to your sides (Figure 17.39) and re-connect your palms back at your heart center (Figure 17.40).
- Repeat a few times to prepare the muscles for the Cow Face Stretch.

Description of therapeutic yoga forms

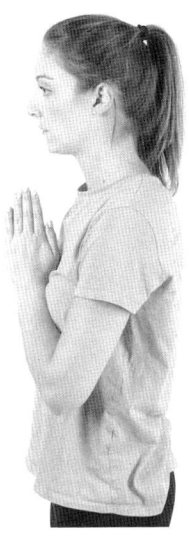

Figure 17.34
Warm-Up Stretch 1

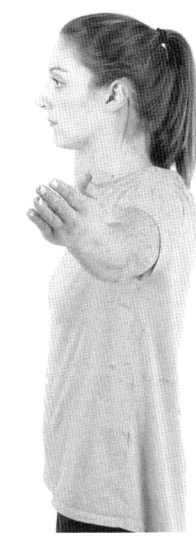

Figure 17.35
Warm-Up Stretch 2

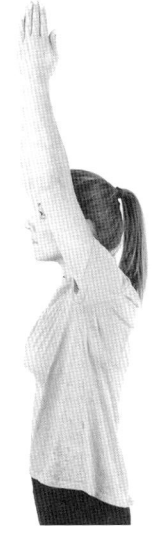

Figure 17.36
Warm-Up Stretch 3

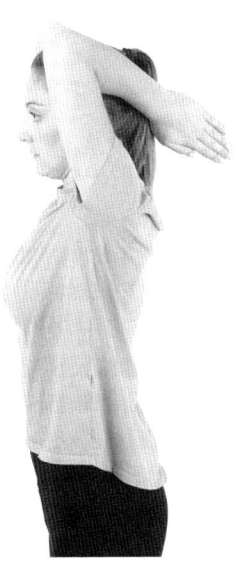

Figure 17.37
Warm-Up Stretch 4

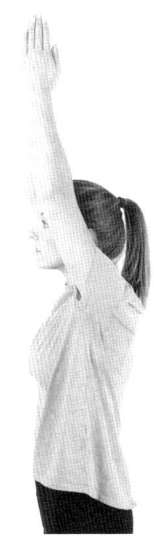

Figure 17.38
Warm-Up Stretch 5

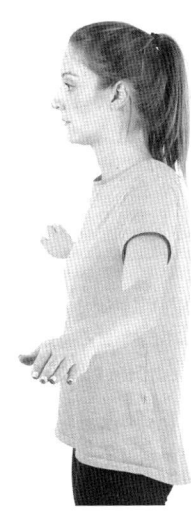

Figure 17.39
Warm-Up Stretch 6

Chapter 17

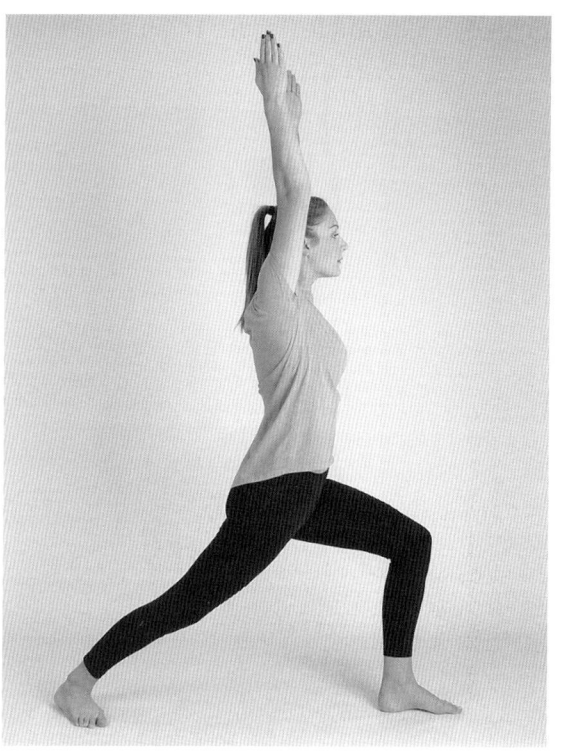

Figure 17.44

Dynamic Warrior I – static hold

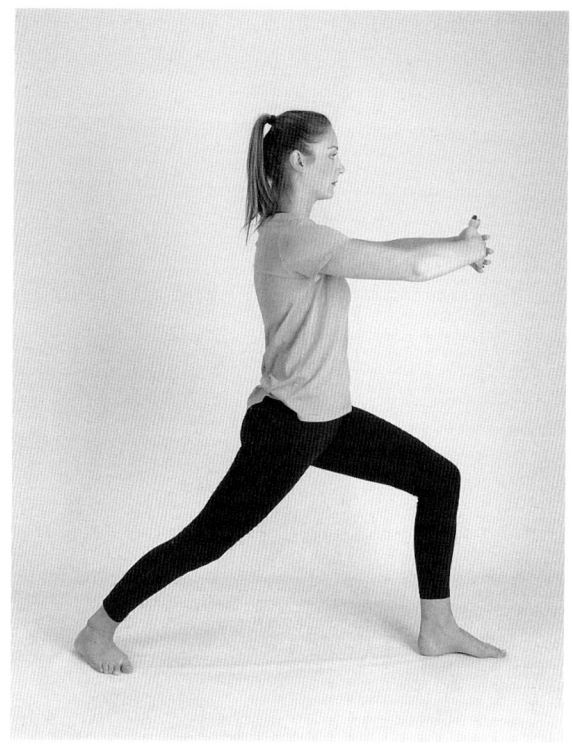

Figure 17.45

Dynamic Warrior I – with Vajrapradama mudra

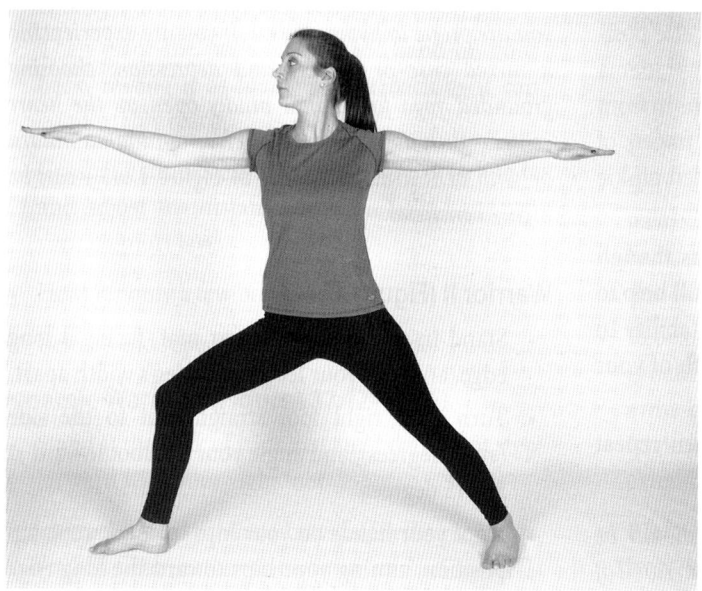

Figure 17.46

Warrior II

Description of therapeutic yoga forms

of the mat without torqueing your right knee out of alignment. (Due to body mechanics, your hips will actually be positioned somewhat diagonally.)
- Bend your right knee until your knee is directly over (but does not bend past) your ankle.
- Raise your arms to out to the sides at shoulder height.
- Turn your head to the left to check that your left arm, wrist and fingers are straight and parallel to the floor.
- Then turn your head to the right to gaze over your right fingertips.
- Hold Warrior II for several breaths, and then repeat the steps on the other side.

With practice, you may find that you are able to adjust your right foot further away from your body so your hips sink further, allowing the right thigh to approach a position more parallel to the floor.

Extended Side Angle (Figure 17.47)
- Assume Warrior II with your left leg forward.
- Laterally bend your torso toward your bent leg and rest your left proximal forearm (the area close to your elbow) on your left thigh with your palm facing upward.
- Place the back of your right wrist against your lower back and draw your right shoulder back to facilitate rotating your torso so your heart center is facing forward.
- Once your torso and shoulder are aligned, raise your right arm overhead until it comes parallel to your left ear with your palm facing downward.
- Gaze upward and toward the right, past your armpit.
- Hold for several breaths, then switch sides.

Reverse Warrior (Figure 17.48)
- Assume Warrior II with your left leg forward.
- Turn your left palm up.

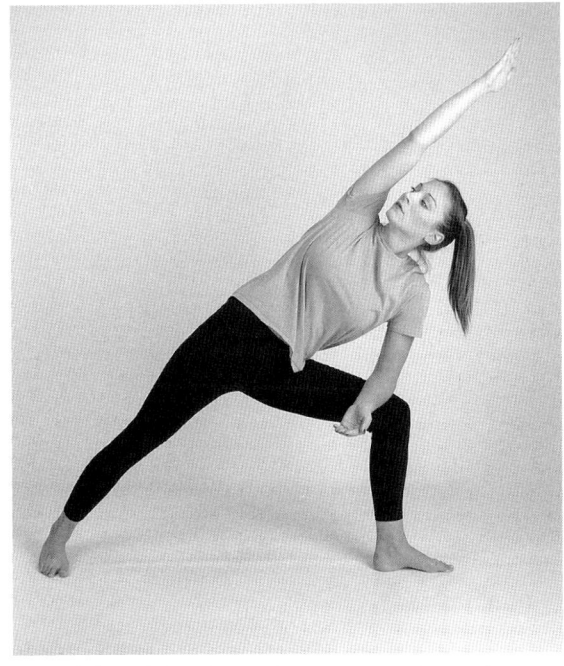

Figure 17.47
Extended Side Angle

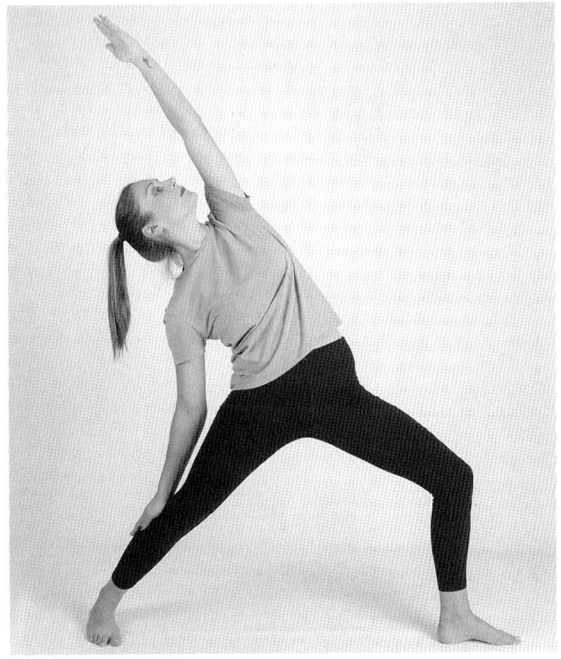

Figure 17.48
Reverse Warrior

Chapter 17

- Lower your right arm down to the back of your right thigh as you raise your right arm overhead with your palm facing toward you.
- As you move your arms, laterally bend your torso to the right and slide your right hand down your right leg as far as it will comfortably go.
- Gaze past your upper arm.
- Stay for approximately four breaths, focusing your awareness on the breath as it stretches and releases tension in your left ribcage.
- Repeat on the other side.

Follow Warrior forms (or a series of Warrior forms) with a Standing Wide-Legged Forward Fold (or a standard Standing Forward Fold, Figure 17.51).

Standing Wide-Legged Forward Fold with Block (Figure 17.49)

- Position a block within close reach before beginning Warrior forms.
- *(Following completion of any Warrior form)* Keeping your wide-legged Warrior stance, turn both feet to face the long edge of your mat with toes pointing slightly outward.
- Place your hands on your hips and take a nice long inhale, lengthening up through the crown of your head.
- As you exhale, slightly bend your knees to protect your lower back, and hinge forward from your hips. When your back is horizontal, lower your arms to the floor.
- Find your block and place it at its tallest height in the perfect spot to allow you to rest the crown of your head on it.
- Stay here for several breaths, and if it is helpful, imagine tension rolling off your back with each exhalation.

Standing Forward Fold (Figures 17.50 and 17.51)

- Stand in Mountain, with your feet hip distance apart, and place your hands on your hips. Lengthen up through the crown of your head.
- Soften the knees, and hinge at the hips until your back is horizontal. Avoid rounding the back (Figure 17.50).
- Once the back is horizontal, release your hands to the ground, allowing your head and arms to hang like a rag doll (Figure 17.51)

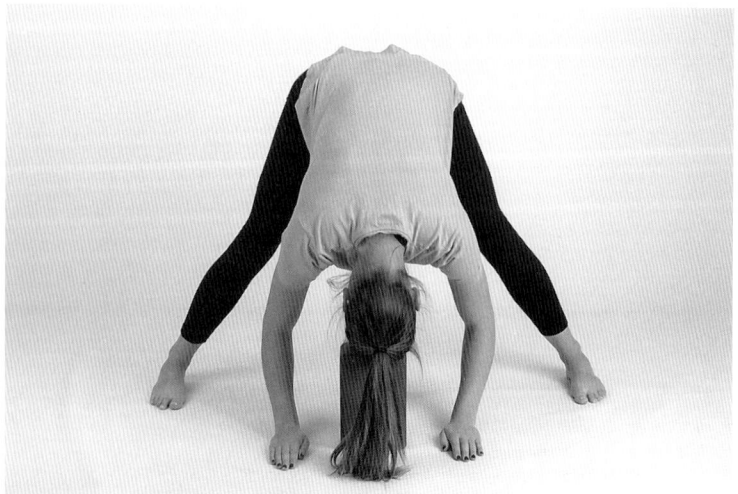

Figure 17.49

Standing Wide-Legged Forward Fold with Block

Description of therapeutic yoga forms

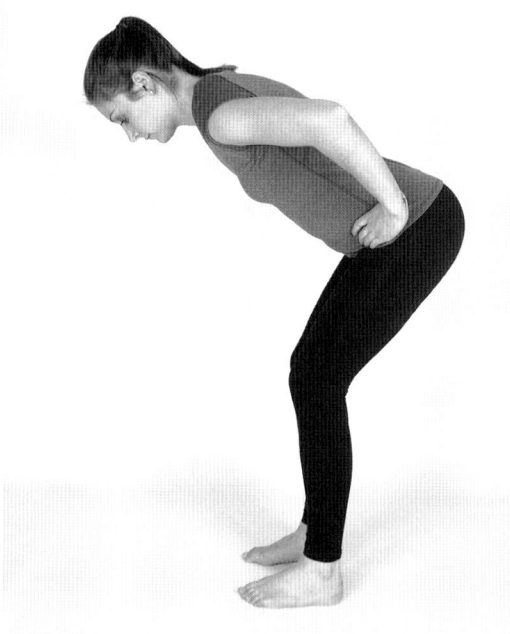

Figure 17.50
Standing Forward Fold

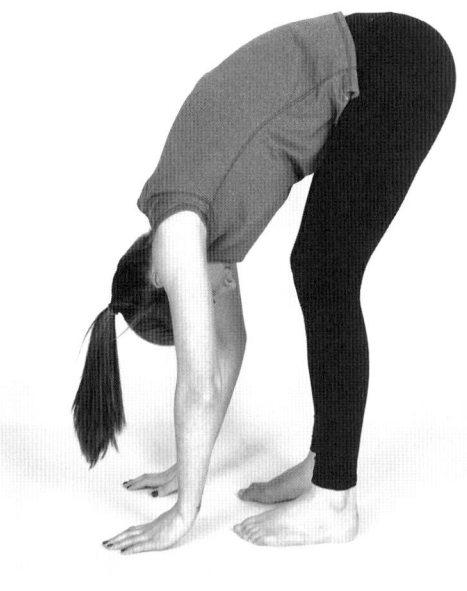

Figure 17.51
Standing Forward Fold

- Shake the arms a bit, then rock your head slowly back and forth, to release any tension.
- Stay for several breaths, and then return to standing by bending the knees, placing the hands back on the hips (or on the thighs), and coming back up with a straight back without rounding.

The above version is less stressful for the back. *If you are certain your client does not have any back issues, you may invite him or her to do the following:*

- Circle the arms out to the sides and up toward the ceiling (on an inhalation), then soften the knees, hinge at the hips, and swan dive forward with the arms coming out to the sides before reaching the ground next to the feet (on an exhalation).
- To rise back up, *bend the knees* (to protect the back), and as you inhale and turn your palms outward, raise the arms out to the sides and up overhead (palms now facing each other), then exhale the arms back down to your sides.

Tree (Figures 17.52–17.54)

- Stand arm distance away from a wall, so that when you raise your left arm out to your side at shoulder level, your palm lies flat on the wall without leaning toward or away from the wall. (*This step is optional, though beginners especially benefit from having a wall nearby to reach toward if they begin to completely lose their balance.*)
- Then remove your hand from the wall and assume Mountain with your palms together at the heart center (Namaste position).
- Find a non-moving focal point straight in front of you (not another person).

243

Chapter 17

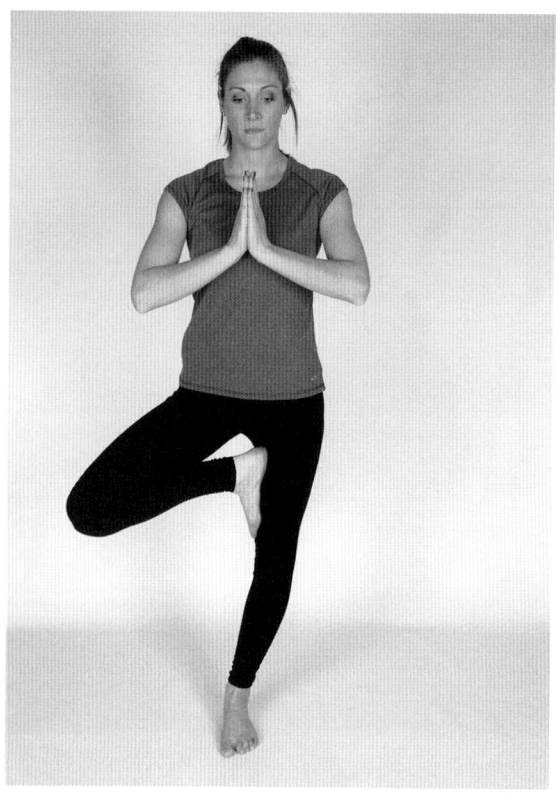

Figure 17.52
Tree 1

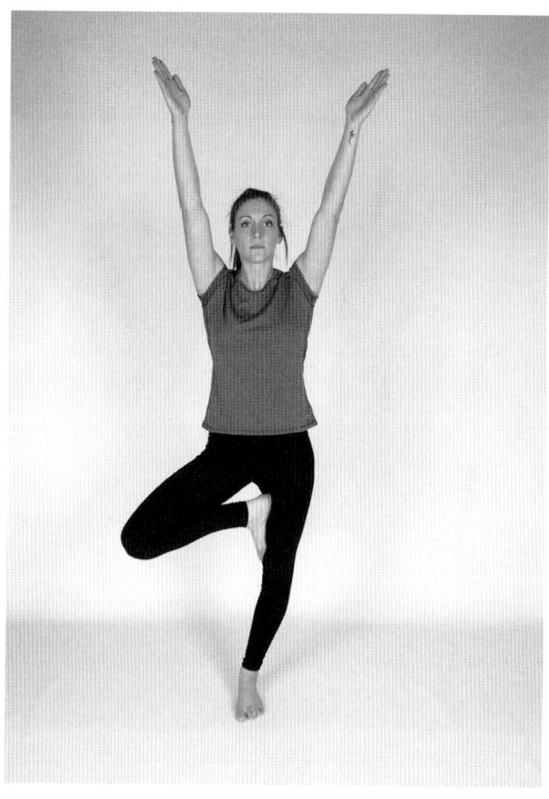

Figure 17.53
Tree 2

- Shift your weight to your left foot and turn your right foot so the heel is up on the left ankle and you are up on the toes of the right foot.
- You may wish to stay right here, or if you'd like more of a challenge, you may lift your right foot up onto your calf or onto your thigh (but not directly on the knee) (Figure 17.52).
- Keep your hips facing forward while aiming your right knee straight out to the side.
- If you wish to take it even further, you may slowly raise your arms overhead, stretching the arms and fingers upward with palms facing each other (Figure 17.53).

- To come out of **Tree**, slowly lower the arms and then place your right foot back on the floor.
- Repeat on the other side.
- *Modification*: Position a chair as shown in Figure 17.54 and hold onto it with one hand.

Crocodile (Figure 17.55)

- Lie on your stomach with your feet a bit apart and toes turned out.
- Cross the arms, holding the upper arms near the elbows.
- Pull the arms a bit closer to you so your chest is lifted.

Description of therapeutic yoga forms

- Then rest your forehead on your arms.
- Focus on your breath and the movement of your belly against the floor.

Baby Cobra (Figure 17.56)

- Lie on your stomach, keeping your legs together or slightly apart.
- Place your hands on the mat just beyond your head, touching your thumbs together and index fingers together.
- Engage the muscles of your legs and root the front of the hips and feet into the floor.
- Lift your head and chest, pressing your forearms into the mat.
- Pressing through the arms, lift your ribcage, and draw your shoulder blades down away from the ears.
- Stay for several breaths.

Cobra (Figure 17.57)

- Lie on your stomach keeping your legs together or slightly apart.
- Place your hands with fingers spread under your shoulders with your elbows close to your sides. Allow your forehead to rest on the floor.

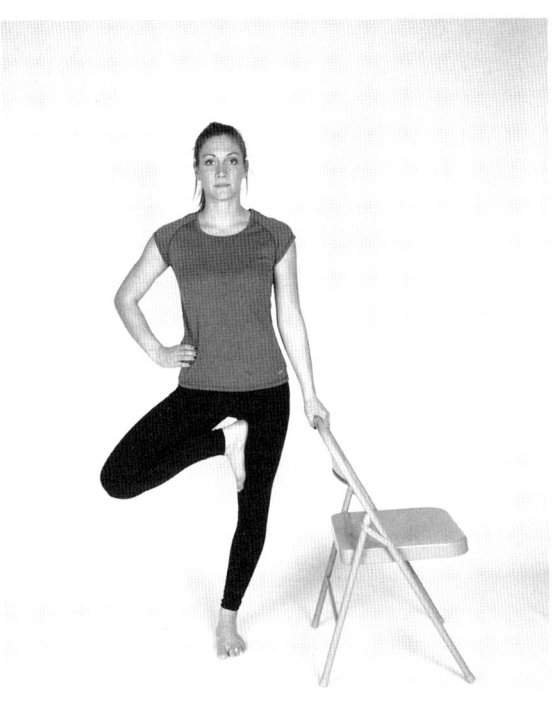

Figure 17.54
Tree 3

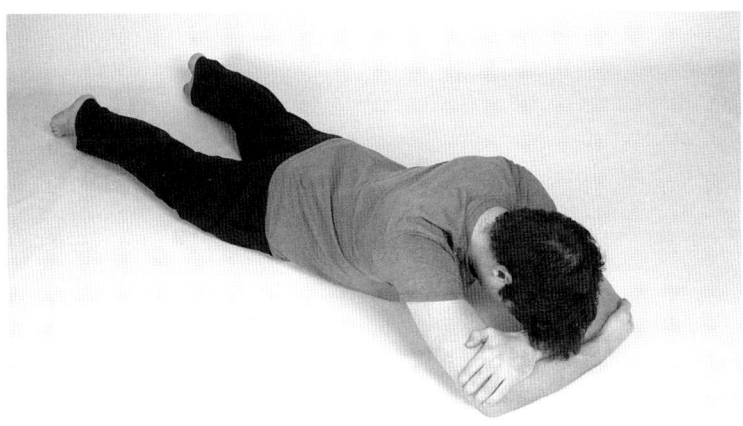

Figure 17.55
Crocodile

Chapter 17

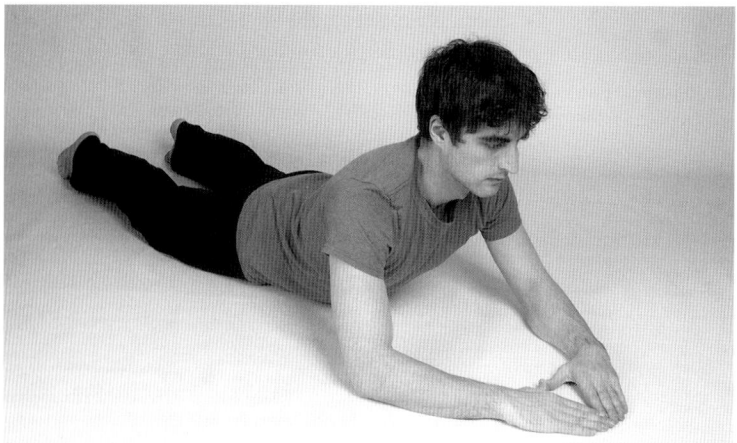

Figure 17.56
Baby Cobra

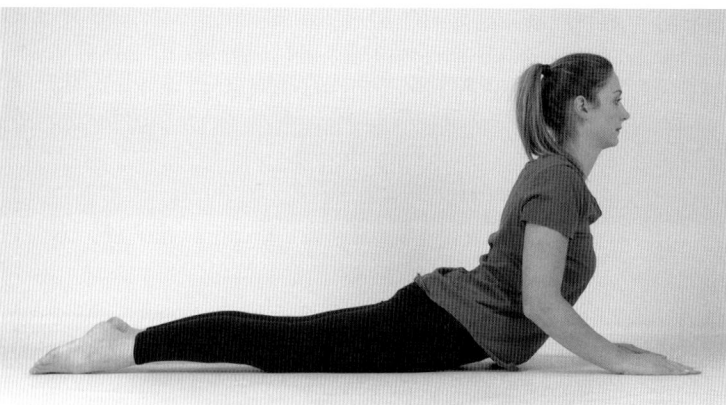

Figure 17.57
Cobra

- Engage the muscles of your legs and root the front of the hips and feet into the floor.

Tip: Lift your pubic bone upward toward your navel as you release your tailbone downward to lengthen your lower back.

- Inhale as you lift your head and chest off the floor, only rising as far as you can *without* pressing your hands into the floor; then exhale as you release back down to the floor.
- Repeat on the next inhalation, and after you have risen as far as you can just by using your back muscles, press through your palms and fingers to lift your ribcage off the floor, drawing your shoulder blades down and away from the ears, and pull the floor toward you with your palms to keep your back lengthened.
- Stay for several breaths, then release back down to the floor.
- Bend your knees and "windshield wipe" your lower legs to release any tension from your lower back.

Dynamic Head to Knee (Figures 17.58–17.60)

- Sit on the edge of a folded blanket to support the pelvis in a neutral position. (Do not sit on your sacrum; imagine you have a tail and lift it out from underneath you.)

Description of therapeutic yoga forms

- Extend both legs parallel to each other.
- Press your hands into the floor next to your hips, and take several breaths, lengthening up through the crown of your head with each inhalation and maintaining that length during each exhalation.
- Position the sole of your left foot against the inner surface of your upper right thigh.
- Maintaining a slight bend in your right knee, inhale your arms out to your sides and up overhead (Figure 17.58).
- As you exhale, bend your torso forward, hinging at the hips, as you draw your arms back with bent elbows (Figure 17.59). (This maintains expansion of the chest and prevents excessive rounding of the thoracic spine.)
- As you inhale, return to an upright position as you raise your arms back up overhead.
- Repeat this flow a few times with the breath, then on your next exhalation bend forward and hold onto your foot, leg, or a strap placed around the foot (Figure 17.60).
- Stay for at least 30 seconds, sensing your breath stretching the back of your body on each inhalation, and releasing muscle tension on each exhalation.
- Repeat on the other side.

Yoga forms using a chair

Seated Mountain (Figure 17.61)

- Sit a bit forward in your chair so your back is away from the backrest.
- Position your feet directly under your knees and rest your palms on your lower thighs (Figure 17.61).

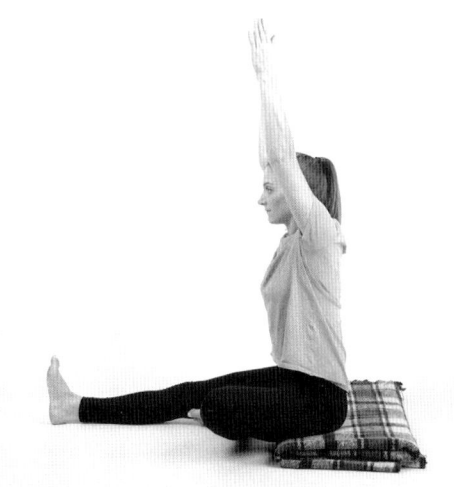

Figure 17.58
Dynamic Head to Knee 1

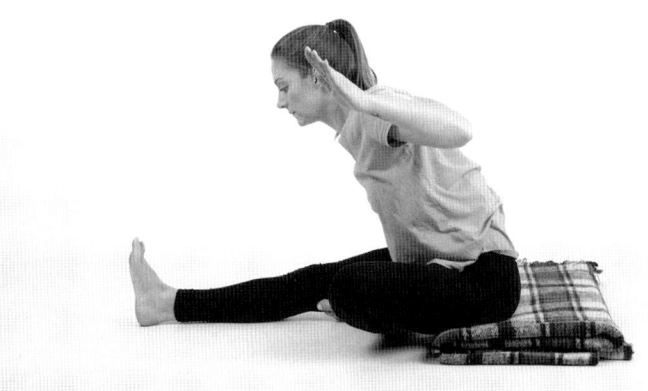

Figure 17.59
Dynamic Head to Knee 2

Chapter 17

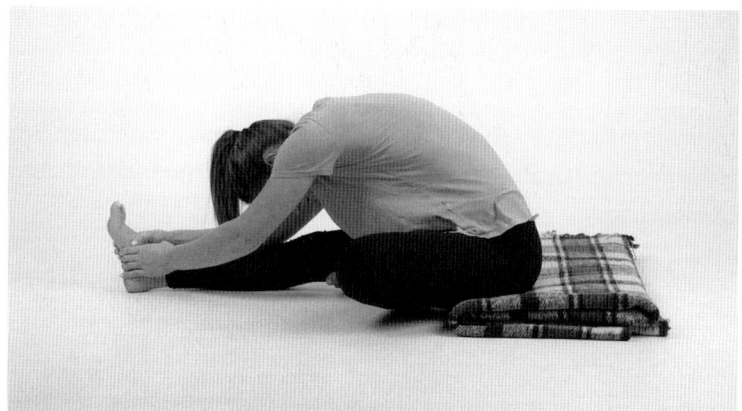

Figure 17.60
Dynamic Head to Knee 3

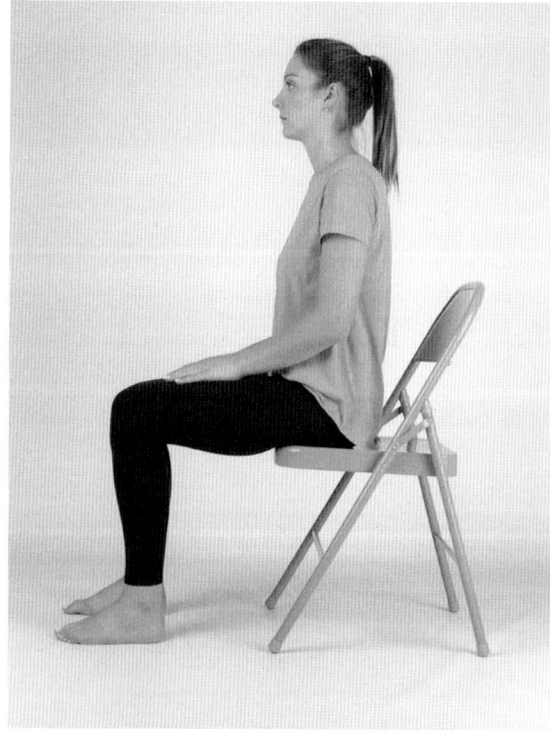

Figure 17.61
Seated Mountain

- Press your sitting bones into the seat surface and lengthen the spine all the way up through the crown of your head.
- Drop your shoulders down away from the ears.
- Draw your chin back to align your head over your torso (*not shown*).
- You may close your eyes or use a soft gaze.
- Focus on your breath.

Sun Breaths (Figures 17.62–17.64)

- Assume Seated Mountain with your arms hanging by your sides. (Be sure to press the sitting bones down into the chair as you lengthen up through the spine.)
- As you inhale, turn your palms up (Figure 17.62) as you raise your arms overhead (Figure 17.63).
- As you exhale, turn your palms down as you lower your arms back down toward your sides (Figure 17.64).
- Repeat 4–6 times, coordinating the movements with your breath.

This is a good substitution for Symmetrical Stretch on the mat.

Description of therapeutic yoga forms

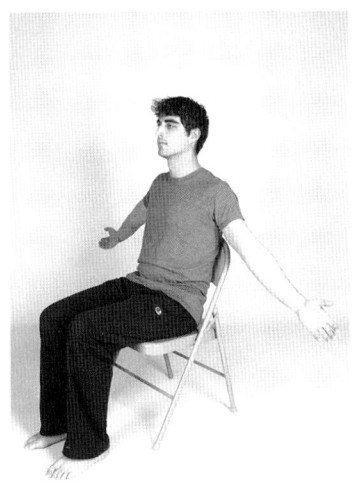

Figure 17.62
Sun Breaths 1

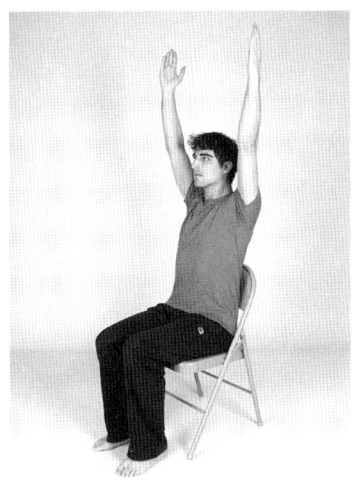

Figure 17.63
Sun Breaths 2

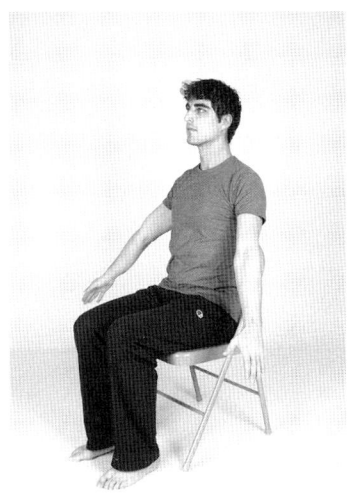

Figure 17.64
Sun Breaths 3

Seated Half-Moon Stretch (Figure 17.65)

- Assume Seated Mountain.
- Prepare for the stretch by holding onto the side edge of the chair with your left hand to help keep you stable.
- Turn your right palm up as you raise your arm overhead, and lean toward the left without collapsing the left side of your torso.
- Stretch up through the right side of your torso and all the way through to the fingertips of your right hand.
- Allow your head to release downward toward your left ear.
- *Direct your breath into the right ribcage*, sensing the small muscles between the ribs expand with each inhalation and release more and more with each exhalation.
- After 3–4 breaths, return to center and repeat these steps on the other side.

This is a good substitution for Supine Half-Moon Stretch.

Dynamic Knee to Chest to Extended Leg (Figures 17.66 and 17.67)

- Sit a bit forward in your chair and assume Seated Mountain.
- Inhale, and as you exhale, clasp your hands over your right knee as you raise it up toward your chest.
- As you inhale, extend your leg in front of you, supporting your leg by clasping your hands under your thigh.
- Repeat this flow around five times on the same side, exhaling as your flex your leg and inhaling as you extend your leg.
- *Optional*: Then maintain your leg extended as you flex and extend your ankle and/or make circles with your ankle in one direction and then the other.
- Slowly release your leg back to the floor and repeat this process with your other leg.

This is a good substitution for Knees to Chest on the mat.

249

Chapter 17

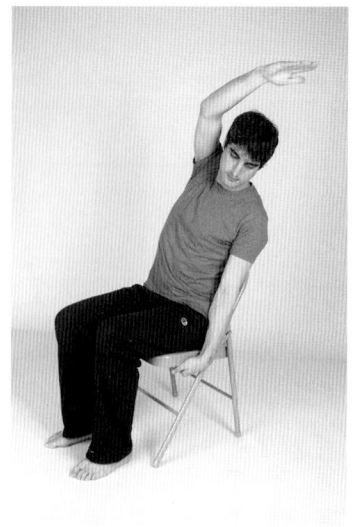

Figure 17.65
Seated Half-Moon Stretch

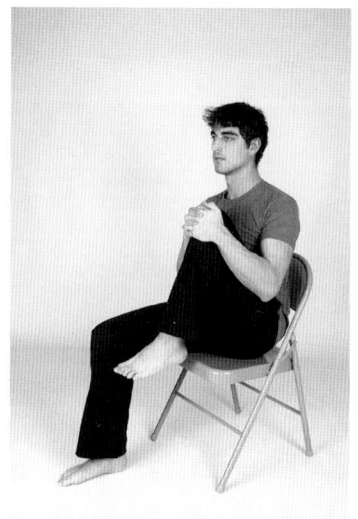

Figure 17.66
Dynamic Knee to Chest to Extended Leg 1

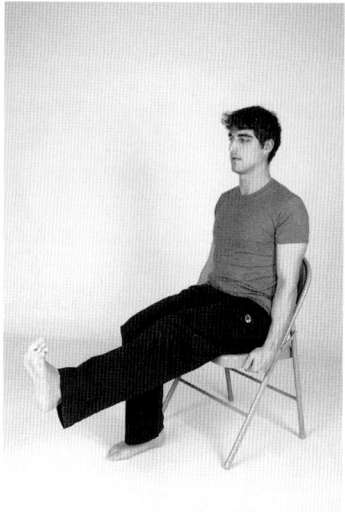

Figure 17.67
Dynamic Knee to Chest to Extended Leg 2

Leg Stretches in the Chair (Figures 17.68 and 17.69)

- If you would like to use a yoga strap with these stretches, prepare a small loop in the strap first. If you choose not to use a strap, you may find it helpful to hold your thigh with your hands to help support your leg during the stretches.
- Sit close to the front edge of your chair and assume Seated Mountain.
- Place the loop of the strap over the ball of your right foot, and extend your leg forward, holding the strap as close to your feet as you can to enable your arms to also receive a good stretch while maintaining a fully upright posture.
- Press through your heel and take several breaths in this position.
- If you would like to, you may make circles with your leg as you support it with the strap, to loosen up the muscles of your right hip.
- Then, if you wish, straighten out your left leg and cross your right leg over your left until you feel a good stretch through your right hip.
- Return your leg to center, bend your knee to remove the strap and place your foot back on the floor.
- Repeat this sequence with your other leg.

This is a good substitute for Leg Stretches with a yoga strap on a mat.

Sun Breath Twists (Figure 17.70)

- Assume Seated Mountain Position, with your hands down by your sides.
- As you inhale, turn your palms upward and raise your arms out to your sides and overhead.
- As you exhale, maintain length in your spine as you twist your torso to your right, placing your left hand on the outside of your right knee and your right arm to the chair.

Description of therapeutic yoga forms

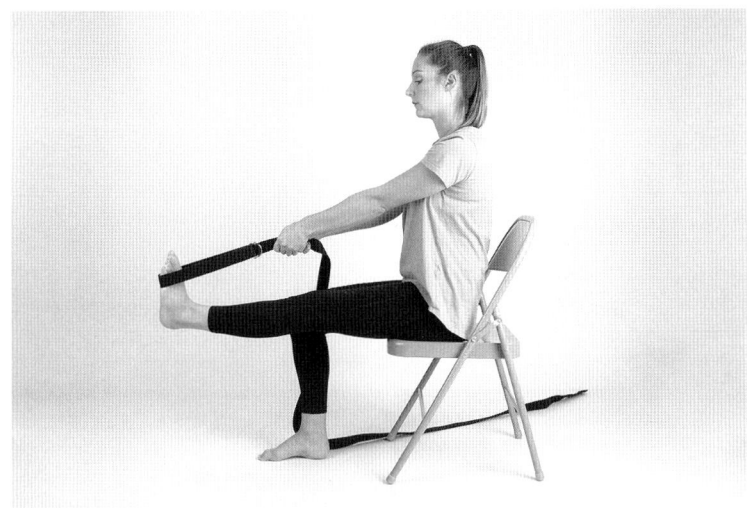

Figure 17.68
Leg Stretches in the Chair 1

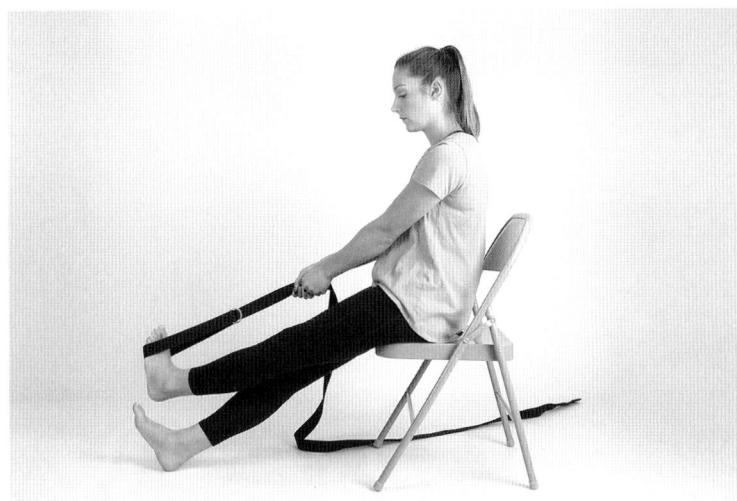

Figure 17.69
Leg Stretches in the Chair 2

- As you inhale, bring your arms back up overhead as you untwist back to center.
- Exhale as you twist to the left side.
- Repeat this flow from side to side, moving with your breath, then hold the twist for three breaths on each side.
- Slowly unwind and feel the effects.

Seated Cat/Cow (Figures 17.71 and 17.72)

- Assume Seated Mountain closer to the front edge of your chair with your palms on your lower thighs.
- Inhale as you lengthen up through the crown of your head and draw your shoulder blades closer together.
- As you exhale, tuck your tailbone under as you round your whole back and allow your head to hang. You may wish to pull in your abdominal muscles at the end of the exhalation.
- Continue with this flow, inhaling into Cow and exhaling into Cat, focusing on sensation and breath.
- Repeat at least six times, then assume Seated Mountain and feel the effects.

251

Chapter 17

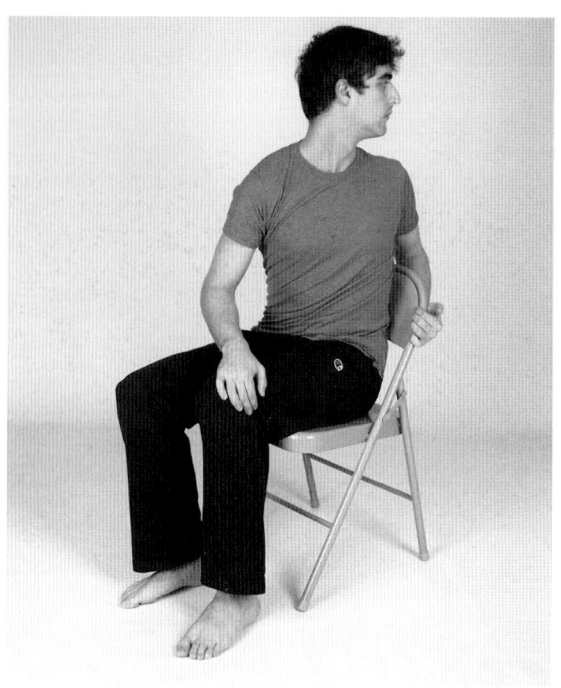

Figure 17.70
Sun Breath Twists

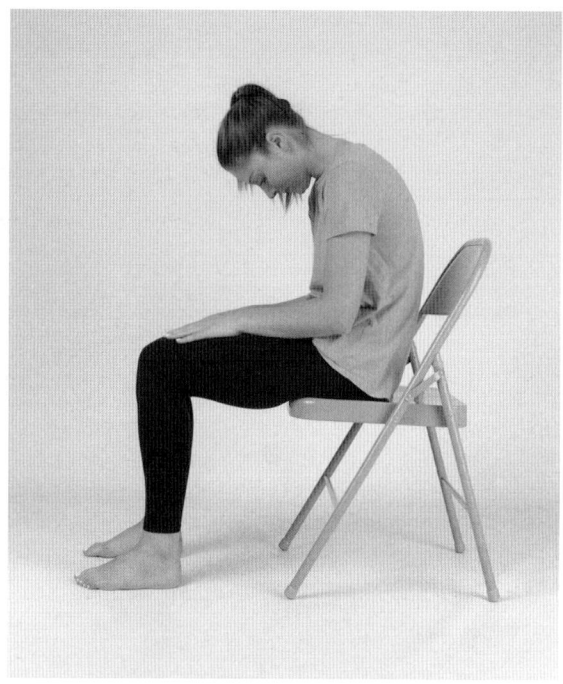

Figure 17.71
Seated Cat

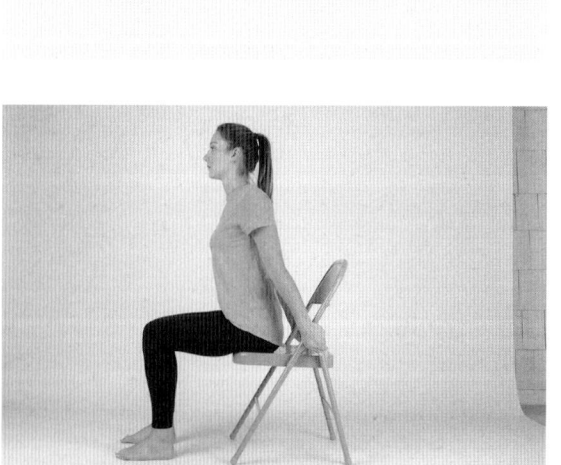

Figure 17.72
Seated Cow

Setting Sun (Figures 17.73 and 17.74)

- Assume Seated Mountain.
- On an inhale, sweep your arms out to the sides and overhead.
- On an exhale, turn your palms down and swan dive forward, hinging at the hips, placing your palms on your lower thighs to protect the back.
- Repeat this flow about six times, slowly and rhythmically with your breath.
- Then assume Seated Mountain and feel the effects.

Seated Thread the Needle (Figure 17.75 and 17.76)

- Assume Seated Mountain with your palms on your lower thighs.

Description of therapeutic yoga forms

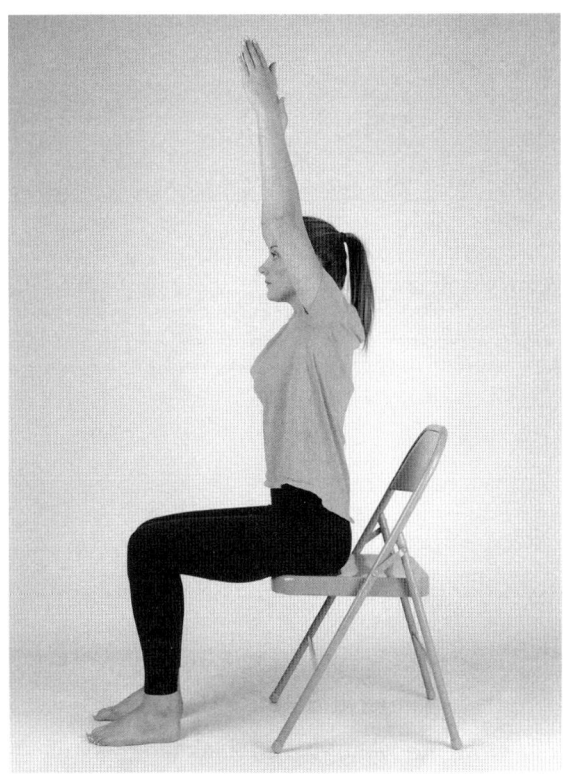

Figure 17.73
Setting Sun 1

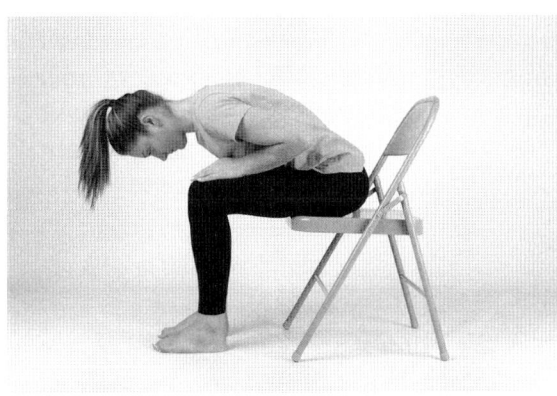

Figure 17.74
Setting Sun 2

- As you inhale, turn your right palm up as you raise your arm out to the side and overhead, allowing your gaze to follow your hand.
- As you exhale, turn your palm down and lower your arm to thread it between your left arm and torso, again allowing your head and eyes to follow your hand.
- Do not rest your forearm on your leg just yet, but instead, as you inhale, unthread your arm and raise it back up overhead.
- Continue this flow slowly with your breath several times, inhaling your arm up, and exhaling as you "thread the needle."
- Then rest your forearm or upper arm on your left thigh as you hold and breathe into the twist.
- Slowly return to an upright position and then repeat the steps on the other side.

This flow is a good substitution for Thread the Needle on the mat.

Seated Warrior I (Figure 17.77)

- Sit on the corner of your chair or so your right thigh is parallel to the front of the chair.
- Position your ankle directly under your knee.
- Stretch your left (back) leg out behind you, finding a position that is comfortable and *allows you to maintain a neutral pelvis*, in which you aren't sitting on your tailbone or overarching your back. (For some people, the leg will need to be bent.)
- Place your hands on your hips to gently guide them to face toward your front bent knee.
- On an inhalation, lengthen your spine up through the crown of your head. Exhale, maintaining that length.
- On your next inhalation, stretch your arms up overhead, palms facing each other.
- Stay for several breaths, then switch to the other side.

Chapter 18

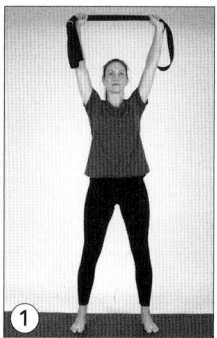

Inhale to **Extended Mountain** Pose

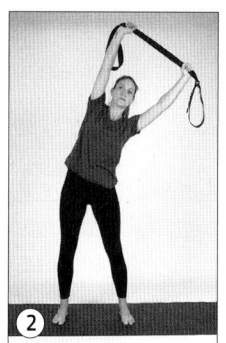

Exhale as you stretch to the left

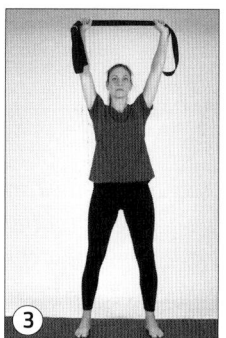

Inhale back to center

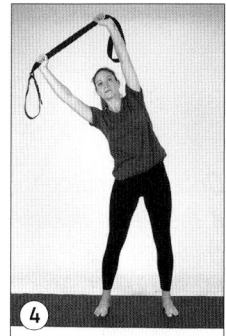

Exhale as you stretch to the right

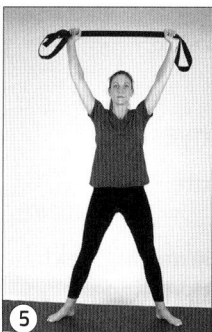

Inhale to **Five-Pointed Star** (stepping legs further apart and widening the space between the hands)

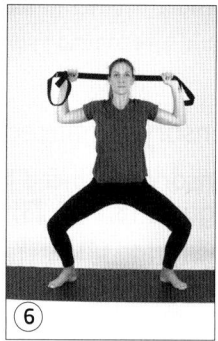

Bend your knees and elbows as you **exhale** into **Victory Squat**, lowering the strap behind your head

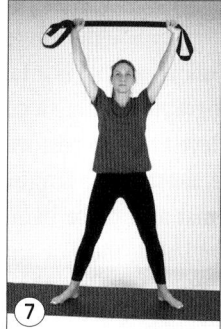

Inhale back to **Five-Pointed Star**

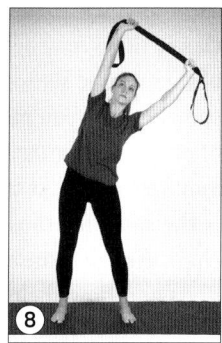

Exhale as you lean toward the left (left hand reaches downward, right upward)

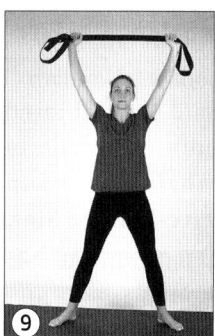

Inhale to **Five-Pointed Star**

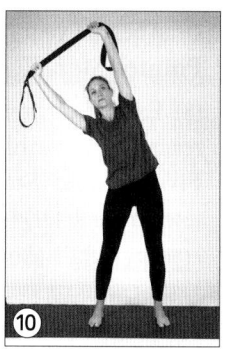

Exhale as you lean toward the right

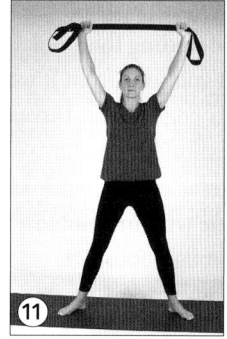

Inhale to **Five-Pointed Star**

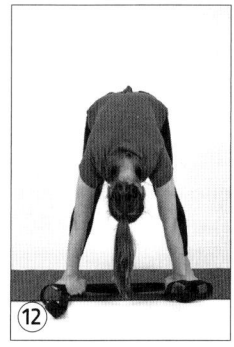

Exhale into **Forward Fold.** *In the split second in which the strap is on the floor, walk your feet in a bit closer and position your hands a bit closer on the strap, then ...*

Sensory-Enhanced Yoga® vinyasas

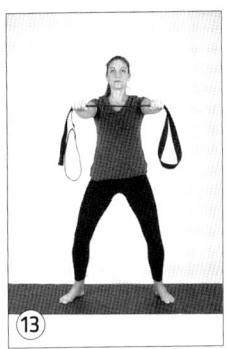

Inhale upright, raising strap to shoulder height (knees bent)

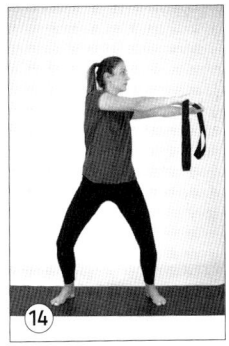

Exhale as you twist to the left, eyes follow the left hand

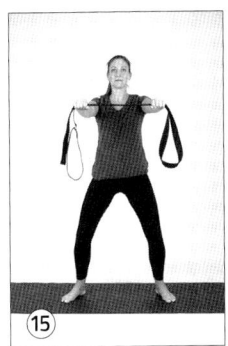

Inhale to center

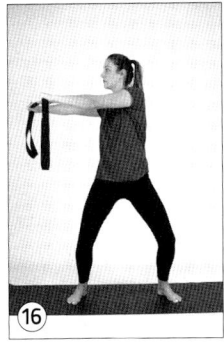

Exhale as you twist to the right, eyes follow the right hand

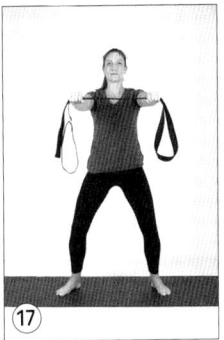

Inhale back to center (then let go of the strap with one hand and re-grasp the strap behind your back)

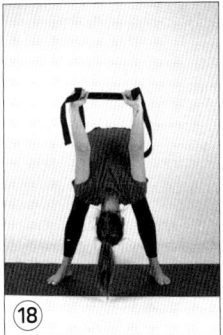

Exhale, fold, lifting strap up behind your back (knees stay soft or bent)

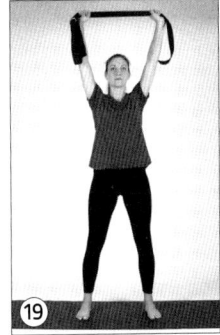

Inhale all the way into **Extended-Mountain**, flipping the strap around to the front once your trunk is upright

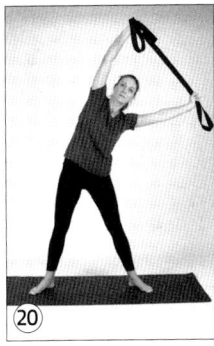

Exhale as you stretch to the left

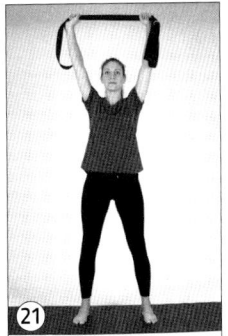

Inhale to center

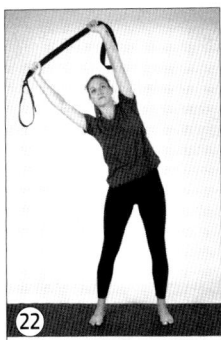

Exhale as you stretch to the right
(Move from here back into step 2 shown in Figure 18.5 to repeat the flow 1–3 more times)

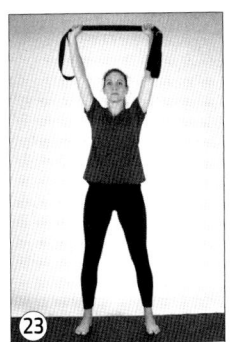

Inhale to center, then slowly **exhale** arms down, drop the strap to the floor and sense the effects of the practice

Figures 18.1–18.23

Chapter 18

6. **(17) Inhale** back to center (then let go of the strap with one hand and re-grasp the strap behind your back); **(18) exhale**, fold, lifting strap up behind your back (knees stay soft or bent); **(19) inhale** all the way into **Extended Mountain**, flipping the strap around to the front once your trunk is upright.
7. **(20) Exhale** as you stretch to the L; **(21) inhale** to center; **(22) exhale** as you stretch to the R. (Move from here back into step 2 to repeat the flow 1–3 more times.)
8. **(23) Inhale** to center, then slowly **exhale** arms down, drop the strap to the floor and sense the effects of the practice.

Benefits of the Sensory-Enhanced Moon Salute

- Lengthens and stretches the spine in various directions to release deep muscle tension around the vertebrae, which may help to release nerve constrictions and improve blood flow.
- Includes forward folds/inversions and a spinal twist, which tend to be calming.
- Performing this series using a strap provides enhanced proprioceptive (muscle and joint) input, which helps to relieve anxiety and also improves body awareness in space.

The enhanced body sensation produced by this practice helps to drop the mind back into the body, which may be especially helpful for individuals who are experiencing symptoms of numbing/dissociation.

Sun Salutation using a chair
(Figures 18.24–18.43; Table 18.1)

This version of **Sun Salutation** is a dynamic flow emphasizing integration of movement with the breath, but in addition, it incorporates a static muscle-loading form (**Warrior I**) as well as the option of a slow, rhythmic flow (**Down Dog to Plank**).

1. **(24)** Bring your palms together at the heart center, and take a nice **inhale and exhale.**
2. **(25)** On your next **inhale**, circle your arms up; hands connect overhead.
3. **(26)** Soften the knees, and hinge at the hips as you **exhale** into a swan dive *(hands may hold the chair or touch the ground).*
4. **(27) Inhale** to a flat back *(sliding hands up the shins or still holding the chair).*

   Tip: Think about just drawing your shoulders up and back without moving at the hips.
5. **(28) Exhale**, fold, keeping the knees soft.
6. **(29) Inhale** your right leg back.
7. **(30)** As you **exhale**, bend your front knee directly over *(but not past)* the ankle.
8. **(31) Inhale** arms overhead into **Warrior I**.
9. *For at least the first time on each side, add the following*: Take several nice easy breaths here as you find your center, rise up through your core, lengthen the spine, and feel the reach of your arms toward the sky.
10. **On your next exhale**, return your hands to the chair.
11. **(32) Inhale** your right foot forward and left foot back, coming into a comfortable **Plank**. (*Position your hips to form your body into a long straight line, extend through the heels, and support your weight on your straight arms.*) Note: you may go straight from Plank to Down Dog, omitting steps 12 and 13, to modify this flow.
12. **Exhale**, keeping elbows close to the body as you lower toward the chair.
13. **(33)** Lift the chest through the arms as you **inhale** into **Cobra** *(drawing the shoulders down away from the ears)*.
14. **(34) Exhale**, lifting the hips back into **Down Dog**. *(Bend the knees, lift the tail, and drop the chest.)*
15. *First time, add the following*: Continue to breathe as we make some adjustments: (i) keep your knees at least slightly bent so you are hinging at the hips and not rounding the back.

(ii) Lengthen your tail away from the chair, elongating the spine and creating a good stretch in the shoulders and arms. (iii) If your hamstrings are flexible enough, you can then slowly press your heels toward the floor as long as you can still keep the length in the spine.

16. *If desired*, incorporate a rhythmic flow here: **Down Dog to Plank**, or **Down Dog to Up Dog** (more advanced).
17. (35) From Down Dog, **inhale** the **R** foot forward and **L** foot back.
18. (36) As you **exhale**, bend your front knee directly over (*but not past*) the ankle.
19. (37) **Inhale** arms overhead into **Warrior I** *(but this time the right leg is forward)*.

Warrior I—static version: "Continue to breathe here. Lift the heart and experience the receptivity of the form … what would you like to receive?" This positive suggestion is presented within a heart-opening form that embodies its essence, bringing the power of the thought into the full "mind-body" experience.

20. **As you exhale**, return hands to the chair.
21. (38) **Inhale** your **L** foot forward and **R** foot back into **Mountain**.
22. (39) **Exhale**, fold.
23. (40) **Inhale** to a flat back.
24. (41) **Exhale** fold.
25. (42) **Inhale** as you circle the arms up (*hands connect overhead*).
26. (43) **Exhale**, returning palms to the heart center.

Take a few moments to notice the effects of the Sun Salutation.

Repeat on the other side, and if desired, you can repeat the whole routine one or more times.

Sensory-Enhanced Sun Salutations can also be performed *behind* the chair as long as all chair legs are on the mat and the front chair legs are securely positioned against a wall. This works well for many individuals who find reaching down to a chair seat too much of a stretch.

Chapter 18

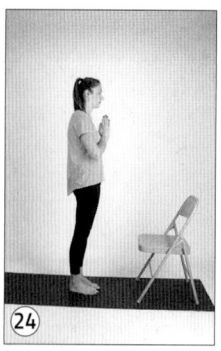

㉔ Bring your palms together at the heart center, and take a nice **inhale and exhale**

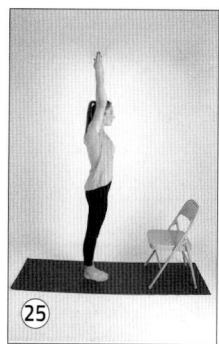

㉕ On your next **inhale**, circle your arms up; hands connect overhead

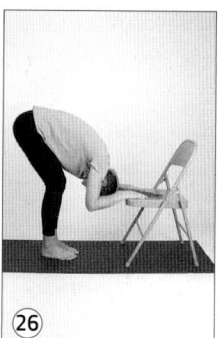

㉖ Soften the knees, and hinge at the hips as you **exhale** into a swan dive (*hands may hold the chair or touch the ground*)

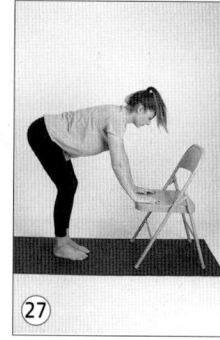

㉗ **Inhale** to a flat back (*sliding hands up the shins or still holding the chair*)

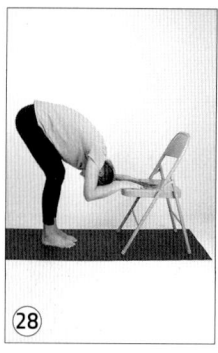

㉘ **Exhale**, fold, keeping the knees soft

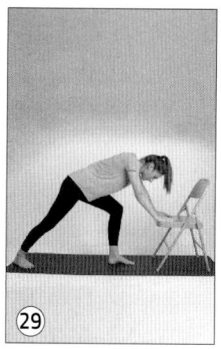

㉙ **Inhale** your right leg back

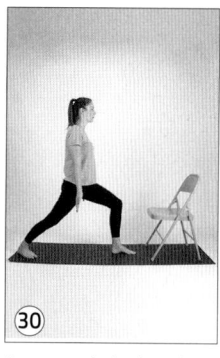

㉚ As you **exhale**, bend your front knee directly over (*but not past*) the ankle

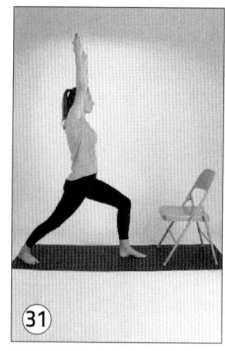

㉛ **Inhale** arms overhead into **Warrior I**

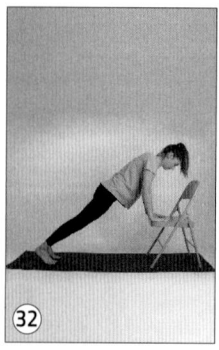

㉜ **Inhale** your right foot forward and left foot back, coming into a comfortable **Plank**. (*Position your hips to form your body into a long straight line, extend through the heels, and support your weight on your straight arms.*)

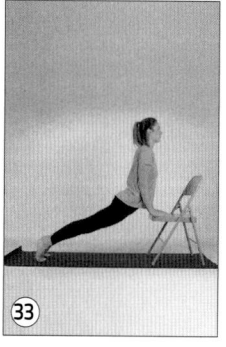

㉝ Lift the chest through the arms as you **inhale** into **Cobra** (*drawing the shoulders down away from the ears*)

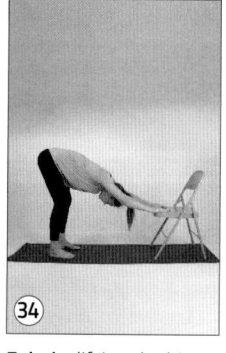

㉞ **Exhale**, lifting the hips back into **Down Dog.** (*Bend the knees, lift the tail, and drop the chest.*)

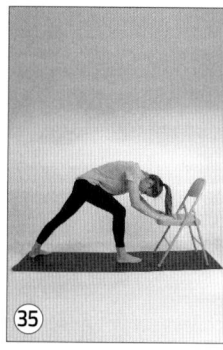

㉟ From Down Dog, **inhale** the **R** foot forward and **L** foot back

Sensory-Enhanced Yoga® vinyasas

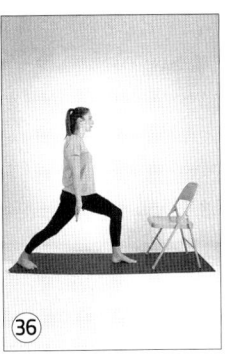

36

As you **exhale**, bend your front knee directly over (*but not past*) the ankle

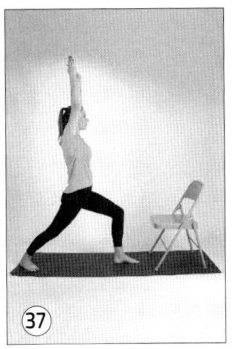

37

Inhale arms overhead into **Warrior I** (*but this time the right leg is forward*)

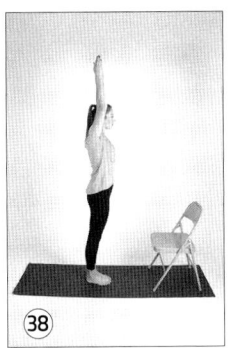

38

Inhale your **L** foot forward and **R** foot back into **Mountain**

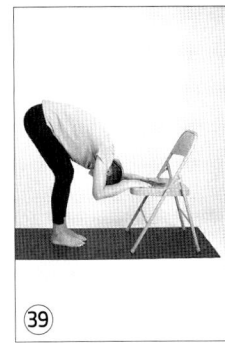

39

Exhale, fold

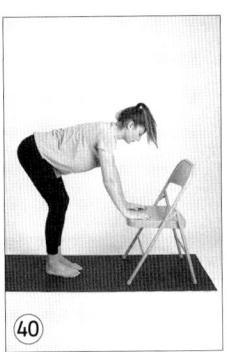

40

Inhale to a flat back

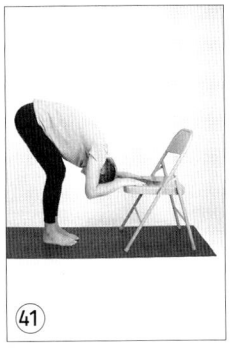

41

Exhale fold

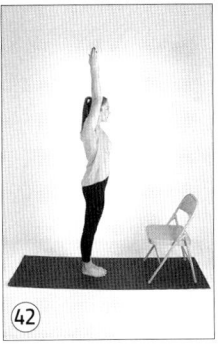

42

Inhale as you circle the arms up (*hands connect overhead*)

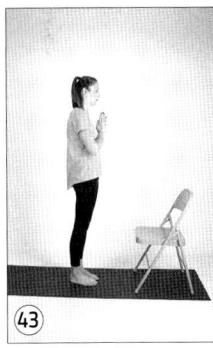

43

Exhale, returning palms to the heart center

Figures 18.24–18.43

Chapter 18

Table 18.1 Choreographed Sun Salutation

Sequence/languaging	Traditional—on mat	Student faces chair seat (or stands behind the chair)*
Bring your palms together at the heart center, and take a **nice inhale and exhale**		
On your next **inhale**, circle the arms up, hands connect overhead		
As you **exhale**, soften the knees and hinge at the hips as you swan dive forward. Fingertips touch the ground or the seat of the chair	(Fingertips touch the ground)	(Hands are placed on chair seat or grasp back of chair)
Inhale to a flat back, *sliding the hands up the shins or hold the chair***		
Exhale, fold, *placing hands on either side of your feet or hold the chair*		
Inhale as you step the right leg back	b. If on the mat, you may lower the right knee to the floor or keep it raised	a. Let go of the chair and rotate your back foot outward a bit
As you **exhale**, position the left knee directly over (but not past) the ankle		
On your next **inhale**, raise the arms up overhead, palms facing one another	(Low or High Lunge)	(Warrior I position)
Take several nice easy breaths here as you find your center … rise up through your core … lengthen the spine … and feel the reach of your arms toward the sky		
Inhale, and on your next exhale, return the hands to the floor or the chair		
Inhale as you step your left foot back next to your right, coming into a comfortable plank. *Position your hips to form your body into a long straight line and extend through the heels*		
Exhale, *bending elbows close to your sides* as you lower your body downward		
Inhale as you sink the hips and lift the chest through the arms into **Up Dog**. *Drop the shoulders down away from the ears*		
Exhale, lifting the hips back into **Down Dog**		
(First run through) Continue to breathe while we work on some adjustments here, which apply to everyone: –Keep your knees at least slightly bent so you are hinging at the hips and not rounding the back –Lengthen your tailbone away from the floor or the chair, elongating the spine and creating a good stretch in the shoulders and arms –Press the floor or chair forward and away from you –If your hamstrings are flexible enough, then slowly press your heels toward the floor as long as you can still keep the length in the spine		
(Optional: Move into a Down Dog/Up Dog OR Down Dog/Plank Flow)		

continued

Table 18.1 (Continued)

On your next inhale (from Down Dog), step your right foot and then your left foot forward
Exhale, **fold**
Inhale to a flat back, *sliding the hands up the shins, or still hold onto the chair*
Exhale, **fold**
Inhale, keeping the knees bent, circle the arms up, hands connect overhead
Exhale, returning the palms to the heart center
*If using a chair please note that all four legs of the chair must always be placed on the mat. If the student is standing behind the chair, it must also be placed carefully against the wall to prevent tipping. **Wording in *italics* is presented during the initial learning process.

APPENDICES

Appendix A

Number of Vietnam era (or older) combat veterans diagnosed with PTSD who "frequently" or "always"* agree with these Adolescent/Adult Sensory Profile items from Stoller, C. & Cimini, L. (2008). [Sensory Profiles of Older Veterans Diagnosed with PTSD.] Unpublished raw data.

Number of veterans	AASP item	AASP Category
	Taste/smell processing	
9/12	I only eat familiar foods	SA
4/12	I go over to smell fresh flowers when I see them	SK
	Movement processing	
5/12	I become dizzy easily (for example, after bending over, getting up too fast)	SS
5/11	I enjoy how it feels to move about (for example, dancing, running)	SK
4/11	I trip or bump into things	LR
4/12	I'm afraid of heights	SS
4/12	I choose to engage in physical activities	SK
	Visual processing	
10/12	I become frustrated when trying to find something in a crowded drawer or messy room	SS
9/12	I am bothered by lots of movement around me (for example, at a busy mall, parade, carnival)	SS
7/12	I miss the street, building, or room signs when trying to go somewhere new	LR
5/12	I keep the shades down at home when at home	SA
4/12	I am bothered by unsteady or fast moving images in movies or TV	SS
	Touch processing	
7/12	I get scrapes or bruises but don't remember how I got them	LR
6/12	I like how it feels to get my hair cut	SK

Appendix A *continued*		
Number of veterans	AASP item	AASP Category
6/12	I avoid standing in lines or standing close to other people because I don't like to get too close to others	SA
6/12	I move away when others get too close to me	SA
Activity level		
11/12	I avoid situations where unexpected things may happen (for example, going to unfamiliar places or being around people I don't know	SA
9/12	I find it hard to concentrate for the whole time when sitting in a long class or a meeting	SS
8/11	I stay away from crowds	SA
5/11	I find time to get away from my busy life and spend time by myself	SA
5/12	It takes me more time than other people to wake up in the morning	LR
Auditory processing		
9/12	I startle easily at unexpected or loud noises (for example, vacuum cleaner, dog barking, telephone ringing)	SS
8/12	I am distracted if there is a lot of noise around	SS
8/12	I find it difficult to work with background noise (for example, fan, radio)	SS
9/12	I stay away from noisy settings	SA
8/12	I have trouble following what people are saying when they talk fast or about unfamiliar topics	LR
6/12	I have to ask people to repeat things	LR

*Note: This chart reorganizes unpublished raw data from Stoller, C. & Cimini, L. (2008). [Sensory profiles of older veterans diagnosed with PTSD.] This informal presentation of results reports only items in which at least four out of the 12 veterans reported "frequently" or "always."

APPENDICES *continued*

Appendix B
Sensory qualities of selected yoga forms and rhythmic flows Lynn Stoller, OT, MS, OTR, C-IAYT, RYT 500/E-RYT200
© 2013–2019

Supine and table-based forms						
Form	Breath	Deep Pressure	Enhanced Proprioception	Slow, Rhythmic Movement	Balance/ Integration	Comments
Reclined Cat Stretch	●		●			
Reclined Half-Moon Stretch	●		●			
Knees to Chest	●	●				Roll over tight areas in sacral area and lower back
Leg Stretch with Strap		● Soles of feet	● + Arms and legs			
Dynamic Reclined Twist (lower body)	●	●				Releases abdominal tension. Follow flow with "stay" for deep muscle release
Dynamic Reclined Twist * (upper body)	●	●		●		
Cat-Cow*	●	● Hands		●		
Sun Bird* (Cat-Cow with Knee-Head)	●	● Hands		●	●	
Spinal Balance					●+	Excellent balance and integrative form
Down Dog		●	●+			Inversion (calming); proprioceptive input through entire body
Down Dog to Up Dog Flow*	●	●	●+	●+		Very powerful and integrating

271

Appendix B continued

Supine and table-based forms continued

Form	Breath	Deep Pressure	Enhanced Proprioception	Slow, Rhythmic Movement	Balance/ Integration	Comments
Hare to Up Dog Flow*	●	● Hands	●	●+		Less challenging (and less powerful) than Down Dog flow
Knee-Down Lunge			●+		●+	Both grounding and receptive

Standing-based postures

Form	Breath	Deep Pressure	Enhanced Proprioception	Slow, Rhythmic Movement	Balance/ Integration	Comments
Mountain	Frees the breath		● (Via mindfulness)		● (via mindfulness)	Postural alignment; point of reference for other standing asanas
Extended Mountain with Strap	●	●	●+		●	
Standing Side Stretch with Strap	●		●+		●	Use of strap provides enhanced proprioceptive input, which is calming and increases sense of grounding
Standing Twist with Strap			●+		●	
Five-Star to Victory Squat w/ Stay	●		●+	●		Very powerful and calming when performed with Ujjayi breath. May not be suitable for MST
Cow Face (arm version, with strap)	Frees the breath		●+			Chest opener presented in a "secure" position

Appendix B continued

Standing-based postures continued

Form	Breath	Deep Pressure	Enhanced Proprioception	Slow, Rhythmic Movement	Balance/ Integration	Comments
Warrior I		● (Feet: ground and press apart)	●+		●	Grounding, receptive
Warrior I to Pyramid Flow*	●	● (Feet: ground and press apart)	●	●+	●	A more challenging flow balance-wise. Use chair if necessary
Warrior II	● (If using breath to enhance qualities of the form)	● (Feet: ground and press apart)	●+		●	Draw attention to the strength/power qualities of the form
Side Angle		●+	●+		●	Enhanced proprioceptive input offsets dizziness that may be produced by head off center of gravity
Triangle			●		●	If presented, move into Triangle directly from Side Angle to reduce dizziness/anxiety. This chest opener is presented in a less secure position than the Cow Face stretch
Standing Forward Fold						Important counterform for many standing postures. Releases muscle tension. If prone to dizziness, try resting head on stacked blocks, or do a chair version
Reverse Warrior			●	●		Look straight ahead, and keep back hand on leg to enhance security and reduce anxiety/dizziness

Appendix B continued

Standing-based postures continued

Form	Breath	Deep Pressure	Enhanced Proprioception	Slow, Rhythmic Movement	Balance/Integration	Comments
Tree			● (via mindfulness)		●+	Head is upright and within center of gravity, therefore less apt to increase arousal than other balance forms
Eagle		●+	●+		●+	
Chair form		● (feet)	●+		●	Intense muscle loading posture; sense of grounding (Good prep for Eagle)

Prone or supine back bends

Form	Breath	Deep Pressure	Enhanced Proprioception	Slow, Rhythmic Movement	Balance/Integration	Comments
Crocodile	● (Belly)	● (Belly)	● (Upper body)			Good mild back bends for a balanced practice. Less likely to elicit anxiety than strong back bends (e.g. Camel)
Sphinx	●		●			
Baby Cobra	● (Belly)	● (Belly)	●			
Cobra			●+			
Bow	● (Belly)	● (Belly)	●+			Strong backbend but head is upright, so less apt to cause dizziness or anxiety
Bridge	●	●	●+			May not be suitable for those who have experienced sexual trauma, though some are fine with this yoga form if offered a blanket to drape over themselves

APPENDICES continued

Appendix B continued

Restorative forms

Form	Breath	Deep Pressure	Enhanced Proprioception	Slow, Rhythmic Movement	Balance/ Integration	Comments
Weighted Child's Form		●+				
Supported Savasana (Version 1)	● Via chest expansion	●				
Supported Savasana (Version 2)		●				Restorative forms encourage deep release of muscle tension, some of which may be trauma-based
Mental Tension Reliever		●				
Weighted Spinal Twist over a Bolster		●+				
Weighted Legs Up the Wall		●+	●			

Seated positions
Many seated postures and movement flows can be just as therapeutic but are simply not listed in this chart. The chair forms/flows in the manual can be used with individuals who cannot perform the full forms or flows on the mat, or are performing the practice in a room with limited space (e.g. a counselor's office).

Proceed with caution
The following is a partial list of forms that may increase arousal and/or stimulate protective reactions. Avoid if are anxious, experiencing active symptoms of combat stress or PTSD, or prone to dizziness.
Warrior III, Crow, Standing Half-Moon, Fish, Camel, Handstand, Headstand, Triangle, and revolved standing forms.

Also, if the yoga student may have experienced sexual trauma, I suggest avoiding certain wide-legged or otherwise vulnerable positions, including Bound Angle, Happy Baby, Victory Squat (aka Goddess), Bridge, Frog, Lizard, or Reclined Tree. However, some students who have experienced sexual trauma have been willing to try certain forms such as Bridge or Bound Angle if the teacher offers to place a blanket over them while in the form.

REFERENCES

References

Chapter 1

1. van der Kolk BA, McFarlane AC, Weisaeth L (eds). Traumatic stress: the effects of overwhelming experience on mind, body, and society. New York: Guilford; 1996.

2. Kessler RC, Berglund PA, Demler O, Jin R, Walters EE. Lifetime prevalence and age-of-onset distributions of DSM-IV disorders in the National Comorbidity Survey Replication (NCS-R). Archives of General Psychiatry. 2005;62(6):593–602.

3. Kessler RC, Chiu WT, Demler O, Walters EE. Prevalence, severity, and comorbidity of twelve-month DSM-IV disorders in the National Comorbidity Survey Replication (NCS-R). Archives of General Psychiatry. 2005;62(6):617–27.

4. American Psychiatric Association. Diagnostic and statistical manual of mental disorders DSM-III. 3rd ed. Washington, DC: APA; 2008.

5. RAND Center for Military Health Policy Research. Invisible wounds: mental health and cognitive care needs of America's returning veterans; 2008 [accessed 22 May 2009]. Available from: www.rand.org/pubs/monographs/MG720/.

6. Marmar CR, Schlenger W, Henn-Haase C et al. Course of posttraumatic stress disorder 40 years after the Vietnam War: findings from the National Vietnam Veterans Longitudinal Study. JAMA Psychiatry. 2015;72:875–81.

7. Fulton JJ, Calhoun PS, Wagner HR et al. The prevalence of posttraumatic stress disorder in Operation Enduring Freedom/Operation Iraqi Freedom (OEF/OIF) veterans: a meta-analysis. Journal of Anxiety Disorders. 2015;31:98–107. doi: 10.1016/j.janxdis.2015.02.003.

8. National Center for PTSD. (Author: MJ Friedman.) History of PTSD in veterans: Civil War to DSM-5, n.d. [accessed 11 February 2018]. Available from: https://www.ptsd.va.gov/public/PTSD-overview/basics/history-of-ptsd-vets.asp.

9. Yoga Alliance. Highlights from the 2016 Yoga in America Study; 2016 [accessed 31 May 2018]. Available from: https://www.yogaalliance.org/Learn/About_Yoga/2016_Yoga_in_America_Study/Highlights.

10. Libby D, Reddy F, Pilver C, Desai R. The use of yoga in specialized VA PTSD treatment programs. International Journal of Yoga Therapy. 2012;22(1): 79–88.

11. Stoller CC, Greuel JH, Cimini LS, Fowler MS, Koomar JA. Effects of sensory enhanced yoga on symptoms of combat stress in deployed military personnel. American Journal of Occupational Therapy. 2012;66(1):59–68.

12. Cimini L, Stoller C. General principles of the Yoga Warrior method. West Boylston, MA: Lucy Cimini; 2009.

13. Kessler RC, Sonnega A, Bromet E, Hughes M, Nelson CB. Posttraumatic stress disorder in the National Comorbidity Survey. Archives of General Psychiatry. 1995;52(12):1048–60.

14. National Center for PTSD. Traumatic effects of specific types of disasters; 2016 [accessed 25 November 2017]. Available from: https://www.ptsd.va.gov/professional/trauma/disaster-terrorism/traumatic-effects-disasters.asp.

15. National Center for PTSD. Community violence; 2016 [accessed 15 January 2017]. Available from: https://www.ptsd.va.gov/professional/trauma/other/community-violence.asp.

16. Lui K. A record 65.6 million people are now displaced worldwide, says UNHCR. Time Magazine; 2017 [accessed 1 January 2018]. Available from: http://time.com/4823271/unhcr-displaced-people-conflict-refugees/.

17. Widom CS, Maxfield MG. An update on the "cycle of violence." Washington, DC: National Institute of Justice; 2001 [accessed 31 May 2018]. Available from: http://www.ncjrs.gov/pdffiles1/nij/184894.pdf.

Chapter 2

1. Rothschild B. The body remembers: the psychophysiology of trauma and trauma treatment. New York: WW Norton; 2000.

2. American Psychiatric Association. Diagnostic and statistical manual of mental disorders, DSM-5. 5th ed. Washington, DC: APA; 2013.

3. Roberts AL, Dohrenwend BP, Aiello A, Wright RJ, Maercker A, Galea S, Koenen KC. The stressor criterion for posttraumatic stress disorder: does it matter? Journal of Clinical Psychiatry. 2012;73(2):e264–e270. Available from: http://doi.org/10.4088/JCP.11m07054.

4. Dohrenwend BP. The stressor criterion A in posttraumatic stress disorder: issues, evidence, and implications. In Simpson HB, Lewis-Fernandez R, Neria Y, Schneier F, editors. Anxiety disorders: theory, research and clinical perspectives. Cambridge: Cambridge University Press; 2010, p. 216–26.

5. Brewin CR, Lanius RA, Novac A, Schnyder U, Galea S. Reformulating PTSD for DSM-V: life after criterion A. Journal of Traumatic Stress. 2009;22:366–73. Available from: http://dx.doi.org/10.1002/jts.20443.

6. Anders S, Frazier P, Frankfurt S. Variations in criterion A and PTSD rates in a community sample of women. Journal of Anxiety Disorders. 2011;25(2):176–84. Available from: http://doi.org/10.1016/j.janxdis.2010.08.018.

REFERENCES continued

7. Schore AN. The science of the art of psychotherapy. New York: WW Norton; 2012.

8. Calati R, Bensassi I, Courtet P. The link between dissociation and both suicide attempts and non-suicidal self-injury: meta-analyses. Psychiatry Research. 2017;251:103–14.

9. Ball C, Little J. A comparison of involuntary autobiographical memory retrievals. Applied Cognitive Psychology. 2006;20:1167–79.

10. Van der Kolk BA, Fisler R. Dissociation and the fragmentary nature of traumatic memories: overview and exploratory study. Journal of Traumatic Stress. 1995;8(4):505–25.

11. Hirsch CR, Holmes EA. Mental imagery in anxiety disorders. Psychiatry. 2007;6(4):165 [accessed 17 July 2011]. Available from: http://www.psychiatry.ox.ac.uk/epct/emily_holmes/articles/hirsch_holmes.

12. Lanius RA, Brand B, Vermetten E, Frewen PA, Spiegel D. The dissociative subtype of posttraumatic stress disorder: rationale, clinical and neurobiological evidence, and implications. Depression and Anxiety. 2012;29:701–8. doi:10.1002/da.21889.

13. Wolf EJ. The dissociative subtype of PTSD: rationale, evidence, and future directions. PTSD Research Quarterly. 2013;24(4):1050–1835.

14. Lanius RA, Bluhm R, Lanius U, Pain C. A review of neuroimaging studies in PTSD: heterogeneity of response to symptom provocation. Journal of Psychiatric Research. 2006;40:709–29.

15. Schell TL, Marshall GN, Jaycox LH. All symptoms are not created equal: the prominent role of hyperarousal in the natural course of posttraumatic psychological distress. Journal of Abnormal Psychology. 2004;113(2):189–97.

16. Thompson KE, Vasterling JJ, Benotsch EG et al. Early symptom predictors of chronic distress in Gulf War veterans. Journal of Nervous and Mental Disease. 2004;192(2):146–52.

17. Solomon Z, Horesh D, Ein-Dor T. The longitudinal course of posttraumatic stress disorder symptom clusters among war veterans. Journal of Clinical Psychiatry. 2009;70(6):837–43.

18. Rothschild B. Post-traumatic stress disorder: identification and diagnosis. Invited article for Soziale Arbeit Schweiz (The Swiss Journal of Social Work), February 1998 [accessed 25 May 2009]. Available from: http://home.webuniverse.net/babette/PTSD.html.

19. Newport DJ, Nemeroff CB. Neurobiology of post traumatic stress disorder. Current Opinions in Neurobiology. 2000;10:211–18.

20. van der Kolk BA. The psychobiology of posttraumatic stress disorder. Journal of Clinical Psychiatry. 1997;58:16–24.

21. van der Kolk BA. The body keeps the score: brain, mind, and body in the healing of trauma. New York: Viking (Penguin Random House); 2014.

22. Stewart LP, White PM. Sensory filtering phenomenology in PTSD. Depression and Anxiety. 2008;25:38–45.

23. Johnson MR, Adler LE (1993), cited in Stewart LP, White PM. Sensory filtering phenomenology in PTSD. Depression and Anxiety. 2008;25:39.

24. White and Yee (1997), cited in Stewart LP, White PM. Sensory filtering phenomenology in PTSD. Depression and Anxiety. 2008;25:39.

25. Adler et al. (1994), cited in Stewart LP, White PM. Sensory filtering phenomenology in PTSD. Depression and Anxiety. 2008;25:39.

26. Kardiner A. The traumatic neuroses of war. Psychosomatic Medicine Monographs. 1941;1(2/3).

27. van der Kolk BA. Psychobiology of posttraumatic stress disorder. In Panksepp J (ed.), Biological psychiatry. Hoboken, NJ: Wiley-Liss; 2004.

28. Dunnigan JF, Nofi AA. Dirty little secrets of the Vietnam War: military information you're not supposed to know. New York: St Martin's Press; 1999.

29. Institute of Medicine (IOM). Gulf War and health, Vol. 6: Physiologic, psychologic, and psychological effects of deployment-related stress. Washington, DC: National Academies Press; 2008.

30. Balaban CD. A sense of balance: understanding the balance-anxiety-migraine linkage. Journal of Korean Balance Society. 2006;5(1):99–107.

31. Carey J, Amin N. Evolutionary changes in the cochlea and labyrinth: solving the problem of sound transmission to the balance organs of the inner ear. Anatomical Record, Part A. 2006;288A(4):482–90.

32. Haber YO, Chandler HK, Serrador JM. Symptoms associated with vestibular impairment in veterans with posttraumatic stress disorder. PLoS ONE. 2016;11(12):e0168803. Available from: http://doi.org/10.1371/journal.pone.0168803.

33. Hunt SC, Jakupcak M, McFall M, Orsborn M, Felker B, Larson S, Klevens M. Re: chronic multisymptom illness complex in Gulf War I veterans 10 years later. American Journal of Epidemiology. 2006;164:706–10.

34. van der Kolk BA, McFarlane AC, Weisaeth L (eds). Traumatic stress: the effects of overwhelming experience on mind, body, and society. New York: Guilford; 1996.

35. Clancy K, Ding M, Bernat E, Schmidt NB, Li W. Restless "rest": intrinsic sensory hyperactivity and disinhibition in post-traumatic stress disorder. Brain. 2017;140(7):2041–50. Available from: https://doi.org/10.1093/brain/awx116.

36. Shalev et al. (1992), cited in van der Kolk BA, McFarlane AC, Weisaeth L (eds). Traumatic stress: the effects of overwhelming experience on mind, body, and society. New York: Guilford; 1996, p. 221.

37. Ornitz and Pynoos (1989), cited in van der Kolk BA, McFarlane AC, Weisaeth L (eds). Traumatic stress: the effects of overwhelming experience on mind, body, and society. New York: Guilford; 1996, p. 221.

38. Butler et al. (1990), cited in van der Kolk BA, McFarlane AC, Weisaeth L (eds). Traumatic stress: the effects of overwhelming experience on mind, body, and society. New York: Guilford; 1996, p. 221.

39. Ross et al. (1989), cited in van der Kolk BA, McFarlane AC, Weisaeth L (eds). Traumatic stress: the effects of overwhelming experience on mind, body, and society. New York: Guilford; 1996, p. 221.

40. Bundy A, Lane S, Murray E. Sensory integration: theory and practice. 2nd ed. Philadelphia: FA Davis; 2002.

41. Engel-Yeger B, Palgy-Levin D, Lev-Wiesel R. The sensory profile of people with post-traumatic stress symptoms. Occupational Therapy in Mental Health. 2013;29:266–78.

42. Stoller C, Cimini L. [Sensory profiles of older veterans diagnosed with PTSD.] Unpublished raw data; 2008.

43. Porges SW. The polyvagal theory: neurophysiological foundations of emotions, attachment communication, and self-regulation. New York: WW Norton; 2011.

44. Bergmann U. The neurobiology of EMDR: exploring the thalamus and neural integration. Journal of EMDR Practice and Research. 2008;2(4):300–14. Available from: http://dx.doi.org/10.1891/1933-3196.2.4.300.

45. Javanbakht A, Liberzon I, Amirsadri A, Gjini K, Boutros NN. Event-related potential studies of post-traumatic stress disorder: a critical review and synthesis. Biology of Mood and Anxiety Disorders. 2011;1:5. Available from: http://doi.org/10.1186/2045-5380-1-5.

46. Petroff OAC. Book review: GABA and glutamate in the human brain. The Neuroscientist. 2002;8(6):562–73. Available from: https://doi.org/10.1177/1073858402238515.

47. Prager EM, Bergstrom HC, Wynn GH, Braga MFM. The basolateral amygdala GABAergic system in health and disease. Journal of Neuroscience Research. 2016;94(6):548–67. Available from: http://doi.org/10.1002/jnr.23690.

48. Ayres AJ. Sensory integration and learning disorders. Los Angeles: Western Psychological Services; 1972.

49. Streeter CC, Gerbarg P, Saper RB, Ciraulo DA, Brown RP. Effects of yoga on the autonomic nervous system, gamma-aminobutyric-acid, and allostasis in epilepsy, depression, and post-traumatic stress disorder. Medical Hypotheses. 2012;78(5):571–9.

50. Thayer JF, Lane RD. A model of neurovisceral integration in emotion regulation and dysregulation. Journal of Affective Disorders. 2000;61:201–16.

51. Thayer JF, Lane RD. Claude Bernard and the heart-brain connection: further elaboration of a model of neurovisceral integration. Neuroscience and Biobehavioral Reviews 2009;33(2):81–8. doi: 10.1016/j.neubiorev.2008.08.004.

52. Knight et al. (1999), cited in Thayer JF, Lane RD. Claude Bernard and the heart-brain connection: further elaboration of a model of neurovisceral integration. Neuroscience and Biobehavioral Reviews 2009;33(2):81–8, p. 83.

53. Thayer (2006), cited in Thayer JF, Lane RD. Claude Bernard and the heart-brain connection: further elaboration of a model of neurovisceral integration. Neuroscience and Biobehavioral Reviews 2009;33(2):81–8, p. 83.

54. Thayer and Lane (2005), cited in Thayer JF, Lane RD. Claude Bernard and the heart-brain connection: further elaboration of a model of neurovisceral integration. Neuroscience and Biobehavioral Reviews 2009;33(2):81–8, p. 83..

55. Azevedo FA, Carvalho LR, Grinberg LT, Farfel JM, Ferretti RE, Leite RE, Jacob Filho W, Lent R, Herculano-Houzel S. Journal of Comparative Neurology. 2009;513(5):532–41.

56. Javanbakht A, Liberzon I, Amirsadri A, Gjini K, Boutros NN. Event-related potential studies of post-traumatic stress disorder: a critical review and synthesis. Biology of Mood and Anxiety Disorders. 2011;1:5. Available from: http://doi.org/10.1186/2045-5380-1-5.

57. Lanius RA, Frewen PA, Vermetten E, Yehuda R. Fear conditioning and early life vulnerabilities: two distinct pathways of emotional dysregulation and brain dysfunction in PTSD. European Journal of Psychotraumatology. 2010;1(1):5467. DOI: 10.3402/ejpt.v1i0.5467.

58. Yehuda R, Hoge CW, McFarlane AC, Vermetten E, Lanius RA, Nievergelt CM, Hobfoll SE, Koenen KC, Nevlan TC, Hyman SE. Post-traumatic stress disorder. Nature Reviews Disease Primers. 2015;1:15057. doi: 10.1038/nrdp.2015.57.

Chapter 3

1. Levine PA. Waking the tiger; healing trauma. Berkeley: North Atlantic Books; 1997.

2. van der Kolk BA. The body keeps the score: brain, mind, and body in the healing of trauma. New York: Viking (Penguin Random House); 2014.

3. LeDoux J. The amygdala is NOT the brain's fear center. Blog post; 2015. Available from: https://www.psychologytoday.com/blog/i-got-mind-tell-you/201508/the-amygdala-is-not-the-brains-fear-center.

4. LeDoux J. Anxious. New York: Penguin Random House LLC; 2015.

5. Roxo MR, Franceschini PR, Zubaran C, Kleber FD, Sander JW. The limbic system conception and its historical evolution.

REFERENCES continued

Scientific World Journal. 2011;11:2428–41. Available from: http://doi.org/10.1100/2011/157150.

6. Porges SW. The polyvagal theory: neurophysiological foundations of emotions, attachment communication, and self-regulation. New York: WW Norton; 2011.

7. Damasio AR. The feeling of what happens: body and emotion in the making on consciousness. New York: Harcourt Brace; 1999.

8. Damasio AR, Grabowski TJ, Bechara A, Damasio H, Ponto LLB, Parvizi J, Hichwa RD. Subcortical and cortical brain activity during the feeling of self-generated emotions. Nature Neuroscience. 2000;3:1049–56.

9. Hopper JW, Frewen PA, vanderKolk BA, Lanius RA. Neural correlates of reexperiencing, avoidance, and dissociation in PTSD: symptom dimensions and emotion dysregulation in responses to script-driven trauma imagery. Journal of Traumatic Stress. 2007;20(5):713–25.

10. Lanius RA, Vermetten E, Loewenstein RJ, Brand B, Schmahl C, Bremner JD, Spiegel D. Emotion modulation in PTSD: clinical and neurobiological evidence for a dissociative subtype. American Journal of Psychiatry. 2010;167(6):640-7. doi:10.1176/appi.ajp.2009.09081168.

11. Ayres AJ. Sensory integration and learning disorders. Los Angeles: Western Psychological Services; 1972.

12. Cozolino L. The neuroscience of psychotherapy: healing the social brain. 2nd ed. New York: WW Norton; 2010.

13. Bundy A, Lane S, Murray E. Sensory integration: theory and practice. 2nd ed. Philadelphia: FA Davis; 2002.

14. Wingate DS. Healing brain injury with Chinese medical approaches: integrative approaches for practitioners. Philadelphia: Singing Dragon; 2018.

15. Fast CD, McGann JP. Amygdalar gating of early sensory processing through interactions with locus coeruleus. Journal of Neuroscience. 2017;37(11):3085–101. doi: 10.1523/JNEUROSCI.2797-16.2017.

16. McGann JP. Associative learning and sensory neuroplasticity: how does it happen and what is it good for? Learning and Memory. 2015;22:567–76. doi:10.1101/lm.039636.115.

17. Technical University of Munich (TUM). Sensory function: thalamus enhances, stores sensory information: important brain network for processing sensory perceptions elucidated. ScienceDaily, 21 January 2016. Available from: www.sciencedaily.com/releases/2016/01/160121110929.htm.

18. Menon V. Large-scale brain networks and psychopathology: a unifying triple network model. Trends in Cognitive Sciences. 2011;15:483–506.

19. Lanius RA, Frewen PA, Tursich M, Jetly R, McKinnon MC. Restoring large-scale brain networks in PTSD: a proposal for neuroscientifically-informed treatment interventions. European Journal of Psychotraumatology. 2015;6:27313. doi: 10.3402/ejpt.v6.2731.

20. Yehuda R, Hoge CW, McFarlane AC, Vermetten E, Lanius RA, Nievergelt CM, Hobfoll SE, Koenen KC, Nevlan TC, Hyman SE. Post-traumatic stress disorder. Nature Reviews Disease Primers. 2015;(1)15057:1–22.

21. Benarroch EE. The locus ceruleus norepinephrine system: functional organization and potential clinical significance. Neurology. 2009;73(20):1699–704. Doi: 10.1212/WNL.0b013e3181c2937c.

22. Atzori M, Cuevas-Olguin R, Esquivel-Rendon E, Garcia-Oscos F, Salgado-Delgado RC, Saderi N et al. Locus ceruleus norepinephrine release: a central regulator of CNS spatio-temporal activation? Frontiers in Synaptic Neuroscience. 2016;8:25. Available from: http://doi.org/10.3389/fnsyn.2016.00025.

23. Harricharan S, Rabellino D, Frewen PA, Densmore M, Théberge J, McKinnon MC et al. fMRI functional connectivity of the periaqueductal gray in PTSD and its dissociative subtype. Brain and Behavior. 2016;6(12):e00579. Available from: http://doi.org/10.1002/brb3.579.

24. Bandler R, Keay KA, Floyd N, Price J. Central circuits mediating patterned autonomic activity during active vs. passive emotional coping. Brain Research Bulletin. 2000;53:95–104.

25. Shin LM, Liberzon I. The neurocircuitry of fear, stress, and anxiety disorders. Neuropsychopharmacology. 2010;35(1):169–91. doi: 10.1038/npp.2009.83.

26. Stephens MA, Wand G. Stress and the HPA axis. Alcohol Research. 2012;34(4):468–83.

27. van der Werff SJA, van den Berg SM, Pannekoek JN, Elzinga BM, van der Wee NJA. Neuroimaging resilience to stress: a review. Frontiers in Behavioral Neuroscience. 2013;7:39. Available from: http://doi.org/10.3389/fnbeh.2013.00039.

28. Ten Donkelaar HJ, Hori A. The hypothalamus and hypothalamohypophysial systems. In Clinical Neuroanatomy, pp. 603–31. Berlin, Heidelberg: Springer-Verlag; 2011 [accessed 14 July 2018]. Doi: 10.1007/978-3-642-19134-3_13. Available from: https://canlabweb.colorado.edu/brainstemwiki/lib/exe/fetch.php/fulltext_25_.pdf.

29. Jiang Z, Rajamanickam S, Justice NJ. Local corticotropin-releasing factor signaling in the hypothalamic paraventricular nucleus. Journal of Neuroscience. 2018;38(8):1874–90. DOI:10.1523/JNEUROSCI.1492-17.2017.

30. Chapman IM (n.d.). Overview of the pituitary gland. Merck Manual Online [accessed 14 July 2018]. Available from: https://www.merckmanuals.com/home/hormonal-and-metabolic-disorders/pituitary-gland-disorders/overview-of-the-pituitary-gland.

31. Pocock G, Richards CD, Richards D. Human physiology. 4th ed. UK: Oxford University Press; 2016 [accessed 14 July 2018]. Available from: http://global.oup.com/fdscontent/academic/pdf/he/9780199574933_Ch15.pdf.

32. Hwang K, Bertolero MA, Liu WB, D'Esposito M. The human thalamus is an integrative hub for functional brain networks. Journal of Neuroscience. 2017;37(23):5594–607.

33. Courtiol E, Wilson DA. The olfactory thalamus: unanswered questions about the role of the mediodorsal thalamic nucleus in olfaction. Frontiers in Neural Circuits. 2015;9:49. doi:10.3389/fncir.2015.00049.

34. Saalmann Y, Kastner S. The cognitive thalamus. Frontiers in Systems Neuroscience. 2015;9:39. doi: 10.3389/fnsys.2015.00039.

35. Coulon P, Budde T, Pape HC. The sleep relay—the role of the thalamus in central and decentral sleep regulation. Pflugers Archiv – European Journal of Physiology. 2012;463(1):53–71. Available from: https://doi.org/10.1007/s00424-011-1014-6.

36. Wijesinghe R, Protti DA, Camp AJ. Vestibular interactions in the thalamus. Frontiers in Neural Circuits. 2015;9:79. Available from: http://doi.org/10.3389/fncir.2015.00079.

37. Nagata (1986), cited in Wijesinghe R, Protti DA, Camp AJ. Vestibular interactions in the thalamus. Frontiers in Neural Circuits. 2015;9:79, p. 2.

38. Matesz et al. (2002), cited in Wijesinghe R, Protti DA, Camp AJ. Vestibular interactions in the thalamus. Frontiers in Neural Circuits. 2015;9:79, p. 2.

39. Vertes RP, Hoover WB, Szigeti-Buck K, Leranth C. Nucleus reuniens of the midline thalamus: link between the medial prefrontal cortex and the hippocampus. Brain Research Bulletin. 2007;71(6):601–9.

40. Jin J, Maren S. Prefrontal-hippocampal interactions in memory and emotion. Frontiers in Systems Neuroscience. 2015;9:170. doi:10.3389/fnsys.2015.00170.

41. Sridharan D, Levitin DJ, Menon V. A critical role for the right fronto-insular cortex in switching between central-executive and default-mode networks. Proceedings of the National Academy of Sciences. 2008;105(34):12569–74.

42. Menon V, Uddin LQ. Saliency, switching, attention and control: a network model of insula function. Brain Structure and Function. 2010;214(5–6):655–67. Available from: http://doi.org/10.1007/s00429-010-0262-0.

43. Craig A.D. How do you feel? Interoception: the sense of the physiological condition of the body. Nature Reviews Neuroscience. 2002;3:655–66.

44. Craig AD. Interoception: the sense of the physiological condition of the body. Current Opinion in Neurobiology. 2003;13:500-5.

45. Gilbertson MW, Shenton ME, Ciszewski A, Kasai K, Lasko NB, Orr SP, Pitman RK. Smaller hippocampal volume predicts pathologic vulnerability to psychological trauma. Nature Neuroscience. 2002;5(11):1242–7. Available from: http://doi.org/10.1038/nn958.

46. Feder A, Nestler EJ, Charney DS (2009), cited in van der Werff SJA, van den Berg SM, Pannekoek JN, Elzinga BM, van der Wee NJA. Neuroimaging resilience to stress: a review. Frontiers in Behavioral Neuroscience. 2013;7:39. Available from: http://doi.org/10.3389/fnbeh.2013.00039.

47. Zeidman P, Maguire EA. Anterior hippocampus: the anatomy of perception, imagination and episodic memory. Nature Reviews Neuroscience. 2016;17(3):173–82.

48. Mahmutyazıcıoğlu K, Konuk N, Hüseyin Özdemir H, Atasoy N, Atik L, Gündoğdu S. Evaluation of the hippocampus and the anterior cingulate gyrus by proton MR spectroscopy in patients with post-traumatic stress disorder. Diagnostic and Interventional Radiology. 2005;11:125–9.

49. Radley JJ, Sawchenko PE. A common substrate for prefrontal and hippocampal inhibition of the neuroendocrine stress response. Journal of Neuroscience. 2011;31:9683–95.

50. Fanselow MS, Dong HW. Are the dorsal and ventral hippocampus functionally distinct structures? Neuron. 2010;65(1):7–19.

51. Stevens FL, Hurley RA, Taber KH, Hayman LA, Taber KH. Anterior cingulate cortex: unique role in cognition and emotion. Journal of Neuropsychiatry and Clinical Neurosciences. 2011;23(2):121–5.

52. Blini E, Tilikete C, Farnè A, Hadj-Bouziane F. Probing the role of the vestibular system in motivation and reward-based attention. Cortex. 2018;103:82–99. Available from: http://doi.org/10.1016/j.cortex.2018.02.009.

53. Lanius RA, Williamson PC, Bluhm RL, Densmore M, Boksman K, Gupta M, et al. Functional connectivity of dissociative responses in posttraumatic stress disorder: a functional magnetic resonance imaging investigation. Biological Psychiatry. 2005;57:873–84.

54. Lavin C, Melis C, Mikulan E, Gelormini C, Huepe D, Ibañez A. The anterior cingulate cortex: an integrative hub for human socially-driven interactions. Frontiers in Neuroscience. 2013;7:64. Available from: http://doi.org/10.3389/fnins.2013.00064.

55. Etkin A, Egner T, Kalisch R. Emotional processing in anterior cingulate and medial prefrontal cortex. Trends in Cognitive Sciences. 2011;15(2):85–93. Available from: http://doi.org/10.1016/j.tics.2010.11.004.

56. Klavir O, Genud-Gabai R, Paz R. Functional connectivity between amygdala and cingulate cortex for adaptive aversive learning. Neuron. 2013;80:1290–300.

REFERENCES *continued*

57. Leech R, Braga R, Sharp DJ. Echoes of the brain within the posterior cingulate cortex. Journal of Neuroscience. 2012;32(1):215–22.

58. Cavanna AE, Trimble MR. The precuneus: a review of its functional anatomy and behavioral correlates. Brain. 2006;129(3):564–83. Available from: https://doi.org/10.1093/brain/awl004.

59. Zhang S, Li CR. Functional connectivity mapping of the human precuneus by resting state fMRI. Neuroimage. 2012;59(4):3548–62. Available from: http://doi.org/10.1016/j.neuroimage.2011.11.023.

60. Bluhm RL, Williamson PC, Osuch EA, Frewen PA, Stevens TK, Boksman K et al. Alterations in default network connectivity in posttraumatic stress disorder related to early-life trauma. Journal of Psychiatry and Neuroscience . 2009;34(3):187–94.

61. Vogt BA, Laureys S. Posterior cingulate, precuneal and retrosplenial cortices: cytology and components of the neural network correlates of consciousness. Progress in Brain Research. 2005;150:205–17. Available from: http://doi.org/10.1016/S0079-6123(05)50015-3.

62. Sato W, Kochiyama T, Uono S, Kubota Y, Sawada R, Yoshimura S et al. The structural neural substrates of subjective happiness. Scientific Reports. 2015;5:16891 [accessed 30 July 2018]. Available from: https://www.nature.com/articles/srep16891.

63. Filimon F, Nelson JD, Huang R-S, Sereno MI. Multiple parietal reach regions in humans: cortical representations for visual and proprioceptive feedback during on-line reaching. Journal of Neuroscience. 2009;29(9):2961–71. Available from: http://doi.org/10.1523/JNEUROSCI.3211-08.2009.

64. Funahashi S. Working memory in the prefrontal cortex. Brain Sciences. 2017;7(5):49. Available from: http://doi.org/10.3390/brainsci7050049.

65. Wimmer RD, Schmitt LI, Davidson TJ, Nakajima M, Deisseroth K, Halassa MM. Thalamic control of sensory selection in divided attention. Nature. 2015;526:705–9. doi:10.1038/nature15398.

66. Shin LM, Rauch SL, Pitman RK. Amygdala, medial prefrontal cortex, and hippocampal function in PTSD. Annals of the New York Academy of Sciences. 2006;1071:67–79. Available from: https://doi.org/10.1196/annals.1364.007.

67. Roy M, Shohamy D, Wager TD. Ventromedial prefrontal-subcortical systems and the generation of affective meaning. Trends in Cognitive Sciences. 2012;16(3):147–56. Available from: http://doi.org/10.1016/j.tics.2012.01.005.

68. Fogel A. Body sense. New York: WW Norton; 2009.

69. Hayes JP, Hayes SM, Mikedis AM. Quantitative meta-analysis of neural activity in posttraumatic stress disorder. Biology of Mood and Anxiety Disorders. 2012;2:9. Available from: http://doi.org/10.1186/2045-5380-2-9.

70. Hayes JP, VanElzakker MB, Shin LM. Emotion and cognition interactions in PTSD: a review of neurocognitive and neuroimaging studies. Frontiers in Integrative Neuroscience. 2012;6:89. Available from: http://doi.org/10.3389/fnint.2012.00089.

71. Goldman-Rakic PS, Selemon L, Schwartz ML. Dual pathways connecting the dorsolateral prefrontal cortex with the hippocampal formation and parahippocampal cortex in the rhesus monkey. Neuroscience. 1984;12(3):719–43. Available from: https://doi.org/10.1016/0306-4522(84)90166-0.

72. Cohen YE. Multimodal activity in the parietal cortex. Hearing Research. 2009;258(1–2):100–5. Available from: http://doi.org/10.1016/j.heares.2009.01.011.

73. Vingerhoets G. Contribution of the posterior parietal cortex in reaching, grasping, and using objects and tools. Frontiers in Psychology. 2014;5:151. Available from: http://doi.org/10.3389/fpsyg.2014.00151.

74. Berryhill ME, Olson IR. Is the posterior parietal lobe involved in working memory retrieval? Evidence from patients with bilateral parietal lobe damage. Neuropsychologia. 2008;46(7):1767–74. doi:10.1016/j.neuropsychologia.2008.01.009.

75. Katsuki F, Constantinidis C. Unique and shared roles of the posterior parietal and dorsolateral prefrontal cortex in cognitive functions. Frontiers in Integrative Neuroscience. 2012;6:17. Available from: http://doi.org/10.3389/fnint.2012.00017.

76. Ruben J, Schweimann J, Deuchert M, Meyer R, Krause T, Curio G et al. Somatotopic organization of human secondary somatosensory cortex. Cerebral Cortex. 2001;11(5):463–73. Available from: https://doi.org/10.1093/cercor/11.5.463.

77. Cunningham DA, Machado A, Yue G H, Carey JR, Plow EB. Functional somatotopy revealed across multiple cortical regions using a model of complex motor task. Brain Research. 2013;153:25–36.

78. LeDoux J. The emotional brain. New York: Simon and Shuster International; 1998.

79. Jänig W. The integrative action of the autonomic nervous system: neurobiology of homeostasis. New York: Cambridge University Press; 2006.

80. Siegel DJ. The developing mind. New York: Guilford; 1999.

81. Wilbarger P, Wilbarger J. Sensory defensiveness and related social/emotional and neurological problems. Conference, October 13–14, 1990, Hartford CT.

82. Wilbarger P, Wilbarger J. Sensory defensiveness and related social/emotional and neurological problems; 1990. Follow-up workshop, circa 1997.

83. Scaer RC. The body bears the burden: trauma, dissociation and disease. New York: Taylor and Francis Group (Routledge); 2007.
84. Bremner JD. Acute and chronic responses to psychological trauma: where do we go from here? American Journal of Psychiatry. 1999;56:349–51.
85. Lanius RA, Bluhm R, Lanius U, Pain C. A review of neuroimaging studies in PTSD: heterogeneity of response to symptom provocation. Journal of Psychiatric Research. 2006;40:709–29.
86. Heim C, Nemeroff CB. Neurobiology of traumatic stress disorder. CNS Spectrum. 2009;14(1)(Suppl 1):13–24.
87. Swenson R. Chapter 10: Thalamic organization. In Swenson R (ed.), Review of clinical and functional neuroscience. Dartmouth Medical School (online); 2006 [accessed July 28, 2018]. Available from: https://www.dartmouth.edu/~rswenson/NeuroSci/chapter_10.html.
88. Herman JP, McKlveen JM, Ghosal S, Kopp B, Wulsin A, Makinson R et al. Regulation of the hypothalamic-pituitary-adrenocortical stress response. Comprehensive Physiology. 2016;6(2):603–21. Available from: http://doi.org/10.1002/cphy.c150015.
89. Cooper O, Bonert V, Moser F, Mirocha J, Melmed S. Altered pituitary gland structure and function in posttraumatic stress disorder. Journal of the Endocrine Society. 2017;1(6):577–87. Available from: http://doi.org/10.1210/js.2017-00069.
90. 90. Yehuda R, Golier JA, Halligan SL, Meaney M, Bierer LM. The ACTH response to dexamethasone in PTSD. American Journal of Psychiatry. 2004;161(8):1397–403.
91. Vyas A, Mitra R, Rao S, Chattarji S. Chronic stress induces contrasting patterns of dendritic remodeling in hippocampal and amygdaloid neurons. Journal of Neuroscience. 2002;22(15):6810–18.
92. Pascoe MC, Thompson DR, Ski CF. Yoga, mindfulness-based stress reduction and stress-related physiological measures: a meta-analysis. Psychoneuroendocrinology. 2017;86:152–68. doi: 10.1016/j.psyneuen.2017.08.008.

Chapter 4

1. Scaer R. The trauma spectrum: hidden wounds and human resiliency. New York: WW Norton; 2005.
2. Bremner JD. Neuroimaging in posttraumatic stress disorder and other stress-related disorders. Neuroimaging Clinics of North America. 2007;17(4):523–38, ix. doi:10.1016/j.nic.2007.07.003..
3. University of California San Diego Center for Functional MRI. What is fMRI? (n.d.) [accessed 16 September 2018]. Available from: http://fmri.ucsd.edu/Research/whatisfmri.html.
4. Mayo Clinic. Positron emission tomography scan. Mayo Clinic; 27 March 2018. Available from: https://www.mayoclinic.org/tests-procedures/pet-scan/about/pac-20385078.
5. Mayo Clinic. Suicide: what to do when someone is suicidal. Mayo Clinic; 31 January 2018. Available from: https://www.mayoclinic.org/diseases-conditions/suicide/in-depth/suicide/art-20044707.
6. Mayo Clinic. SPECT scan. May Clinic; 23 December 2016. Available from: https://www.mayoclinic.org/tests-procedures/spect-scan/about/pac-20384925.
7. National Institute of Biomedical Imaging and Bioengineering. Nuclear medicine. NIBIB; July 2016. Available from https://www.nibib.nih.gov/sites/default/files/Nuclear%20Medicine%20Fact%20Sheet%202016-english_FINAL.pdf.
8. Hughes KC, Shin LM. Functional neuroimaging studies of post-traumatic stress disorder. Expert Reviews in Neurotherapy. 2011;11(2):275–85.
9. Huang MX, Yurgil KA, Robb A et al. Voxel-wise resting-state MEG source magnitude imaging study reveals neurocircuitry abnormality in active-duty service members and veterans with PTSD. NeuroImage: Clinical. 2014;5:408–19. Available from: https://doi.org/10.1016/j.nicl.2014.08.004.
10. Massachusetts Institute of Technology. Basic principles of magnetoencephalography; n.d. [accessed 16 September 2018]. Available from: http://web.mit.edu/kitmitmeg/whatis.html.
11. Rauch et al. (1998), cited in Rauch SL, Shin LM, Phelps EA. Neurocircuitry models of posttraumatic stress disorder and extinction: human neuroimaging research—past, present, and future. Biological Psychiatry. 2006;60(4):376–82. Available from: https://doi.org/10.1016/j.biopsych.2006.06.004.
12. Rauch SL, Shin LM, Phelps EA. Neurocircuitry models of posttraumatic stress disorder and extinction: human neuroimaging research—past, present, and future. Biological Psychiatry. 2006;60(4):376–82. Available from: https://doi.org/10.1016/j.biopsych.2006.06.004.
13. Shin L, Rauch S, Pitman R. Structural and functional anatomy of PTSD. In Vasterling B (ed.), Neuropsychology of PTSD. New York: Guilford Press; 2005.
14. Shin LM, Liberzon I. The neurocircuitry of fear, stress, and anxiety disorders. Neuropsychopharmacology. 2010;35(1):169–91. doi: 10.1038/npp.2009.83.
15. Hayes JP, Hayes S M, Mikedis AM. Quantitative meta-analysis of neural activity in posttraumatic stress disorder. Biology of Mood and Anxiety Disorders. 2012;2:9. Available from: http://doi.org/10.1186/2045-5380-2-9.

REFERENCES continued

16. Bremner J, Staib L, Kaloupek D, Southwick S, Soufer R, Charney D. Neural correlates of exposure to traumatic pictures and sound in Vietnam combat veterans with and without posttraumatic stress disorder: a positron emission tomography study. Biological Psychiatry. 1999;45:806–16.

17. Etkin A, Wager TD. Functional neuroimaging of anxiety: a meta-analysis of emotional processing in PTSD, social anxiety disorder, and specific phobia. American Journal of Psychiatry. 2007;164(10):1476–88.

18. Kim SJ, Lyoo IK, Lee YS, Kim J, Sim ME, Bae SJ et al. (2007). Decreased cerebral blood flow of thalamus in PTSD patients as a strategy to reduce reexperience symptoms. Acta Psychiatrica Scandinavica. 2007;116:145–53.

19. Lanius RA, Williamson PC, Densmore M, Boksman K, Gupta M, Neufield RW et al. Neural correlates of traumatic memories in posttraumatic stress disorder: a functional MRI investigation. American Journal of Psychiatry. 2001;158:1920–22.

20. Lanius RA, Williamson PC, Hopper J, Densmore M, Boksman K, Gupta MA et al. Recall of emotional states in posttraumatic stress disorder: an fMRI investigation. Biological Psychiatry. 2003;53:204–10. doi: 10.1016/S0006-3223(02)01466-X.

21. Liberzon I, Taylor SF, Amdur R, Jung TD, Chamberlain KR, Minoshima S et al. Brain activation in PTSD in response to trauma-related stimuli. Biological Psychiatry. 1999;45:817–26. doi: 10.1016/S0006-3223(98)00246-7.

22. Ayres AJ. Sensory integration and learning disorders. Los Angeles: Western Psychological Services; 1972.

23. Krystal JH, Bennett AL, Bremner JD, Southwick SM, Charney DS. Toward a cognitive neuroscience of dissociation and altered memory functions in post-traumatic stress disorder. Neurobiological and clinical consequences of stress. In Friedmen MJ, Charney DS, Deutsch AY (eds). Normal adaptions to PTSD. New York: Raven Press; 1995, pp. 239–68.

24. Bergmann U. The neurobiology of EMDR: exploring the thalamus and neural integration. Journal of EMDR Practice and Research. 2008;2(4):300–14. Available from: http://dx.doi.org/10.1891/1933-3196.2.4.300.

25. VanElzakker MB, Dahlgren MK, Davis FC, Dubois S, Shin LM. From Pavlov to PTSD: the extinction of conditioned fear in rodents, humans, and in anxiety disorders. Neurobiology of Learning and Memory. 2014;113:3–18. Available from: http://doi.org/10.1016/j.nlm.2013.11.014.

26. Lanius RA, Vermetten E, Loewenstein RJ, Brand B, Schmahl C, Bremner JD et al. Emotion modulation in PTSD: clinical and neurobiological evidence for a dissociative subtype. American Journal of Psychiatry. 2010;167(6):640–7. doi: 10.1176/appi.ajp.2009.09081168.

27. Lanius RA, Williamson PC, Bluhm RL, Densmore M, Boksman K, Gupta M et al. Functional connectivity of dissociative responses in posttraumatic stress disorder: a functional magnetic resonance imaging investigation. Biological Psychiatry. 2005;57:873–84.

28. Lanius RA, Williamson PC, Boksman K, Densmore M, Gupta M, Neufeld RW et al. Brain activation during script-driven imagery induced dissociative responses in PTSD: a functional magnetic resonance imaging investigation. Biological Psychiatry. 2002;52:305–11.

29. Hopper J.W., Frewen P.A., van der Kolk B.A., Lanius R.A. (2007). Neural correlates of reexperiencing, avoidance, and dissociation in PTSD: Symptom dimensions and emotion dysregulation in responses to script-driven trauma imagery. Journal of Traumatic Stress, 20(5), p. 713–725.

30. Yehuda, R., Hoge, C.W., McFarlane, A.C., Vermetten, E., Lanius, R.A., Nievergelt, C.M., Hobfoll, S.E., Koenen, K.C., Nevlan, T.C., & Hyman, S.E. (2015). Post-traumatic stress disorder. Nature Reviews Disease Primers (1)15057, p. 1-22.

31. Bluhm RL, Williamson PC, Osuch EA, Frewen PA, Stevens TK, Boksman K et al. Alterations in default network connectivity in posttraumatic stress disorder related to early-life trauma. Journal of Psychiatry and Neuroscience. 2009;34(3):187–94.

32. van der Kolk BA. The body keeps the score: brain, mind, and body in the healing of trauma. New York: Viking (Penguin Random House); 2014.

33. Lanius RA, Frewen PA, Tursich M, Jetly R, McKinnon MC. Restoring large-scale brain networks in PTSD: a proposal for neuroscientifically-informed treatment interventions. European Journal of Psychotraumatology. 2015;6:27313. doi: 10.3402/ejpt.v6.27313.

34. Stark EA, Parsons CE, Van Hartevelt TJ, Charquero-Ballester M, McManners H, Ehlers A et al. Post-traumatic stress influences the brain even in the absence of symptoms: a systematic, quantitative meta-analysis of neuroimaging studies. Neuroscience and Biobehavioral Reviews. 2015;56:207–21. doi: 10.1016/j.neubiorev.2015.07.007.

35. Sridharan D, Levitin DJ, Menon V. A critical role for the right fronto-insular cortex in switching between central-executive and default-mode networks. Proceedings of the National Academy of Sciences. 2008;105(34):12569–74.

36. Menon V. Large-scale brain networks and psychopathology: a unifying triple network model. Trends in Cognitive Sciences 2011;15:483–506.

37. Patel R, Spreng RN, Shin LM, Girard TA. Neurocircuitry models of posttraumatic stress disorder and beyond: a meta-analysis of functional neuroimaging studies. Neuroscience and Biobehavioral Reviews 2012;36(9):2130–42. doi: 10.1016/j.neubiorev.2012.06.003.

38. Seeley WW, Menon V, Schatzberg AF, Keller J, Glover GH, Kenna, H et al. Dissociable intrinsic connectivity networks for salience processing and executive control. Journal of Neuroscience. 2007;27(9):2349–56. Available from: http://doi.org/10.1523/JNEUROSCI.5587-06.2007.

39. Beaty RE, Benedek M, Barry Kaufman S, Silvia PJ. Default and executive network coupling supports creative idea production. Scientific Reports. 2015;5:10964. Available from: http://doi.org/10.1038/srep10964.

40. Akiki TJ, Averill CL, Abdallah CG. A network-based neurobiological model of PTSD: evidence from structural and functional neuroimaging studies. Current Psychiatry Reports. 2017;19(11):81. DOI 10.1007/s11920-017-0840-4.

41. Sripada RK, King AP, Welsh RC, Garfinkel SN, Wang X, Sripada CS et al. Neural dysregulation in posttraumatic stress disorder: evidence for disrupted equilibrium between salience and default mode brain networks. Psychosomatic Medicine. 2012;74(9):904–11. Available from: http://doi.org/10.1097/PSY.0b013e318273bf33.

42. Nicholson AA, Ros T, Frewen PA, Densmore M, Théberge J, Kluetsch RC et al. Alpha oscillation neurofeedback modulates amygdala complex connectivity and arousal in posttraumatic stress disorder. NeuroImage: Clinical. 2016;12:506–16. Available from: http://doi.org/10.1016/j.nicl.2016.07.006.

43. Zhang Y, Chen H, Long Z, Cui Q, Chen H. Altered effective connectivity network of the thalamus in post-traumatic stress disorder: a resting-state FMRI study with Granger causality method. Applied Informatics. 2016;3(1):1–8.

44. Damasio AR, Grabowski TJ, Bechara A, Damasio H, Ponto LLB, Parvizi J et al. Subcortical and cortical brain activity during the feeling of self-generated emotions. Nature Neuroscience. 2000;3:1049–56.

45. Cisler JM, Bush K, James GA, Smitherman S, Kilts CD. Decoding the traumatic memory among women with PTSD: implications for neurocircuitry models of PTSD and real-time fMRI neurofeedback. PLoS ONE. 2015;10(8):e0134717. Available from: https://doi.org/10.1371/journal.pone.0134717.

46. Clancy K, Ding M, Bernat E, Schmidt NB, Li W. Restless "rest": intrinsic sensory hyperactivity and disinhibition in post-traumatic stress disorder. Brain. 2017;140(7):2041–50. Available from: https://doi.org/10.1093/brain/awx116.

47. Abdou AM, Higashiguchi S, Horie K, Kim M, Hatta H, Yogogoshi H. Relaxation and immunity enhancement effects of gamma-aminobutyric acid (GABA) administration in humans. Biofactors. 2006;26(3):201–8.

48. Fox JJ, Snyder AC. The role of alpha-band brain oscillations as a sensory suppression mechanism during selective attention. Frontiers in Psychology. 2011;2(154):1–13. Available from: https://doi.org/10.3389/fpsyg.2011.00154.

49. Klimesch W. Alpha-band oscillations, attention, and controlled access to stored information. Trends in Cognitive Sciences. 2012;16(12):606–17. Available from: http://doi.org/10.1016/j.tics.2012.10.007.

50. Kerr CE, Sacchet MD, Lazar SW, Moore CI, Jones SR. Mindfulness starts with the body: somatosensory attention and top-down modulation of cortical alpha rhythms in mindfulness meditation. Frontiers in Human Neuroscience. 2013;7:12. Available from: http://doi.org/10.3389/fnhum.2013.00012.

51. Freyer F et al. (2011), cited in Huang MX, Yurgil KA, Robb A, Angeles A, Diwakar M, Risbrough VB et al. Voxel-wise resting-state MEG source magnitude imaging study reveals neurocircuitry abnormality in active-duty service members and veterans with PTSD. NeuroImage: Clinical. 2014;5:415.

52. Hindriks R, van Putten MJ (2013), cited in Huang MX, Yurgil KA, Robb A, Angeles A, Diwakar M, Risbrough VB et al. Voxel-wise resting-state MEG source magnitude imaging study reveals neurocircuitry abnormality in active-duty service members and veterans with PTSD. NeuroImage: Clinical. 2014;5:415.

53. Lopes da Silva FH, Pijn JP, Velis D, Nijssen PC (1997), cited in Huang MX, Yurgil KA, Robb A, Angeles A, Diwakar M, Risbrough VB et al. Voxel-wise resting-state MEG source magnitude imaging study reveals neurocircuitry abnormality in active-duty service members and veterans with PTSD. NeuroImage: Clinical. 2014;5:415.

54. Falconer E, Bryant R, Felmingham KL, Kemp AH, Gordon E, Peduto A et al. The neural networks of inhibitory control in posttraumatic stress disorder. Journal of Psychiatry and Neuroscience. 2008;33(5):413–22.

55. Sripada RK, King AP, Welsh RC, Garfinkel SN, Wang X, Sripada CS et al. Neural dysregulation in posttraumatic stress disorder: evidence for disrupted equilibrium between salience and default mode brain networks. Psychosomatic Medicine. 2012;74(9):904–11. Available from: http://doi.org/10.1097/PSY.0b013e318273bf33.

56. Lanius RA, Frewen PA, Tursich M, Jetly R, McKinnon MC. Restoring large-scale brain networks in PTSD: a proposal for neuroscientifically-informed treatment interventions. European Journal of Psychotraumatology. 2015;6:27313. doi: 10.3402/ejpt.v6.27313.

57. Kamei T, Toriumi Y, Kimura H, Ohno S, Kumano H, Kimura, K. Decrease in serum cortisol during yoga exercise is correlated with alpha wave activation. Perceptual and Motor Skills. 2000;90:1027–32.

58. Cahn BR, Polich J. Meditation states and traits: EEG, ERP, and neuroimaging studies. Psychological Bulletin. 2006;132(2):180–211.

59. Streeter CC, Jensen JE, Perlmutter RM, Cabral HJ, Tian H, Terhune DB et al. Yoga asana sessions increase brain GABA levels: a pilot study. Journal of Alternative and Complementary Medicine. 2007;13(4):419–26. DOI: 10.1089/acm.2007.6338.

REFERENCES continued

108. Creswell J, Way B, Eisenberger N, Lieberman M. Neural correlates of dispositional mindfulness during affect labeling. Psychosomatic Medicine. 2007;69:560–5.

109. Lutz A, McFarlin DR, Perlman DM, Salomons TV, Davidson RJ. Altered anterior insula activation during anticipation and experience of painful stimuli in expert meditators. NeuroImage. 2012;64:538–46.

110. Herwig U, Kaffenberger T, Jancke L, Brühl A. Self-related awareness and emotion regulation. NeuroImage. 2010;50:734–41.

111. Hölzel BK, Carmody J, Evans KC, Hoge EA, Dusek JA, Morgan L et al. Stress reduction correlates with structural changes in the amygdala. Social Cognitive and Affective Neuroscience. 2009;5(1):11–17.

112. Lazar SW, Bush G, Gollub RL, Fricchione GL, Khalsa G, Benson H. Functional brain mapping of the relaxation response and meditation. NeuroReport. 2000;11(7):581–5.

113. Hölzel BK, Ott U, Hempel H, Hackl A, Wolf K, Stark R et al. Differential engagement of anterior cingulate and adjacent medial frontal cortex in adept meditators and non-meditators. Neuroscience Letters. 2007;42:16–21.

114. Hölzel BK, Ott U, Gard T, Hempel H, Weygandt M, Morgen K et al. Investigation of mindfulness meditation practitioners with voxel-based morphometry. Social Cognitive and Affective Neuroscience. 2008;3(1):55–61. Available from: http://doi.org/10.1093/scan/nsm038.

115. Holzel BK, Carmody J, Vangel M, Congleton C, Yerramsetti SM, Gard T et al. Mindfulness practice leads to increases in regional brain gray matter density. Psychiatry Research: Neuroimaging 2011;191:36–43.

116. Luders E, Toga AW, Lepore N, Gaser C. The underlying anatomical correlates of long-term meditation: larger hippocampal and frontal volumes of gray matter. NeuroImage. 2009;45:672–8.

117. Froeliger B, Garland EL, McClernon FJ. Yoga meditation practitioners exhibit greater gray matter volume and fewer reported cognitive failures: results of a preliminary voxel-based morphometric analysis. Evidence-Based Complementary and Alternative Medicine: eCAM. 2012;821307. Available from: http://doi.org/10.1155/2012/821307.

118. Courtiol E, Wilson DA. The olfactory thalamus: unanswered questions about the role of the mediodorsal thalamic nucleus in olfaction. Frontiers in Neural Circuits. 2015;9:49. doi:10.3389/fncir.2015.00049.

119. Menon V, Uddin LQ. Saliency, switching, attention and control: a network model of insula function. Brain Structure and Function. 2010;214(5–6):655–67. Available from: http://doi.org/10.1007/s00429-010-0262-0.

120. Craig AD. How do you feel? Interoception: the sense of the physiological condition of the body. Nature Reviews Neuroscience. 2002;3:655–66.

121. Craig AD. Interoception: the sense of the physiological condition of the body. Current Opinion in Neurobiology. 2003;13:500-5.

122. Shucard W, Fetter H, Chung C, Ramasamy D, Violanti J. Symptoms of posttraumatic stress disorder and exposure to traumatic stressors are related to brain structural volumes and behavioral measures of affective stimulus processing in police officers. Psychiatry Research: Neuroimaging. 2012;204(1):25–31.

123. Geuze E, van Berckel BN, Lammertsma AA, Boellaard R, deKloet CS, Vermetten E et al. Reduced GABA benzodiazepine receptor binding in veterans with post-traumatic stress disorder. Molecular Psychiatry. 2008;13:74–83.

124. Frewen and Lanius (2006), cited in Lanius RA, Frewen PA, Tursich M, Jetly R, McKinnon MC. Restoring large-scale brain networks in PTSD: a proposal for neuroscientifically-informed treatment interventions. European Journal of Psychotraumatology. 2015;6:27313. doi: 10.3402/ejpt.v6.27313.

125. Lanius, Vermetten et al. (2010), cited in Lanius RA, Frewen PA, Tursich M, Jetly R, McKinnon MC. Restoring large-scale brain networks in PTSD: a proposal for neuroscientifically-informed treatment interventions. European Journal of Psychotraumatology. 2015;6:27313. doi: 10.3402/ejpt.v6.27313.

126. Osuch EA, Benson B, Geraci M, Podell D, Herscovitch P, McCann UD. Regional cerebral blood flow correlated with flashback intensity in patients with posttraumatic stress disorder. Biological Psychiatry. 2001;50:246–53.

127. Whalley MG, Farmer E, Brewin CR. Pain flashbacks following the July 7th 2005 London bombings. Pain. 2007;132:332–6. doi: 10.1016/j.pain.2007.08.011.

128. Whalley MG, Kroes MCW, Huntley Z, Rugg MD, Davis SW, Brewin CR. An fMRI investigation of posttraumatic flashbacks. Brain and Cognition. 2013;81(1):151–9. Available from: http://doi.org/10.1016/j.bandc.2012.10.002.

129. Rosso IM, Weiner MR, Crowley DJ, Silveri MM, Rauch SL, Jensen JE. Insula and anterior cingulate GABA levels in post-traumatic stress disorder: preliminary findings using magnetic resonance spectroscopy. Depression and Anxiety. 2014;31(2):115–23. Available from: http://doi.org/10.1002/da.22155.

130. Newberg A, Alavi A, Baime M, Pourdehnad M, Santanna J, d'Aquili E. The measurement of regional cerebral blood flow during the complex cognitive task of meditation: a preliminary SPECT study. Psychiatry Research. 2001;106(2):113–22.

131. Bremner JD, Mishra S, Campanella C, Shah M, Kasher N, Evans S, et al. A pilot study of the effects of mindfulness-based stress reduction on post-traumatic stress disorder symptoms and brain response to

traumatic reminders of combat in Operation Enduring Freedom/Operation Iraqi Freedom combat veterans with post-traumatic stress disorder. Frontiers in Psychiatry. 2017;8:157. Available from: http://doi.org/10.3389/fpsyt.2017.00157.

132. Lazar SW, Kerr CE, Wasserman RH, Gray JR, Greve DN, Treadway MT et al. Meditation experience is associated with increased cortical thickness. Neuroreport. 2005;16(17):1893–7.

133. Villemure C, Čeko M, Cotton VA, Bushnell MC. Neuroprotective effects of yoga practice: age-, experience-, and frequency-dependent plasticity. Frontiers in Human Neuroscience. 2015;9:281. Available from: http://doi.org/10.3389/fnhum.2015.00281.

134. Farb NAS, Segal ZV, Mayberg H, Bean J, McKeon D, Fatima Z et al. Attending to the present: mindfulness meditation reveals distinct neural modes of self-reference. Social Cognitive and Affective Neuroscience. 2007;2(4):313–22. http://doi.org/10.1093/scan/nsm030.

135. Bromis K, Calem M, Reinders AATS, Williams SCR, Kempton MJ. Meta-analysis of 89 structural MRI studies in posttraumatic stress disorder and comparison with major depressive disorder. American Journal of Psychiatry. 2018;175(10):989–98. DOI: 10.1176/appi.ajp.2018.17111199.

136. Corbo V, Clément MH, Armony JL, Pruessner JC, Brunet A. Size versus shape differences: contrasting voxel-based and volumetric analyses of the anterior cingulate cortex in individuals with acute posttraumatic stress disorder. Biological Psychiatry. 2005;58(2):119–24.

137. Corbo V, Salat DH, Amick MM, Leritz EC, Milberg WP, McGlinchey RE. Reduced cortical thickness in veterans exposed to early life trauma. Psychiatry Research. 2014;223(2):53–60.

138. Chen S, Xia W, Li L, Liu J, He Z, Zhang Z, Yan L, Zhang J, Hu D. Gray matter density reduction in the insula in fire survivors with posttraumatic stress disorder: a voxel-based morphometric study. Psychiatry Research. 2006;146:65–72.

139. Chen S, Li L, Xu B, Liu J. Insular cortex involvement in declarative memory deficits in patients with post-traumatic stress disorder. BMC Psychiatry. 2009;9(39):1–9.

140. Herringa R, Phillips M, Almeida J, Insana S, Germain A. Post-traumatic stress symptoms correlate with smaller subgenual cingulate, caudate, and insula volumes in unmedicated combat veterans. Psychiatry Research. 2012;203(2–3):139–45.

141. Kasai K, Yamasue H, Gilbertson MW, Shenton ME, Rauch SL, Pitman RK. Evidence for acquired pregenual anterior cingulate gray matter loss from a twin study of combat-related posttraumatic stress disorder. Biological Psychiatry. 2008;63:550–6.

142. Perez DL, Matin N, Barsky A, Costumero-Ramos V, Makaretz SJ, Young SS et al. Cingulo-insular structural alterations associated with psychogenic symptoms, childhood abuse and PTSD in functional neurological disorders. Journal of Neurology, Neurosurgery, and Psychiatry. 2017;88(6):491–7.

143. Lindemer ER, Salat DH, Leritz EC, McGlinchey RE, Milberg WP. Reduced cortical thickness with increased lifetime burden of PTSD in OEF/OIF veterans and the impact of comorbid TBI. NeuroImage: Clinical. 2013;2:601–11. Available from: http://doi.org/10.1016/j.nicl.2013.04.009.

144. Clausen AN, Billinger SA, Sisante JV, Suzuki H, Aupperle RL. Preliminary evidence for the impact of combat experiences on gray matter volume of the posterior insula. Frontiers in Psychology. 2017;8:2151. doi:10.3389/fpsyg.2017.02151.

145. Zeidan F, Martucci KT, Kraft RA, McHaffie JG, Coghill RC. Neural correlates of mindfulness meditation-related anxiety relief. Social Cognitive and Affective Neuroscience. 2014;9(6):751–9. Available from: https://doi.org/10.1093/scan/nst041.

146. Gard T, Hölzel BK, Sack AT, Hempel H, Lazar SW, Vaitl D et al. Pain attenuation through mindfulness is associated with decreased cognitive control and increased sensory processing in the brain. Cerebral Cortex. 2011;22(11):2692–702.

147. Grant JA, Courtemanche J, Rainville P. A non-elaborative mental stance and decoupling of executive and pain-related cortices predicts low pain sensitivity in Zen meditators. Pain. 2011;152:150–6.

148. Stevens FL, Hurley RA, Taber KH. Anterior cingulate cortex: unique role in cognition and emotion. Journal of Neuropsychiatry and Clinical Neurosciences. 2011;23(2):121–5.

149. Blini E, Tilikete C, Farnè A, Hadj-Bouziane F. Probing the role of the vestibular system in motivation and reward-based attention. Cortex. 2018;103:82–99. Available from: http://doi.org/10.1016/j.cortex.2018.02.009.

150. Etkin A, Egner T, Kalisch R. Emotional processing in anterior cingulate and medial prefrontal cortex. Trends in Cognitive Sciences. 2011;15(2):85–93. Available from: http://doi.org/10.1016/j.tics.2010.11.004.

151. Shin LM, Rauch SL, Pitman RK. Amygdala, medial prefrontal cortex, and hippocampal function in PTSD. Annals of the New York Academy of Sciences. 2006;1071:67–79. Available from: https://doi.org/10.1196/annals.1364.007.

152. Shin LM, Bush G, Whalen PJ, Handwerger K, Cannistraro PA, Wright CI et al. Dorsal anterior cingulate function in posttraumatic stress disorder. Journal of Traumatic Stress. 2007;20:701–12.

19. Stoller CC, Greuel JH, Cimini LS, Fowler MS, Koomar JA. Effects of sensory enhanced yoga on symptoms of combat stress in deployed military personnel. American Journal of Occupational Therapy. 2012;66(1):59–68. Available from: http://ajot.aota.org/article.aspx?articleid=1851541.

20. US Census. Percentage of veterans among the adult population, 3 November 2017. https://www.census.gov/library/visualizations/2017/comm/veterans-day.html.

21. Yoga Service Council, Horton C (ed.). Best practices for yoga with veterans. Available from: https://yogaservicecouncil.org/best-practices-for-yoga-with-veterans.

22. Gutman SA. Reporting standards for intervention effectiveness studies. American Journal of Occupational Therapy. 2010;64:523–7.

23. Stoller C, Greuel J, Cimini L. Quality of Life Survey [unpublished]; 2009.

24. Engel-Yeger B, Palgy-Levin D, Lev-Wiesel R. The sensory profile of people with post-traumatic stress symptoms. Occupational Therapy in Mental Health. 2013;29:266–78.

25. Stoller C, Cimini L. [Sensory profiles of older veterans diagnosed with PTSD]. Unpublished raw data; 2008.

Chapter 6

1. Kilpatrick D, Resnick H, Ruggiero K, Conoscenti L, Cauley J. Drug-facilitated, incapacitated, and forcible rape: a national study; 2007 [accessed 11 December 2017]. Available from: http://www.ncjrs.gov/pdffiles1/nij/grants/219181.pdf.

2. Perry SW. American Indians and crime—a BJS statistical profile 1992–2002. Bureau of Justice Statistics, US Department of Justice, Office of Justice Programs; 1 December 2004. Available from: http://bjs.ojp.usdoj.gov/index.cfm?ty=pbdetail&iid=386.

3. Crenshaw K. Mapping the margins: intersectionality, identity politics, and violence against women of color. Stanford Law Review. 1991;43(6):1241–99.

4. Moraga C (ed.). This bridge called my back. 4th ed. Albany: State University of New York; 2015.

5. Herman J. Trauma and recovery: the aftermath of violence—from domestic abuse to political terror. New York: Basic Books; 1997.

6. Rothschild B. The body remembers: the psychophysiology of trauma and trauma treatment. New York: WW Norton; 2000.

7. Rothschild B. The body remembers casebook: unifying methods and models in the treatment of trauma and PTSD (Norton Professional Books). New York: WW Norton; 2003.

8. Clark CJ, Lewis-Dmello A, Anders D, Parsons A, Nguyen-Feng V, Henn L et al. Trauma-sensitive yoga as an adjunct mental health treatment in group therapy for survivors of domestic violence: a feasibility study. Complementary Therapies in Clinical Practice. 2014;20(3):152–8.

9. Crews DA, Stolz-Newton M, Grant NS. The use of yoga to build self-compassion as a healing method for survivors of sexual violence. Journal of Religion and Spirituality in Social Work: Social Thought. 2016;35(3):139–56.

10. Ong JI. Trauma-sensitive yoga: a collective case study of the trauma recovery of women impacted by intimate partner violence (IPV). Dissertation; directed by Dr. Craig S Cashwell; 2016.

11. Earley MD, Chesney MA, Frye J, Greene PA, Berman B, Kimbrough E. Mindfulness intervention for child abuse survivors: a 2.5-year follow-up: MICAS-II. Journal of Clinical Psychology. 2014;70(10):933–41. doi:10.1002/jclp.22102.

12. Hill JM, Vernig PM, Lee JK, Brown C, Orsillo SM. The development of a brief acceptance and mindfulness-based program aimed at reducing sexual revictimization among college women with a history of childhood sexual abuse. Journal of Clinical Psychology. 2011;67(9):969–80. doi:10.1002/jclp.20813.

13. Impett EA, Daubenmier JJ, Hirschman AL. Minding the body: yoga, embodiment, and well-being. Sexuality Research and Social Policy. 2006;3(4):39–48.

14. Rousseau D, Jackson D. Promoting resilience through yoga: profiling the implementation of trauma-informed integrative mindfulness programming in post-earthquake Haiti. Journal of Yoga Service. 2013;1(1):38–46.

15. yogaHOPE. TIMBo Facilitator Manual; 2014.

16. Van der Kolk BA. The body keeps the score: brain, mind and body in the healing of trauma. New York: Penguin Books; 2015.

17. Helms JE, Nicolas G, Green CE. Racism and ethnoviolence as trauma: enhancing professional training. Traumatology. 2010;16(4):53–62. doi:10.1177/1534765610389595.

Chapter 7

1. Kaeble D, Glaze LE. Correctional populations in the United States, 2015. Bureau of Justice Statistics. US Department of Justice; 2016. Available from: https://www.bjs.gov/content/pub/pdf/cpus15.pdf.

2. Bronson J, Berzofsky M. Indicators of mental health problems reported by prisoners and jail inmates, 2011–12. Bureau of Justice Statistics; 2017. Available from: https://www.bjs.gov/content/pub/pdf/imhprpji1112.pdf.

3. Western B. Punishment and inequality in America. New York: Russell Sage; 2006.

4. Alexander M, West C. The new Jim Crow: mass incarceration in the age of colorblindness. Revised ed. New York: New Press; 2010.

5. Snyder TR. The Protestant ethic and the spirit of punishment. Grand Rapids, MI: WB Eerdmans; 2001.

6. Graber J. The furnace of affliction: prisons and religion in antebellum America. Chapel Hill, NC: University of North Carolina Press; 2011.

7. Colvin M. Penitentiaries, reformatories, and chain gangs: social theory and the history of punishment in nineteenth-century America. New York: St Martin's Press; 1997.

8. Smith C, Hancock H, Blake-Mortimer J, Eckert K. A randomized comparative trial of yoga and relaxation to reduce stress and anxiety. Complementary Therapies in Medicine. 2007;15(2):77–83.

9. Somerstein L. Together in a room to alleviate anxiety: yoga breathing and psychotherapy. Procedia – Social and Behavioral Sciences. 2010;5:267–71.

10. Cramer H, Lauche R, Langhorst J, Dobos G. Yoga for depression: a systematic review and meta-analysis. Depression and Anxiety. 2013;30(11):1068–83.

11. Pilkington K, Kirkwood G, Rampes H, Richardson J. Yoga for depression: the research evidence. Journal of Affective Disorders. 2005;89(1):13–24.

12. van der Kolk BA, Stone L, West J, Rhodes A, Emerson D, Suvak M et al. Yoga as an adjunctive treatment for posttraumatic stress disorder: a randomized controlled trial. Journal of Clinical Psychiatry. 2014;75(6).

13. Baer RA. Mindfulness training as a clinical intervention: a conceptual and empirical review. Clinical Psychology: Science and Practice. 2003;10(2):125–43.

14. Carmody J, Baer R. Relationships between mindfulness practice and levels of mindfulness, medical and psychological symptoms and well-being in a mindfulness-based stress reduction program. Journal of Behavioral Medicine. 2008;31(1):23–33. DOI: 10.1007/s10865-007-9130-7.

15. Impett EA, Daubenmier JJ, Hirschman AL. Minding the body: yoga, embodiment, and well-being. Sexuality Research and Social Policy. 2006;3(4):39–48.

16. Mitchell KS, Dick AM, DiMartino DM, Smith BN, Niles B, Koenen KC et al. A pilot study of a randomized controlled trial of yoga as an intervention for PTSD symptoms in women. Journal of Traumatic Stress. 2014;27(2):121–8.

17. Rhodes A, Spinazolla J, van der Kolk B. Yoga for adult women with chronic PTSD: a long-term follow-up study. Journal of Alternative and Complementary Medicine New York. 2016;22(3):189–96.

18. Price M, Spinazzola J, Musicaro R, Turner J, Suvak M, Emerson D et al. Effectiveness of an extended yoga treatment for women with chronic posttraumatic stress disorder. Journal of Alternative and Complementary Medicine. 2017;23 (4):300–9.

19. Bilderbeck AC, Farias M, Brazil IA, Jakobowitz S, Wikholm C. Participation in a 10-week course of yoga improves behavioural control and decreases psychological distress in a prison population. Journal of Psychiatric Research. 2013;47(10):1438–45.

20. Duncombe E, Komorosky D, Wong-Kim E, Turner W. Free inside: a program to help inmates cope with life in prison at Maui Community Correctional Center. Californian Journal of Health Promotion. 2005;3(4):48–58.

21. Epstein R, González T. Gender and trauma: somatic interventions for girls in juvenile justice: implications for policy and practice. Washington, DC: Center on Poverty and Inequality, Georgetown Law, Georgetown University; 2017. Available from: http://www.traumacenter.org/products/pdf_files/gender_and_trauma_yoga_4.25.2017.pdf.

22. Landau PS, Gross JB. Low reincarceration rate associated with Ananda Marga Yoga and meditation. International Journal of Yoga Therapy. 2008;18(1):43–8.

23. Stern K. Voices from American prisons: faith, education and healing. Abingdon and New York: Routledge; 2014. Available from: http://public.eblib.com/choice/publicfullrecord.aspx?p=1715831.

24. Auty KM, Cope A, Liebling A. A systematic review and meta-analysis of yoga and mindfulness meditation in prison: effects on psychological well-being and behavioural functioning. International Journal of Offender Therapy and Comparative Criminology. 2015;61(6):689–710.

25. Muirhead J, Fortune C. Yoga in prisons: a review of the literature. Aggression and Violent Behavior. 2016;28(1–4):57–63.

26. Barrett CJ. Mindfulness and rehabilitation: teaching yoga and meditation to young men in an alternative to incarceration program. International Journal of Offender Therapy and Comparative Criminology. 2016;61(15):1719–38.

27. Bilderbeck AC, Farias M, Brazil IA, Jakobowitz S, Wikholm C. Participation in a 10-week course of yoga improves behavioural control and decreases psychological distress in a prison population. Journal of Psychiatric Research. 2013;47(10):1438–45.

28. Duncombe E, Komorosky D, Wong-Kim E, Turner W. Free inside: a program to help inmates cope with life in prison at Maui Community

Correctional Center. Californian Journal of Health Promotion. 2005;3(4):48–58.

29. Harner H, Hanlon AL, Garfinkel M. Effect of Iyengar yoga on mental health of incarcerated women: a feasibility study. Nursing Research and Practice. 2010;59(6):389–99.

30. Danielly Y, Silverthorne C. Psychological benefits of yoga for female inmates. International Journal of Yoga Therapy. 2017;27(1):9–14.

31. Horton C (ed.). Best practices for yoga in the criminal justice system. Rhinebeck, NY: YSC-Omega Publications; 2017.

32. Helms JE, Nicolas G, Green CE. Racism and ethnoviolence as trauma: enhancing professional training. Traumatology. 2010;16(4):53–62. doi:10.1177/1534765610389595.

Chapter 8

1. Ginwright S. The future of healing: shifting from trauma informed care to healing centered engagement. Medium, 31 May 2018 [accessed 1 August 2018]. Available from: https://medium.com/@ginwright/the-future-of-healing-shifting-from-trauma-informed-care-to-healing-centered-engagement-634f557ce69c.

2. UNHCR. Global trends: forced displacement in 2016; 2017 [accessed 12 December 2017]. Available from: http://www.unhcr.ch/5943e8a34.pdf.

3. International Institute for Strategic Studies (IISS). Armed Conflict Survey. Global conflict fatalities 2016 [map]; 9 May 2017 [accessed 25 January 2018]. Available from: https://www.iiss.org/-/media//documents/publications/acs/acs%202017/acs-2017-global-conflict-numbers.pdf?la=en4.

4. Internal Displacement Monitoring Centre. Global estimates 2015: people displaced by disasters; 2015 [accessed 28 January 2018]. Available from: http://www.internal-displacement.org/assets/library/Media/201507-globalEstimates-2015/20150713-global-estimates-2015-en-v1.pdf.

5. Center for Research on the Epidemiology of Disasters. The human cost of natural disasters: a global perspective; 2015. Available from: https://www.preventionweb.net/publications/view/42895.

6. Herman J. Trauma and recovery: the aftermath of violence—from domestic abuse to political terror. New York: Basic Books; 1997.

7. Fullilove MT. Psychiatric implications of displacement: contributions from the psychology of place. American Journal of Psychiatry. 1996;153:12; PA Research II Periodicals, 1516–23.

8. Fullilove MT. What is rootshock?; 2017 [accessed 25 January 2018]. Available from: http://www.rootshock.org/.

9. Bogic M, Njoku A, Priebe S. Long-term mental health of war-refugees: a systematic literature review. BMC International Health and Human Rights. 2015;15(29):1–41. Available from: https://doi.org/10.1186/s12914-015-0064-9.

10. Porter M, Haslam N. Predisplacement and postdisplacement factors associated with mental health of refugees and internally displaced persons a meta-analysis. Journal of the American Medical Association. 2005;294(5):602–12. doi:10.1001/jama.294.5.602.

11. Li SSY, Liddell BJ, Nickerson A. The relationship between post-migration stress and psychological disorders in refugees and asylum seekers. Current Psychiatry Reports. 2016;18:82.

12. Hamid AARM, Musa SA. Mental health problems among internally displaced persons in Darfur. International Journal of Psychology. 2010;45:278–85.

13. Coffey GJ, Kaplan I, Sampson RC, Tucci MM. The meaning and mental health consequences of long-term immigration detention for people seeking asylum. Social Science Medicine. 2010;70(12):2070–9.

14. Steel Z, Silove D, Brooks R, Momartin S, Alzuhairi B, Susljik I. Impact of immigration detention and temporary protection on the mental health and temporary protection on the mental health of refugees. British Journal of Psychiatry. 2006;188:58–64.

15. Women's Commission on Refugee Women and Children. Rebuilding Rwanda: "A struggle men cannot do alone." Delegate Report. 2000;(Winter):4.

16. Pham PN, Weinstein HM, Longman T. Trauma and PTSD symptoms in Rwanda: implications for attitudes toward justice and reconciliation. JAMA. 2004;292(5):602–12.

17. Neugebauer R, Fisher PW, Turner JB, Yamabe S, Sarsfield JA, Stehling-Ariza T. Post-traumatic stress reactions among Rwandan children and adolescents in the early aftermath of genocide. International Journal of Epidemiology. 2009;38(4):1033–45.

18. Roberts B, Makhashvili N, Javakhisvili J. Hidden burdens of conflict: issues of mental health and access to services among internally displaced persons in Ukraine; 2017 [accessed 29 January 2018]. Available from: http://www.international-alert.org/sites/default/files/Ukraine_HiddenBurdensConflictIDPs_EN_2017.pdf.

19. Rugema L, Krantz G, Mogren I, Ntaganira J, Persson M. "A constant struggle to receive mental health care": health care professionals' acquired experience of barriers to mental health care services in Rwanda. BMC Psychiatry. 2015;15:314. Available from: http://doi.org/10.1186/s12888-015-0699-z.

20. Antares Foundation. Managing stress in humanitarian workers: guidelines for good practice. Amsterdam: Antares Foundation; 2012.

21. Africa Healing Exchange. Restoring resiliency; 2018 [accessed 25 January 2018]. Available from: http://healingexchange.org/restoring-resiliency/.
22. Elliott S, Edmonson DR. The new science of breath: coherent breathing for autonomic nervous system valance, health, and well-being. Allen, TX: Coherence Press; 2006.
23. Gerbarg PL, Brown RP. Yoga and neuronal pathways to enhance stress response, emotion regulation, bonding, and spirituality. In Horovitz EG, Elgelid S (eds), Yoga therapy: theory and practice. New York: Routledge; 2015, pp. 49–64.
24. Brown RP, Gerbarg P.L. The healing power of the breath: simple techniques to reduce stress and anxiety, enhance concentration, and balance your emotions. Boston, MA: Shambhala Publications; 2012.
25. Brown RP, Gerbarg PL. Sudarshan kriya yogic breathing in the treatment of stress, anxiety, and depression: part 1 – neurophysiologic model. Journal of Alternative and Complementary Medicine. 2005;11(1):189–201.
26. Gerbarg PL, Brown RP. Neurobiology and neurophysiology of breath practices in psychiatric care. Psychiatric Times. 2016;33(11):22–5.
27. Fehmi L, Robbins J. The open-focus brain: harnessing the power of attention to heal mind and body. Boston, MA: Trumpeter Books (Shambhala Publications); 2007.
28. Gerbarg PL, Wallace G, Brown RP. Mass disasters and mind-body solutions: evidence and field insights. International Journal of Yoga Therapy. 2011;21:23–34.
29. Brown RP, Gerbarg PL. Breathing techniques in psychiatric treatment. In Gerbarg PL, Brown RP, Muskin PR (eds), Complementary and integrative treatments in psychiatric practice. Washington, DC: American Psychiatric Association Publishing; 2017.
30. Global Grassroots. July 2017 [2017 Young Women's Academy Endline per Student Analysis]. Unpublished raw data.
31. Anderson MB. Do no harm: how aid can produce peace—or war. Colorado: Lynn Rienner Publishing; 1999.
32. Psychosocial Working Group. Considerations in planning psychosocial programs; 2004.

Chapter 9

1. Van der Kolk BA, Roth S, Pelcovitz D, Sunday S, Spinazzola J. Disorders of extreme stress: the empirical foundation of a complex adaptation to trauma. Journal of Traumatic Stress. 2005;18(5):389–99.
2. Courtois CA, Ford JD. Treating complex traumatic stress disorders: an evidence-based guide. New York: Guildford Press; 2009.
3. Pelcovitz D, van der Kolk BA, Roth S, Mandel FS, Kaplan S, Resick PA. Development of a criteria set and a structures interview for disorders of extreme stress (SIDES). Journal of Traumatic Stress. 1997;10(1):3–17.
4. Herman J. Trauma and recovery: the aftermath of violence—from domestic abuse to political terror. New York: Basic Books; 1997.
5. Cloitre M, Stolbach BC, Herman JL, van der Kolk B, Pynoos R, Wang J et al. Developmental approach to complex PTSD: childhood and adult cumulative trauma as predictors of symptom complexity. Journal of Traumatic Stress. 2009;22(5):399–408.
6. Kessler RC, Berglund PA, Demler O, Jin R, Walters EE. Lifetime prevalence and age-of-onset distributions of DSM-IV disorders in the National Comorbidity Survey Replication (NCS-R). Archives of General Psychiatry. 2005;62(6):593–602.
7. Kessler RC, Chiu WT, Demler O, Walters EE. Prevalence, severity, and comorbidity of twelve-month DSM-IV disorders in the National Comorbidity Survey Replication (NCS-R). Archives of General Psychiatry. 2005;62(6):617–27.
8. Kessler RC, Sonnega A, Bromet E Hughes M, Nelson CB. Posttraumatic stress disorder in the National Comorbidity Survey. Archives of General Psychiatry. 1995;52(12):1048–60.
9. Ford JD, Kidd P. Early childhood trauma and disorders of extreme stress as predictors of treatment outcome with chronic PTSD. Journal of Traumatic Stress. 1998;18:743–61.
10. Edwards VJ, Holden GW, Felitti VJ, Anda RF. Relationship between multiple forms of child maltreatment and adult mental health in community respondents: results from the adverse childhood experiences study. American Journal of Psychiatry. 2003;160:1453–60.
11. Edwards VJ, Anda RF, Dube SR, Dong M, Chapman DF, Felitti VJ. The wide-ranging health consequences of adverse childhood experiences. In Kendall-Tackett K, Giacomoni S (eds). Victimization of children and youth: patterns of abuse, response strategies. Kingston, NJ; Civic Research Institute; 2005.
12. Gilbert LK, Breiding MJ, Merrick MT, Parks SE, Thompson WW, Dhingra SS et al. Childhood adversity and adult chronic disease: an update from ten states and the District of Columbia, 2010. American Journal of Preventive Medicine. 2015;48(3):345–9.
13. Dong M, Anda RF, Felitti VJ, Dube SR, Williamson DF, Thompson TJ et al. The interrelatedness of multiple forms of childhood abuse, neglect, and household dysfunction. Child Abuse and Neglect. 2004;28(7):771–84.
14. Coid J, Petruckevitch A, Feder G, Chung W, Richardson J, Moorey S. Relation between childhood sexual and physical abuse and risk of revictimisation in women: a cross-sectional survey. Lancet. 2001;358(9280):450–45.

REFERENCES *continued*

15. Campbell J, Jones AS, Dienemann J, Kub J, Schollenberger J, O'Campo P et al. Intimate partner violence and physical health consequences. Archives of Internal Medicine. 2002;162(10):1157–63.

16. van der Kolk BA. Clinical implications of neuroscience research in PTSD. Annals of the New York Academy of Sciences. 2006;1071:277–93.

17. Ladwig KH, Marten-Mittag B, Deisenhofer I, Hofmann B, Schapperer J, Weyerbrock S et al. Psychophysiological correlates of peritraumatic dissociative responses in survivors of life-threatening cardiac events. Psychopathology. 2002;35(4):241–8.

18. Lanius RA, Frewen PA, Vermetten E, Yehuda R. Fear conditioning and early life vulnerabilities: two distinct pathways of emotional dysregulation and brain dysfunction in PTSD. European Journal of Psychotraumatology. 2010;1(1):5467. DOI: 10.3402/ejpt.v1i0.5467.

19. Lanius RA, Vermetten E, Loewenstein RJ, Brand B, Schmahl C, Bremner JD et al. Emotion modulation in PTSD: clinical and neurobiological evidence for a dissociative subtype. American Journal of Psychiatry. 2010;167(6):640–7. doi:10.1176/appi.ajp.2009.09081168.

20. Rufer M, Held D, Cremer J, Fricke S, Moritz S, Peter H et al. Dissociation as a predictor of cognitive behavior therapy outcome in patients with obsessive-compulsive disorder. Psychotherapy and Psychosomatics. 2006;75(1):40–6.

21. Michelson L, June K, Vives A, Testa S, Marchione N. The role of trauma and dissociation in cognitive-behavioral psychotherapy outcome and maintenance for panic disorder with agoraphobia. Behaviour Research and Therapy. 1998;36(11):1011–50.

22. Schore JR, Schore AN. Attachment theory: the central role of affect regulation in development and treatment. Clinical Social Work Journal. 2007;36(1):9–20.

23. Emerson D, Hopper E. Overcoming trauma through yoga: reclaiming your body. Berkeley, CA: North Atlantic Books; 2011.

24. Emerson D, Sharma R, Chaudhry S, Turner J. Trauma-sensitive yoga: principles, practice, and research. International Journal of Yoga Therapy. 2009;19:123–8.

25. van der Kolk BA, Stone L, West J, Rhodes A, Emerson D, Suvak M et al. Yoga as an adjunctive treatment for posttraumatic stress disorder: a randomized controlled trial. Journal of Clinical Psychiatry. 2014;75(6):e559–65. doi: 10.4088/JCP.13m08561.

26. Rhodes AM. Claiming peaceful embodiment through yoga in the aftermath of trauma. Complementary Therapies in Clinical Practice. 2015;21(4):247–56.

27. Rhodes A, Spinazolla J, van der Kolk B. Yoga for adult women with chronic PTSD: a long-term follow-up study. Journal of Alternative and Complementary Medicine New York. 2016;22(3):189–96.

28. Emerson D. Trauma-sensitive yoga in therapy: bringing the body into treatment. New York: WW Norton; 2015.

29. van der Kolk BA, Stone L, West J, Rhodes A, Emerson D, Suvak M et al. (2014). Yoga as an adjunctive treatment for posttraumatic stress disorder: a randomized controlled trial. Journal of Clinical Psychiatry. 2014;75(6): e559–65. doi: 10.4088/JCP.13m08561.

30. Price M, Spinazzola J, Musicaro R, Turner J, Suvak M, Emerson D et al. Effectiveness of an extended yoga treatment for women with chronic posttraumatic stress disorder. Journal of Alternative and Complementary Medicine. 2017;23(4):300–9.

31. West J, Liang B, Spinazzola J. Trauma sensitive yoga as a complementary treatment for posttraumatic stress disorder: a qualitative descriptive analysis. International Journal of Stress Management. 2017;24(2):173–95. doi: 10.1037/str0000040.

32. Spinazzola J, Rhodes A, Emerson D, Earle E, Monroe K. Application of yoga in residential treatment of traumatized youth. Journal of the American Psychiatric Nurses Association. 2011;17(6):431–44.

Chapter 10

1. Stone M. The inner tradition of yoga. Boston: Shambhala Publications; 2008.

2. Kremer W. Does doing yoga make you a Hindu? BBC World Service, 21 November 2013 [accessed 28 September 2018]. Available from: https://www.bbc.com/news/magazine-25006926.

3. Ryan T (n.d.). Is yoga a religion? [Web article]; n.d. [accessed 29 September 2018]. Available from: www.christianspractingyoga.com/is-yoga-a-religion/.

4. Sharvananda S. Upanishad Series No. 7: Taittiriya-Upanishad. Mylapore, Madras: The Ramakrishna Math; 1921 [accessed 29 September 2018]. Available from: http://estudantedavedanta.net/Taittiriya%20Upanishad%20-%20Swami%20Sarvanand%20[Sanskrit-English].pdf.

5. Litz BT, Stein N, Delaney E, Lebowitz L, Nash WP, Silva C et al. Moral injury and moral repair in war veterans: a preliminary model and intervention strategy. Clinical Psychology Review. 2009;29:695–706.

6. Maguen S, Litz B. Moral injury in veterans of war. PTSD Research Quarterly. 2012;23(1):1–3.

7. Sathivaseelan A, Balasundaram S. A comparison of Maslow's theory of hierarchy of needs with the pancha kosha theory of Upanishads. Artha Journal of Social Sciences. 2016;15(1):59–68. Available from: https://doi.org 10.12724/ajss.36.4.

8. Maslow A. Toward a psychology of being. Princeton, NJ: Van Nostrand; 1962. Available from: http://dx.doi.org/10.1037/10793-000.

9. Sharvananda S. Upanishad Series No. 7: Taittiriya-Upanishad. Mylapore, Madras: The Ramakrishna Math; 1921 [accessed 29 September 2018]. Available from: http://estudantedavedanta.net/Taittiriya%20 Upanishad%20-%20Swami%20Sarvanand%20[Sanskrit-English].pdf.

10. Bremner JD. Acute and chronic responses to psychological trauma: where do we go from here? American Journal of Psychiatry. 1999;56:349–51.

11. Lanius RA, Bluhm R, Lanius U, Pain C. A review of neuroimaging studies in PTSD: heterogeneity of response to symptom provocation. Journal of Psychiatric Research. 2006;40:709–29.

12. Lanius RA, Vermetten E, Loewenstein RJ, Brand B, Schmahl C, Bremner JD et al. Emotion modulation in PTSD: clinical and neurobiological evidence for a dissociative subtype. American Journal of Psychiatry. 2010;167(6):640–7. doi:10.1176/appi.ajp.2009.09081168.

13. Lanius RA, Frewen PA, Tursich M, Jetly R, McKinnon MC. Restoring large-scale brain networks in PTSD: a proposal for neuroscientifically-informed treatment interventions. European Journal of Psychotraumatology. 2015;6:27313. doi: 10.3402/ejpt.v6.27313.

14. Stark EA, Parsons CE, Van Hartevelt TJ, Charquero-Ballester M, McManners H, Ehlers A et al. Post-traumatic stress influences the brain even in the absence of symptoms: A systematic, quantitative meta-analysis of neuroimaging studies. Neuroscience and Biobehavioral Reviews. 2015;56:207–21. doi: 10.1016/j.neubiorev.2015.07.007.

15. Vermetten E, Bremner JD. Olfaction as a traumatic reminder in posttraumatic stress disorder: case reports and review. Journal of Clinical Psychiatry. 2003;64:202–7.

16. Nivethitha L, Mooventhan A, Manjunath NK. Effects of various pranayama on cardiovascular and autonomic variables. Ancient Science of Life. 2016;36(2):72–7.

17. Le Page J, Le Page L. Mudras for healing and transformation. Sebastopol, CA: Integrative Yoga Therapy; 2013.

Chapter 11

1. Herman J. Trauma and recovery: the aftermath of violence—from domestic abuse to political terror. New York: Basic Books; 1997.

2. Odgen P, Minton K, Pain C. Trauma and the body: a sensorimotor approach to psychotherapy. New York: WW Norton; 2006.

3. van der Kolk BA. The body keeps the score: brain, mind, and body in the healing of trauma. New York: Viking (Penguin Random House); 2014.

4. Porges SW. The polyvagal theory: neurophysiological foundations of emotions, attachment communication, and self-regulation. New York: WW Norton; 2011.

5. Burstow B. Toward a radical understanding of trauma and trauma work. Violence Against Women. 2003;9(11):1293–317. DOI: 10.1177/1077801203255555.

6. Emerson D, Hopper E. Overcoming trauma through yoga: reclaiming your body. Berkeley, CA: North Atlantic Books; 2011.

7. van der Kolk BA. Affect regulation. Lecture presented at a Pre-Conference Institute of the 19th Annual International Trauma Conference, Boston, MA, 25 June 2008.

8. van der Kolk BA. The body keeps the score: brain, mind, and body in the healing of trauma. New York: Viking (Penguin Random House); 2014.

9. Rothschild B. Safe trauma recovery; 2009. [Video file]. Available from: https://www.youtube.com/watch?v=LhuzpUlaX_k. Also available from: http://www.somatictraumatherapy.com/videos/.

10. Caress SM, Steinemann AC. Prevalence of fragrance sensitivity in the American population. Journal of Environmental Health. 2009;71(7):46–50.

11. Steinemann A, Wheeler AJ, Larcombe A. Fragranced consumer products: effects on asthmatic Australians. Air Quality, Atmosphere, and Health. 2018;11(4):365–71. Available from: http://doi.org/10.1007/s11869-018-0560-x.

12. Steinemann A. Fragranced consumer products: exposures and effects from emissions. Air Quality, Atmosphere, and Health. 2016;9(8):861–6. Available from: http://doi.org/10.1007/s11869-016-0442-z.

13. Aloisi et al. (2002), cited in Watanabe E, Kuchta K, Kimura M, Rauwald HW, Kamei T, Imanishi J. Effects of Bergamot Citrus bergamia (Risso) Wright & Arn. Essential oil aromatherapy on mood states, parasympathetic nervous system activity, and salivary cortisol levels in 41 healthy females. Complimentary Medicine Research. 2015;22:44.

14. Barocelli et al. (2004), cited in Watanabe E, Kuchta K, Kimura M, Rauwald HW, Kamei T, Imanishi J. Effects of Bergamot Citrus bergamia (Risso) Wright & Arn. Essential oil aromatherapy on mood states, parasympathetic nervous system activity, and salivary cortisol levels in 41 healthy females. Complimentary Medicine Research. 2015;22:44.

15. Wilkinson et al. (2007), cited in Watanabe E, Kuchta K, Kimura M, Rauwald HW, Kamei T, Imanishi J. Effects of Bergamot Citrus bergamia (Risso) Wright & Arn. Essential oil aromatherapy on mood states, parasympathetic nervous system activity, and salivary cortisol levels in 41 healthy females. Complimentary Medicine Research. 2015;22:44.

16. Lehrner et al. (2000), cited in Watanabe E, Kuchta K, Kimura M, Rauwald HW, Kamei T, Imanishi J. Effects of Bergamot Citrus bergamia (Risso) Wright & Arn. Essential oil aromatherapy on mood states, parasympathetic nervous system activity, and salivary cortisol levels in 41 healthy females. Complimentary Medicine Research. 2015;22:44.

17. Zhang et al. (2007), cited in Watanabe E, Kuchta K, Kimura M, Rauwald HW, Kamei T, Imanishi J. Effects of Bergamot Citrus bergamia (Risso) Wright & Arn. Essential oil aromatherapy on mood states, parasympathetic nervous system activity, and salivary cortisol levels in 41 healthy females. Complimentary Medicine Research. 2015;22:44.

18. Chaiyana & Okonogi (2012), cited in Watanabe E, Kuchta K, Kimura M, Rauwald HW, Kamei T, Imanishi J. Effects of Bergamot Citrus bergamia (Risso) Wright & Arn. Essential oil aromatherapy on mood states, parasympathetic nervous system activity, and salivary cortisol levels in 41 healthy females. Complimentary Medicine Research. 2015;22:44.

19. Komori et al. (1995), cited in Watanabe E, Kuchta K, Kimura M, Rauwald HW, Kamei T, Imanishi J. Effects of Bergamot Citrus bergamia (Risso) Wright & Arn. Essential oil aromatherapy on mood states, parasympathetic nervous system activity, and salivary cortisol levels in 41 healthy females. Complimentary Medicine Research. 2015;22:44.

20. Komiya, Takeuchi, Harada (2006), cited in Watanabe E, Kuchta K, Kimura M, Rauwald HW, Kamei T, Imanishi J. Effects of Bergamot Citrus bergamia (Risso) Wright & Arn. Essential oil aromatherapy on mood states, parasympathetic nervous system activity, and salivary cortisol levels in 41 healthy females. Complimentary Medicine Research. 2015;22:44.

21. Watanabe E, Kuchta K, Kimura M, Rauwald HW, Kamei T, Imanishi J. Effects of Bergamot Citrus bergamia (Risso) Wright & Arn. Essential oil aromatherapy on mood states, parasympathetic nervous system activity, and salivary cortisol levels in 41 healthy females. Complimentary Medicine Research. 2015;22:43–9. doi: 10.1159/000380989.

22. Telles S, Bhardwaj AK, Kumar N, Balkrishna A. Performance in a substitution task and state anxiety following yoga in army recruits. Psychological Reports. 2012;110(3):963–76.

23. Hirsch CR, Holmes EA. Mental imagery in anxiety disorders. Psychiatry. 2007;6(4):165 [accessed 17 July 2011]. Available from: http://www.psychiatry.ox.ac.uk/epct/emily_holmes/articles/hirsch_holmes.

24. Schiraldi G. The post-traumatic stress disorder sourcebook: a guide to healing, recovery, and growth. New York: McGraw-Hill; 2000.

25. Rothschild B. The body remembers: the psychophysiology of trauma and trauma treatment. New York: WW Norton; 2000.

26. van der Kolk BA, McFarlane AC, Weisaeth L (eds). Traumatic stress: the effects of overwhelming experience on mind, body, and society. New York: Guilford; 1996.

27. Lieberman MD, Eisenberger NI, Crockett MJ, Tom SM, Pfeifer JH, Way BM. Putting feelings into words: affect labeling disrupts amygdala activity in response to affective stimuli. Psychological Science. 2007;18(5):421–8.

28. Mayo Clinic. Suicide: what to do when someone is suicidal; 31 January 2018. Available from: https://www.mayoclinic.org/diseases-conditions/suicide/in-depth/suicide/art-20044707.

Chapter 12

1. Saraswati, Swami Niranjanananda. (2009). Prana and pranayama. Yoga Publications Trust, Mungar, Bijar, India.

2. Saoji AA, Raghavendra BR, Manjunath NK. Effects of yogic breath regulation: a narrative review of scientific evidence. Journal of Ayurveda and Integrated Medicine. 2017;10(1):50–8. Available from: http://dx.doi.org/10.1016/j.jaim.2017.07.008.

3. Briggs T. Breathing lessons. [Web Article.] Yoga Journal, 28 August 2007. Available from: https://www.yogajournal.com/practice-section/breathing-lessons-2.

4. Khedikar S, Erande DV, Shukla M. Critical comparison of yogic nadi with nervous system. Journal of Indian System of Medicine. 2016;4(2):108–13 [accessed 7 October 2018]. Available from: https://www.researchgate.net/publication/317664235_Critical_comparison_of_Yogic_Nadi_with_Nervous_System.

5. Koob A. (n.d.). The root of thought: what do glial cells do? Scientific American online, n.d. [accessed 3 November 2018]. Available from: https://www.scientificamerican.com/article/the-root-of-thought-what/.

6. Brockett AT, Kane GA, Monari PK, Briones BA, Vigneron P-A, Barber GA et al. Evidence supporting a role for astrocytes in the regulation of cognitive flexibility and neuronal oscillations through the Ca2+ binding protein S100β. PLoS ONE. 2018;13(4):e0195726. Available from: https://doi.org/10.1371/journal.pone.0195726.

7. Bellot-Saez A, Cohen G, van Shaik A, Ooi L, Morely JW, Buskila Y. Astrocytic modulation of cortical oscillations. Scientific Reports. 2018;8(1):11565. DOI:10.1038/s41598-018-30003-w.

8. Maxwell RW. The physiological foundation of yoga chakra expression. Zygon Journal of Religion and Science. 2009;44(4):807–24.

9. Netter (1975), cited in Werntz DA, Bickford RG, Bloom FE, Shannahoff-Khalsa DS. Alternating cerebral hemispheric activity and the lateralization of autonomic nervous function. Human Neurobiology. 1983;2:42.

10. Saper et al. (1976), cited in Werntz DA, Bickford RG, Bloom FE, Shannahoff-Khalsa DS. Alternating cerebral hemispheric activity and the lateralization of autonomic nervous function. Human Neurobiology. 1983;2:42.

11. Eccles and Lee (1981), cited in Werntz DA, Bickford RG, Bloom FE, Shannahoff-Khalsa DS. Alternating cerebral hemispheric activity

and the lateralization of autonomic nervous function. Human Neurobiology. 1983;2:42.

12. Werntz DA, Bickford RG, Bloom FE, Shannahoff-Khalsa DS (1983). Alternating cerebral hemispheric activity and the lateralization of autonomic nervous function. Human Neurobiology. 1983;2:39–43.

13. Schore AN. Right-brain affect regulation: an essential mechanism of development, trauma, dissociation, and psychotherapy. In Fosha D, Siegal D, Solomon M (eds), The healing power of emotion: affect neuroscience, development, and clinical practice. New York: Norton; 2009, pp. 112–44.

14. Lin SJ, Danahey DG. Nasal aerodynamics. Medscape. Updated 14 May 2015. Available from: https://emedicine.medscape.com/article/874822-overview.

15. Kahana-Zweig R, Geva-Sagiv M, Weissbrod A, Secundo L, Soroker N, Sobel N. Measuring and characterizing the human nasal cycle. PLoS ONE. 2016;11(10):e0162918. Available from: http://doi.org/10.1371/journal.pone.0162918.

16. Price A, Eccles R. Nasal airflow and brain activity: is there a link? Journal of Laryngology and Otology. 2016;130(9):794–9. doi:10.1017/S0022215116008537.

17. Shannahoff-Khalsa DS. Stress technology medicine: a new paradigm for stress and considerations for self-regulation. In Brown M, Rivier C, Koob G (eds), Stress: neurobiology and neuroendocrinology. New York: Marcel Dekker; 1991, pp. 647–86.

18. Shannahoff-Khalsa DS, Kennedy B, Yates FE, Ziegler MG. The ultradian rhythms of autonomic, cardiovascular, and neuroendocrine systems are related in humans. American Journal of Physiology. 1996;270(4/2):R873–87.

19. Shannahoff-Khalsa DS, Kennedy B, Yates FE, Ziegler MG. Low frequency ultradian insulin rhythms are coupled to cardiovascular, autonomic, and neuroendocrine rhythms. American Journal of Physiology. 1997;41:R962–8.

20. Shannahoff-Khalsa DS. Psychophysiological states: the ultradian dynamics of mind-body interactions. International Review of Neurobiology, vol. 80. Cambridge, MA: Academic Press (Elsevier Scientific Publications); 2008, pp. 1–249.

21. Beissner F, Meissner K, Bär KJ, Napadow V. The autonomic brain: an activation likelihood estimation meta-analysis for central processing of autonomic function. Journal of Neuroscience. 2013;33(25):10503–11.

22. Stillman PE, Wilson JD, Denny MJ, Desmarais BA, Bhamidi S, Cranmer SJ et al. Statistical modeling of the default mode brain nsalmaetwork reveals a segregated highway structure. Scientific Reports. 2017;7(1):11694. doi:10.1038/s41598-017-09896-6.

23. Heck DH, McAfee1 SS, Liu Y, Babajani-Feremi A, Rezaie R, Freeman WJ. Cortical rhythms are modulated by respiration. BioRxiv preprint first posted online 16 April 2016 [accessed 15 October 2018]. Available from: https://core.ac.uk/download/pdf/78475708.pdf. doi: http://dx.doi.org/10.1101/049007.

24. Dillbeck and Bronson (1981), cited in Heck DH, McAfee1 SS, Liu Y, Babajani-Feremi A, Rezaie R, Freeman WJ. Cortical rhythms are modulated by respiration. BioRxiv preprint first posted online 16 April 2016 [accessed 15 October 2018]. Available from: https://core.ac.uk/download/pdf/78475708.pdf. doi: http://dx.doi.org/10.1101/049007.

25. Gaylord et al. (1989), cited in Heck DH, McAfee1 SS, Liu Y, Babajani-Feremi A, Rezaie R, Freeman WJ. Cortical rhythms are modulated by respiration. BioRxiv preprint first posted online 16 April 2016 [accessed 15 October 2018]. Available from: https://core.ac.uk/download/pdf/78475708.pdf. doi: http://dx.doi.org/10.1101/049007.

26. Stancak and Kuna (1994), cited in Heck DH, McAfee1 SS, Liu Y, Babajani-Feremi A, Rezaie R, Freeman WJ. Cortical rhythms are modulated by respiration. BioRxiv preprint first posted online 16 April 2016 [accessed 15 October 2018]. Available from: https://core.ac.uk/download/pdf/78475708.pdf. doi: http://dx.doi.org/10.1101/049007.

27. Raghuraj P, Telles S. Immediate effect of specific nostril manipulating yoga breathing practices on autonomic and respiratory variables. Applied Psychophysiological Biofeedback. 2008;33(2): 65–75. Available from: https://doi.org/10.1007/s10484-008-9055-0.

28. Bhavanani AB, Ramanathan M, Balaji R, Pushpa D. Differential effects of uninostril and alternate nostril pranayamas on cardiovascular parameters and reaction time. International Journal of Yoga. 2014;7(1):60–5. Available from: http://doi.org/10.4103/0973-6131.123489.

29. Bhavanani A, Ramanathan M. Immediate effect of alternate nostril breathing on cardiovascular parameters and reaction time. Online International Interdisciplinary Research Journal. 2014;4:297–302.

30. Ramanathan M, Bhavanani AB. Immediate effect of chandra and suryanadi pranayamas on cardiovascular parameters and reaction time in a geriatric population. International Journal of Physiology. 2014;2:59–63. doi: 10.5958/j.2320-608X.2.1.013.

31. Srivastava D, Jain N, Singhal A. Influence of alternate nostril breathing on cardiorespiratory and autonomic functions in healthy young adults. Indian Journal of Physiological Pharmacology. 2005;49(4):475–83.

32. Ghiya S, Lee CM. Influence of alternate nostril breathing on heart rate variability in non-practitioners of yogic breathing. International Journal of Yoga. 2012;5(1):66–9.

REFERENCES continued

33. Gard T, Noggle JJ, Park CL, Vago DR, Wilson A. Potential self-regulatory mechanisms of yoga for psychological health. Frontiers in Human Neuroscience. 2014;8:770. doi:10.3389/fnhum.2014.00770.

34. Billman GE. Heart rate variability – a historical perspective. Frontiers in Physiology. 2011;2:86. Available from: http://doi.org/10.3389/fphys.2011.00086.

35. Singh N, Moneghetti JM, Christle JW, Hadley D, Plews D, Froelicher V. Heart rate variability: an old metric with new meaning in the era of using mhealth technologies for health and exercise training guidance. Part one: physiology and methods. Arrhythmia and Electrophysiology Review. 2018;7(3):193–8.

36. van der Kolk BA. Clinical implications of neuroscience research in PTSD. Annals of the New York Academy of Sciences. 2006;1071:277–93.

37. Russo MA, Santarelli DM, O'Rourke D. The physiological effects of slow breathing in the healthy human. Breathe (Sheffield, England). 2017;13(4):298–309.

38. Dick et al. (2014), cited in Russo MA, Santarelli DM, O'Rourke D. The physiological effects of slow breathing in the healthy human. Breathe (Sheffield, England). 2017;13(4):301.

39. Bordoni and Zanier (2013), cited in Russo MA, Santarelli DM, O'Rourke D. The physiological effects of slow breathing in the healthy human. Breathe (Sheffield, England). 2017;13(4):301.

40. Elliot S. Coherence: the new science of breath; 2006 [accessed 19 May 2013]. Available from: www.coherence.com/science.

41. Gerbarg PL, Brown RP. Neurobiology and neurophysiology of breath practices in psychiatric care. Psychiatric Times, 30 November 2016. 2016;33(11):22–5.

42. Streeter CC, Gerbarg PL, Saper RB, Ciraulo DA, Brown RP. Effects of yoga on the autonomic nervous system, gamma-aminobutyric-acid, and allostasis in epilepsy, depression, and post-traumatic stress disorder. Medical Hypotheses. 2012;78(5):571–9.

43. Streeter CC, Gerbarg PL, Whitfield TH, Owen L, Johnston J, Silveri MM et al. Treatment of major depressive disorder with Iyengar yoga and coherent breathing: a randomized controlled dosing study. Journal of Alternative and Complementary Medicine. 2017;23(3):201–7. Available from: http://doi.org/10.1089/acm.2016.0140.

44. Nyer M, Gerbarg PL, Silveri MM, Johnston J, Scott TM, Nauphal M et al. A randomized controlled dosing study of Iyengar yoga and coherent breathing for the treatment of major depressive disorder: impact on suicidal ideation and safety findings. Complementary Therapies in Medicine. 2018;37:136–42. doi: 10.1016/j.ctim.2018.02.006.

45. Sharma VK, Trakroo M, Subramaniam V, Rajajeyakumar M, Bhavanani AB, Sahai A. Effect of fast and slow pranayama on perceived stress and cardiovascular parameters in young health-care students. International Journal of Yoga. 2013;6(2):104–10.

46. Sovik R. Yoga breathing for beginners: to pause or not to pause with Rolf Sovik; 5 April 2013 [video]. Available from: https://youtu.be/KHw62vz7MaM.

47. Sovik R. Learn diaphragmatic breathing for deep relaxation; 18 July 2013 [video]. Available from: https://www.youtube.com/watch?v=Q82YnmL0Kr8.

48. Sovik R. Are you ready for pranayama? Yoga breathing basics to master before you begin; 14 November 2013 [video]. Available from: https://www.youtube.com/watch?v=iTso-FGi-xw.

49. Evans KC, Dougherty DD, Schmid AM, Scannell E, McCallister A, Benson H et al. Modulation of spontaneous breathing via limbic/paralimbic-bulbar circuitry: an event related fMRI study. NeuroImage. 2009;47(3):961–71. Available from: http://doi.org/10.1016/j.neuroimage.2009.05.025.

50. Zelano C, Jiang H, Zhou G, Arora N, Schuele S, Rosenow J et al. Nasal respiration entrains human limbic oscillations and modulates cognitive function. Journal of Neuroscience. 2016;36(49):12448–67. Available from: http://doi.org/10.1523/JNEUROSCI.2586-16.2016.

51. Wilbarger P, Wilbarger J. Sensory defensiveness and related social/emotional and neurological problems. Conference, 13–14 October 1990, Hartford CT.

52. Wilbarger P, Wilbarger J. Follow-up workshop, circa 1997 (see note 51).

Chapter 13

1. Fogel A. Body sense. New York: WW Norton; 2009.

2. van der Kolk BA. Affect regulation. Lecture presented at a Pre-Conference Institute of the 19th Annual International Trauma Conference, Boston, MA, 25 June 2008.

3. Yehuda R, Hoge CW, McFarlane AC, Vermetten E, Lanius RA, Nievergelt CM et al. Post-traumatic stress disorder. Nature Reviews Disease Primers. 2015;1:15057, 1–22. doi: 10.1038/nrdp.2015.57.

4. Levine PA. Waking the tiger; healing trauma. Berkeley: North Atlantic Books; 1997.

5. Odgen P, Minton K, Pain C. Trauma and the body: a sensorimotor approach to psychotherapy. New York: WW Norton; 2006.

6. Veenstra L, Schneider IK, Koole SL. Embodied mood regulation: the impact of body posture on mood recovery, negative thoughts, and

mood-congruent recall. Cognition and Emotion. 2017;31(7):1361–76, DOI: 10.1080/02699931.2016.1225003.

7. Ayres AJ. Sensory integration and learning disorders. Los Angeles: Western Psychological Services; 1972.

8. Nakajima M, Halassa MM. Thalamic control of functional cortical connectivity. Current Opinion in Neurobiology. 2017;44:127–31.

9. Crandall SR, Cruikshank SJ, Connors BW. A corticothalamic switch: controlling the thalamus with dynamic synapses. Neuron. 2015;86:768–82.

10. Kabat-Zinn J. Wherever you go, there you are: mindfulness meditation in everyday life. New York: Hyperion; 1994.

11. Gard T, Noggle JJ, Park CL, Vago DR, Wilson A. Potential self-regulatory mechanisms of yoga for psychological health. Frontiers in Human Neuroscience. 2014;8:770. doi: 10.3389/fnhum.2014.00770.

12. McCall (2007), cited in Gard T, Noggle JJ, Park CL, Vago DR, Wilson A. Potential self-regulatory mechanisms of yoga for psychological health. Frontiers in Human Neuroscience. 2014;8:770. doi: 10.3389/fnhum.2014.00770.

13. Falconer E, Bryant R, Felmingham KL, Kemp AH, Gordon E, Peduto A et al. The neural networks of inhibitory control in posttraumatic stress disorder. Journal of Psychiatry and Neuroscience. 2008;33(5):413–22.

14. Clancy K, Ding M, Bernat E, Schmidt NB, Li W. Restless "rest": intrinsic sensory hyperactivity and disinhibition in post-traumatic stress disorder. Brain. 2017;140(7):2041–50. Available from: https://doi.org/10.1093/brain/awx116.

15. Kerr CE, Sacchet MD, Lazar SW, Moore CI, Jones SR. Mindfulness starts with the body: somatosensory attention and top-down modulation of cortical alpha rhythms in mindfulness meditation. Frontiers in Human Neuroscience. 2013;7:12. Available from: http://doi.org/10.3389/fnhum.2013.00012.

16. Rood MS. Neurophysiological reactions as a basis for physical therapy. Physical Therapy Review. 1954;34:444–9.

17. Koomar JA, Bundy AC. Creating direct intervention from theory. In Bundy AC, Lane SJ, Murray EA (eds), Sensory integration theory and practice. Philadelphia: FA Davis, Philadelphia; 2002, pp. 261–308.

18. Iyengar BKS. B.K.S. Iyengar yoga: the path to holistic health. London: Dorling Kindersley; 2001.

19. Lasater J. Rest and renewal: restful yoga for stressful times. Berkeley, CA: Rodmell Press; 1995.

20. Lasater J. Rest and renewal: restful yoga for stressful times. 2nd ed. Berkeley, CA: Rodmell Press; 2011.

21. Desikachar TKV. The heart of yoga: developing a personal practice. Rochester, VT: Inner Traditionals International; 1999.

22. Grandin T. Calming effects of deep touch pressure in patients with autistic disorder, college students, and animals. Journal of Child and Adolescent Psychopharmacology. 1992;2(1):63–72.

23. Le Page J, Le Page L. Mudras for healing and transformation. Sebastopol, CA: Integrative Yoga Therapy; 2013.

24. Forbes B. Yoga for emotional balance. Boston, MA: Shambhala Publications; 2011.

25. Iyengar BKS. B.K.S. Iyengar yoga: the path to holistic health. Revised ed. London: Dorling Kindersley; 2008.

26. Blanche E, Schaaf R. Proprioception: a cornerstone of sensory integrative intervention. In Roley S, Blanche E, Schaaf R (eds.), Understanding the nature of sensory integration with diverse populations. San Antonio, TX: Psychological Corporation; 2001, pp. 109–31.

27. Pfeiffer B, Kinnealey M. Treatment of sensory defensiveness in adults. Occupational Therapy International. 2003;10:175–84.

28. Mollo K, Schaaf R, Benevides T. The use of Kripalu yoga to decrease sensory overresponsivity: a pilot study. Special Interest Section Quarterly, Sensory Integration. 2008;31(3).

29. Rosthchild B. The body remembers: casebook. Norton Professional Book. New York: WW Norton; 2003.

30. Kraftsow G. Yoga for wellness. New York: Penguin Putnam; 1999.

31. Yee R. Poetry of the body. New York: Thomas Dunne Books, St Martin's Press; 2012.

32. Rood MS. Neurophysiological reactions as a basis for physical therapy. Physical Therapy Review. 1954;34:444–9.

33. Bordoloi K, Deka RS. Scientific reconciliation of the concepts and principles of Rood approach. International Journal of Health Sciences and Research. 2018;8(9):225–34.

34. Harricharan S, Nicholson AA, Densmore M, Théberge J, McKinnon MC, Neufeld RWJ et al. Sensory overload and imbalance: resting-state vestibular connectivity in PTSD and its dissociative subtype. Neuropsychologia. 2017;106:169–78. doi: 10.1016/j.neuropsychologia.2017.09.010.

35. Lenggenhager B, Lopez C. Vestibular contributions to the sense of body, self, and others. In Metzinger T, Windt JM (eds), Open MIND: 23(T). Frankfurt am Main: MIND Group; 2015. doi: 10.15502/9783958570023.

36. Hitier M, Besnard S, Smith PF. Vestibular pathways involved in cognition. Frontiers in Integrative Neuroscience. 2014;8:59. doi:10.3389/fnint.2014.00059.

in underweight female students – a pilot study. Biomedical Research. 2016;27(3):611–15.

86. Samoudi et al. (2012), cited in Archana R, Sailesh KS, Mukkadan JK. Effect of vestibular stimulation on stress and cardiovascular parameters in healthy college students. Biomedical Research. 2016;27(3):985–90.

87. Mody and Maguire (2011), cited in Archana R, Sailesh KS, Mukkadan JK. Effect of vestibular stimulation on stress and cardiovascular parameters in healthy college students. Biomedical Research. 2016;27(3):985–90.

88. Patatas OHG, Ganança CF, Ganança FF. Quality of life of individuals submitted to vestibular rehabilitation. Brazilian Journal of Otorhinolaryngology. 2009;75(3):387–94.

89. Meli A, Zimatore G, Badaracco C, De Angelis E, Tufarelli D. Vestibular rehabilitation and 6-month follow-up using objective and subjective measures. Acta Oto-Laryngologica. 2006;126(3):259–66. DOI: 10.1080/00016480500388885.

90. Cawthorne T, Cooksey FS. Original Cawthorne Cooksey rehabilitation exercises 1946. Proceedings of the Royal Society of Medicine. 1946;39:270 [accessed 18 February 2018]. Available from: http://entkent.com/original-cawthorne-cooksey-rehabilitation-exercises-1946/.

91. Wilbarger P, Wilbarger J. Sensory defensiveness and related social/emotional and neurological problems. Conference, 13–14 October 1990, Hartford CT.

92. Wilbarger P, Wilbarger J. Follow-up workshop to reference 91, circa 1997.

93. Saman Y, Bamiou DE, Gleeson M, Dutia MB. Interactions between stress and vestibular compensation – a review. Frontiers in Neurology. 2012;3(116). doi:10.3389/fneur.2012.00116.

94. Kohl RL (1985), cited in Saman Y, Bamiou DE, Gleeson M, Dutia MB. Interactions between stress and vestibular compensation – a review. Frontiers in Neurology. 2012;3(116):4. doi: 10.3389/fneur.2012.00116.

95. Dagilas A et al. (2005), cited in Saman Y, Bamiou DE, Gleeson M, Dutia MB. Interactions between stress and vestibular compensation – a review. Frontiers in Neurology. 2012;3(116):4. doi: 10.3389/fneur.2012.00116.

96. Gale S, Prsa M, Schurger A, Gay A, Paillard A, Herbelin B, Guyot JP et al. Oscillatory neural responses evoked by natural vestibular stimuli in humans. Journal of Neurophysiology. 2015;115(3):1228–42.

97. Benedek M, Schickel RJ, Jauk E, Fink A, Neubauer AC. Alpha power increases in right parietal cortex reflects focused internal attention. Neuropsychologia. 2014;56(100):393–400.

98. Brown RP, Gerbarg PL. The healing power of the breath: simple techniques to reduce stress and anxiety, enhance concentration, and balance your emotions. Boston, MA: Shambhala Publications; 2012.

99. Ayres AJ (1974), cited in Randomski MV, Latham CAT. Occupational therapy for physical dysfunction. Philadelphia, PA, London: Lippincott Williams and Wilkins; 2007.

100. Huss J (1971), cited in Randomski MV, Latham CAT. Occupational therapy for physical dysfunction. Philadelphia, PA, London: Lippincott Williams and Wilkins; 2007.

101. Randomski MV, Latham CAT. Occupational therapy for physical dysfunction. Philadelphia, PA, London: Lippincott Williams and Wilkins; 2007.

102. Dougherty P, n.d., Chapter 3: Central control of the autonomic nervous system and thermoregulation [accessed 25 March 2019]. Neuroscience Online. Available from: https://nba.uth.tmc.edu/neuroscience/m/s4/chapter03.html.

Chapter 14

1. Lowen A. The betrayal of the body. Alexander Lowen Foundation (www.lowenfoundation.org), 1852 Texas Hill Road, Hinesburg, VT 05461; 1967.

2. Michalak J, Troje NF, Fischer J, Vollmar P, Heidenreich T, Schulte D. Embodiment of sadness and depression—gait patterns associated with dysphoric mood. Psychosomatic Medicine. 2009;71(5):580–7. doi: 10.1097/PSY.0b013e3181a2515c.

3. Nair S, Sagar M, Sollers J III, Consedine N, Broadbent E. Do slumped and upright postures affect stress responses? A randomized trial. Health Psychology. 2015;34(6):632–41.

4. Veenstra L, Schneider IK, Koole SL. Embodied mood regulation: the impact of body posture on mood recovery, negative thoughts, and mood-congruent recall. Cognition and Emotion. 2017;31(7):1361–76. DOI: 10.1080/02699931.2016.1225003.

5. Dychtwald K. Bodymind. New York: Jeremy P. Tarcher/Penguin Group; 1986.

6. Rolf I. Structural integration. Systematics. 1963;1(1):9–10.

7. Fogel A. Body sense. New York: WW Norton; 2009.

8. Roy M, Shohamy D, Wager TD. Ventromedial prefrontal-subcortical systems and the generation of affective meaning. Trends in Cognitive Sciences. 2012;16(3):147–56. Available from: http://doi.org/10.1016/j.tics.2012.01.005.

9. Yang C, Barrós-Loscertales A, Pinazo D et al. State and training effects of mindfulness meditation on brain networks reflect neuronal mechanisms of its antidepressant effect. Neural Plasticity. 2016; Article ID 9504642, 14 pages. Available from: https://doi.org/10.1155/2016/9504642.

10. Wood JV, Perunovic WQE, Lee JW. Positive self-statements: power for some, peril for others. Psychology of Science. 2009;20(7):860–6.

11. Stankovic L. Transforming trauma: a qualitative feasibility study of integrative restoration (iRest) yoga nidra on combat-related post-traumatic stress disorder. International Journal of Yoga Therapy. 2011;21:23–37.

12. Le Page J, Le Page L. Mudras for healing and transformation. Sebastopol, CA: Integrative Yoga Therapy; 2013.

13. Zeidman P, Maguire EA. Anterior hippocampus: the anatomy of perception, imagination and episodic memory. Nature reviews. Neuroscience. 2016;17(3):173–82.

14. Vieselmeyer J, Holguin J, Mezulis A. The role of resilience and gratitude in posttraumatic stress and growth following a campus shooting. Psychological Trauma: Theory, Research, Practice, and Policy. 2017;9(1):62–9.

15. Lies J, Mellor D, Hong RY. Gratitude and personal functioning among earthquake survivors in Indonesia. Journal of Positive Psychology. 2014;9(4):295–305.

16. Chen G. Does gratitude promote recovery from substance misuse? Addiction Research and Theory. 2017;25(2):121–8. DOI: 10.1080/16066359.2016.1212337.

Chapter 15

1. Judith A. Eastern body Western mind: psychology and the chakra system as a path to the self. Revised ed. Berkeley, CA: Celestial Arts; 2004.

2. Cope S. The great work of your life: a guide for the journey to your true calling. New York: Bantam Books; 2012.

3. Novotney A. Yoga as a practice tool. Monitor on Psychology (American Psychological Association). 2009;40(10):38.

4. Emerson D. Trauma-sensitive yoga in therapy: bringing the body into treatment. New York: WW Norton; 2015.

5. Selye H. The stress of life. New York: McGraw-Hill; 1976.

6. Kupriyanov R, Zhdanov R. The eustress concept: problems and outlooks. World Journal of Medical Sciences. 2014;11(2):179–85.

7. Van der Kolk BA. The body keeps the score: brain, mind, and body in the healing of trauma. New York: Viking; 2014.

8. Rothschild B. The body remembers: the psychophysiology of trauma and trauma treatment. New York: WW Norton; 2000.

9. Baum C, Christiansen C, Bass J. Person-environment-occupational performance (PEOP) model. In Christiansen C, Baum C, Bass J. Occupational therapy: performance, participation, well-being. 4th ed. Thorofare, NJ: Slack; 2015.

10. American Occupational Therapy Association (AOTA). Adults with serious mental illness. AOTA: Critically Appraised Topics and Papers Series (CAT); 2018. Available from: https://www.aota.org/~/media/corporate/files/secure/practice/ccl/mental%20health/relaxation_mh_mini-cat.pdf.

Chapter 16

1. Stephens M. Yoga sequencing: designing transformative yoga classes. Berkeley, CA: North Atlantic Books; 2012.

Chapter 17

1. Iyengar BKS. B.K.S. Iyengar yoga: the path to holistic health. London: Dorling Kindersley; 2001.

2. Iyengar BKS. B.K.S. Iyengar yoga: the path to holistic health. Revised ed. London: Dorling Kindersley; 2008.

3. Trombly CA. Occupational therapy for physical dysfunction. 2nd ed. Baltimore: Williams and Wilkins; 1983.

4. Le Page J, Le Page L. Mudras for healing and transformation. Sebastopol, CA: Integrative Yoga Therapy; 2013.

Chapter 18

1. van der Kolk BA. Clinical implications of neuroscience research in PTSD. Annals of the New York Academy of Sciences. 2006;1071:277–93.

INDEX

Page numbers followed by f and t

A

Adolescent/adult sensory profile (AASP)   13
   quadrant scores of 12 combat veterans on   13f
   term definitions   14t
Adrenocorticotropic hormone (ACTH)   23
Africa Healing Exchange's (AHE) restoring resiliency model   89–90
Altered self-referential processing   39
Alternate body breathing technique   148
Alternate nostril breath   148–149
Amygdala   22, 27, 36, 47t. See also Subcortical structures
Annamaya kosha   125
ANS. See Autonomic nervous system
Antares Foundation   89
Anterior cingulate cortex (ACC)   23, 24–25, 49t. See also Cortical structures
Anterior hippocampus   24
Anterior insula   24
Anterior precuneus   25
Anxiety, attention deficit hyperactivity disorder (ADHD)   205
Asana (forms), choices of practice   146–147
   survivors of sexual trauma   75
   yoga in prison, recovery/empowerment through   85
Auditory sensitivity   14
Auditory startle reflex   12
Autonomic nervous system (ANS)   27–31, 29f, 30f, 31f, 143. See also Post-traumatic stress disorder (PTSD)
   Porges' polyvagal theory   30–31, 30f
   window of tolerance   31, 31f
   yoga on   34

B

Behavioral functioning   79
Behavioral signs of COSR   57
Blood oxygenation level dependent (BOLD) signals   35
Body sense   182, 182f, 210
Bonding   92
Bottom-up sensory inhibition   41
Brain
   dysfunction   17
   imaging techniques   35
   structures, in PTSD   20f, 21f

Brain changes in PTSD and mind-body practices
   brain imaging techniques   35
   brain studies for yoga practice   45–47
   functional MRI (fMRI)   35
   magnetoencephalography (MEG)   36
   mindfulness-based findings   37, 37f
   neurocircuitry model
      expansion of   37–38, 38f
      of PTSD   36
   positron emission tomography (PET)   35
   sensory hypothesis of PTSD   41–43, 42f
      inverse relationship   43–45, 44f, 47t–51t
   SPECT   35–36
   therapeutic sensory input   36
   triple network model of PTSD   38–41, 40f
   yoga   43
Brain studies for yoga practice
   cortical findings   46–47
   insula findings   46
   limbic findings   45
   thalamic findings   45–46
Breath
   awareness   147, 210–211
   counting practices   144
   precautions for breathing exercises   150
   Sitkari   150
   Ujjayi   149–150
   Yogic   148
Breath-Body-Mind (BBM)   92–93. See also Mind-body practices in mass disaster/conflict
Breath-moving visualization   92

C

Capacitar International   90–91
Centers for Disease Control and Prevention (CDC)   89
Central executive network (CEN)   26, 39, 143
Central nucleus   22
Childhood sexual abuse (CSA)   70
Chronic traumatization   99
Class structure, choices of
   for survivors of sexual trauma and   75
   yoga in prison, recovery/empowerment through   85
Climate-related disasters   87
Cognitive signs of COSR   57
Cognitive techniques   133

Coherent breathing method   92, 145
Combat and operational stress reaction (COSR)
   about   55
   etiology and continuum of   56–57, 56f
   frontline treatments and combat stress control teams   57–58
   Iraq yoga study   63–66
   moral injury   58–62
   post-combat operational stress   58
   prevalence of   55–56
   signs and coping strategies   57
Combat neurosis   68
Combat soldiers
   and sensory symptoms of PTSD   12
Combat stress control (CSC), mission of   58
Combat stress reaction   55
Combat veterans, pilot study of   13–15, 13f, 14t. See also Post-traumatic stress disorder (PTSD)
Complex trauma survivors   99
   benefits of yoga for survivors   102
   limitations of current treatment approaches   101
   prevalence of complex trauma   100
   psychobiology of   101–102
   qualitative studies   103
   quantitative studies   102
Comprehensive Soldier and Family Fitness (CSF2)   62
Conceptual self-awareness   26
Correctional officer (CO)   84, 85
Cortical structures. See also Post-traumatic stress disorder (PTSD)
   anterior cingulate cortex (ACC)   24–25
   hippocampus   24
   insula   23–24
   posterior cingulate cortex (PCC)   25
   posterior parietal cortex (PPC)   26
   precuneus (PrCC)   25
   prefrontal cortex (PFC)   25–26
   somatosensory cortex   26
Corticotropin-releasing factor (CRF)   33
Cortisol   33
COSR. See Combat and operational stress reaction
Curricula development
   for yoga in prison   85

D

Default mode network (DMN)   25, 31, 39, 143
Department of Defense (DoD)   55

INDEX continued

Depersonalization 10
Derealization 10
Diagnostic and Statistical Manual of Mental Disorders (DSM-5) 9
Diaphragmatic breath 147–148
Disorders of extreme stress not otherwise recognized (DESNOS) 99
Dissociation, defined 10
Dissociative subtype of PTSD 10, 37, 38f, 99
Distress 193
Dorsal anterior cingulate cortex (dACC) 25, 37, 49t
Dorsal posterior insula 24
Dorsal vagal system 31
Dorsolateral prefrontal cortex (dlPFC) 26, 50t
Dorsomedial prefrontal cortex (dmPFC) 26, 50t
Down Dog 262
Down Dog to Plank 262
Downward-Facing Dog 209

E

Electroencephalograph (EEG) study 13, 17
Embodied mindfulness practices.
    See also Yoga in prison, recovery/empowerment
  in criminal justice system 78–79
  for traumatised people 78
Embodied self-awareness 26
Emotional dysregulation 17
Emotional overmodulation 37
Emotional signs of COSR 57
Emotional undermodulation 38
Endocrine (hormonal) system 27
Environment
  on sexual trauma survivors 75
Episodic (autobiographical) memory 24
Eustress 193
Excitatory transmitters 16

F

Fight-flight response 30, 31, 33
Flashbacks 10–11. See also Post-traumatic stress disorder (PTSD)
Frontline treatments and combat stress control teams 57–58
Functional MRI (fMRI) 35

G

Gamma activity 42
Gamma-aminobutyric acid (GABA) 15, 16
Generalized anxiety disorder (GAD) 41
Global Gratitude Alliance (GGA) 90
Glucocorticoids 33
Glutamate 15
Gratitude meditations 188–189
Grounding techniques 133
Guided meditations 187–188

H

Heart rate variability (HRV) 144
Hippocampus 24, 36, 47t. See also Cortical structures
HPA axis. See Hypothalamic-pituitary-adrenal axis
Hyperarousal. See also Post-traumatic stress disorder (PTSD)
  as core symptom of PTSD 11
  sensory elements of 11–13
Hyperaroused/reexperiencing subtype of PTSD 37, 38, 38f
Hypothalamic-pituitary-adrenal (HPA) axis. See also Post-traumatic stress disorder (PTSD)
  about 31–34, 32f, 33f
  of endocrine system 17
  yoga on ANS and HPA axis 34
Hypothalamus 22, 27. See also Subcortical structures
Hysteria 68

I

Ida 140
Impact measurement methods 96
Impaired cognitive function 39
Initial centering script 210–211
Inner resource script 132
Inner resource technique 131–132
Insula 23–24, 48t. See also Cortical structures
Internally displaced persons (IDP) 88
International Association of Yoga 139
Intimate partner violence (IPV) 69
Intrusive thoughts 13

Iraq yoga study. See also Combat and operational stress reaction (COSR)
  avoidance/numbing 65
  correlation hypothesis 65
  discussion and implications 65–66
  hyperarousal 65
  objectives and methods 63–64
  re-experiencing 65
  results 64–65
  study limitations 66

K

Kanishtha mudra 189
Kosha model 114–118
  anandamaya 117–118
  annanamaya 114
  manomaya 114–115
  pranamaya 114
  vijnanamaya 115–117

L

Language
  barriers 95
  on sexual trauma survivors 75
  yoga in prison and 85
Lateral nucleus 22
Limbic system 20
Local agency, supporting 94
Locus ceruleus 21. See also Subcortical structures

M

Magnetoencephalography (MEG) 36, 43
Mass incarceration 77
Master gland 22
Medial prefrontal cortex (mPFC) 24, 25, 36, 39, 50t
Meditations
  gratitude 188–189
  guided 187–188
Mental health issues 87–89
Mental health stigma minimization 95
Mental tension reliever 162
Military personnel and combat stress 56
Mind-body practices in mass disaster/conflict accessibility, ensuring 95–96

INDEX continued

BreathBodyMind (BBM)   92–93
  common mental health issues   87–89
  immediate efficacy, providing   96
  impact measurement methods   96
  language barriers   95
  local agency, supporting   94
  long-term support   96
  mental health stigma minimization   95
  mind-body modalities   89–94
  overview   87
  personal safety maximization   94–95
  privacy and consent, honoring   94
  religious and cultural differences, respecting   95
  solidarity and community, fostering   94
  transferability, facilitating   96
Mindfulness-based cognitive therapy (MBCT)   43
Mindfulness-based findings   37, 37f
Mindfulness-based stress reduction (MBSR)   43, 45, 182
Model of Well-Being   195, 195f
Model of Well-Doing   195, 196f
Model of Well-Being and Well-Doing   196, 197f
Mohawk of self-awareness   39
Moral injury   58–62. *See also* Combat and operational stress reaction (COSR)
  case study   59–62
  defined   58
Mountain, standing forms   231–233
  baby cobra   245, 246f
  cobra   245–246, 246f
  cow face (arm version)   236, 237f
  crocodile   244–245, 245f
  dynamic warrior   238–241, 238f–240f
  extended mountain   234, 234f
  extended side angle   241, 241f
  reverse warrior   241–242, 241f
  side stretch   235, 235f
  standing forward fold   242–243, 242f
  standing twist with strap   235, 236f
  standing wide-legged forward fold with block   242, 242f
  tree   243–244, 244f–245f
Mudras   189
  for healing and transformation   190
  sampling of mudras for self-regulation and trauma healing   191t–192t
Myelinated vagus   30

N

Nadis   139–141, 142
Negative feedback loop   33
Neurocircuitry model   36. *See also* Brain changes in PTSD and mind-body practices
  expansion of   37–38, 38f
Neuroimaging studies of PTSD   47t–51t
Neurological thresholds   14
Neuronal impulse transmission   16f
Neurons   15
Neurotransmitter serotonin (5-HT)   32
Neurovisceral integration model   15
Norepinephrine-containing neurons   21
Nucleus reuniens   23
Numbing   9, 11

O

Open focus meditation   92
Operation Iraqi Freedom (OIF)   59
Orbital medial PFC   25

P

Parasympathetic nervous system (PNS)   22, 27
Parasympathetic–right hemisphere   142
Paraventricular nucleus   22
Pat Ogden's Sensorimotor Psychotherapy programs   194
PCC. *See* Posterior cingulate cortex
Periaqueductal gray (PAG)   21–22, 27. *See also* Subcortical structures
Personal safety maximization   94–95
Peter Levine's Somatosensory Experiencing program   194
Physical signs of COSR   57
Pingala   140
Pituitary   22–23. *See also* Subcortical structures
Polyvagal theory   14
Porges' polyvagal theory   30–31, 30f
Positron emission tomography (PET)   35
Post-combat operational stress (PCOS)   58
Posterior cingulate cortex (PCC)   25, 39, 40f, 51t, 182. *See also* Cortical structures
Posterior parietal cortex (PPC)   26, 39. *See also* Cortical structures
Post-traumatic checklist (PCL)   12
Post-traumatic growth (PTG)   58
Post-traumatic stress (PTS)   13
Post-traumatic stress disorder (PTSD)
  combat veterans, pilot study of   13–15, 13f, 14t
  defined   9
  dissociative subtype of   10
  flashbacks   10–11
  hyperarousal
    core symptom of PTSD   11
    sensory elements of   11–13
  neurocircuitry model of   36–38, 38f
  neurophysiology of
    autonomic nervous system (ANS)   27–31, 29f, 30f, 31f
    cortical structures   23–26
    HPA axis   31–34, 32f, 33f
    limbic structures   21
    normal stress response   27, 27f, 28f
    overview   19–20
    sensory filters of limbic system   20–21, 20f
    Subcortical structures   21–23
    yoga on ANS and HPA axis   34
  sensory hypothesis of   41–43, 42f
    inverse relationship   43–45, 44f, 47t–51t
  and sensory processing   15–17, 15f, 16f
  symptom of   9–10
  triple network model of   38–41, 40f
Post-Traumatic Stress Disorder Symptom Scale (PSS-SR)   13
PPC. *See* Posterior parietal cortex
Pranayama (breathing exercises), choices of   139, 145
  for survivors of sexual trauma   75
  practices for trauma survivors   144–146
Precuneus (PrCC)   25, 39, 51t. *See also* Cortical structures
Prefrontal cortex (PFC)   25–26, 50t. *See also* Cortical structures
Pregenual ACC   25
Primary somatosensory cortex   26
Prison setting, impacts of   84–85
Privacy and consent, honoring   94
PTSD. *See* Post-traumatic stress disorder

INDEX continued

R

Randomized controlled trial (RCT) of yoga   102
Recommended mudras for PTSD   190t
Re-experiencing of event   9, 11
Regional cerebral blood flow (rCBF)   35
Religious/cultural differences, respecting   95
Resilience, defined   62
Respiratory sinus arrhythmia (RSA)   144
Right anterior insula   24, 39
Right ventrolateral prefrontal cortex (RVLPFC)   134
Root shock   88
Root teaching for sexual trauma survivors   75–76
Rostral anterior cingulate cortex (rACC)   24, 25
Rothschild's flashback halting protocol   134

S

Safety   125
  class segregation   127
  concept of   125
  healing space   126
  inner resource technique   131
  promotion in bodymind   128–129
  sensory precautions   129–131
  triggering flashbacks   132–133
Safety maximization   94–95
Salience network (SN)   39
Savasana
  sample script   214
  short grounding   215
  with 41 points   216
Schore's description of the medial prefrontal cortex   142
Secondary somatosensory cortex   26
Self-awareness and systemic oppression   85
Self-chosen positive affirmations   186
Self-regulation strategies   14
Sensorimotor processes   40
Sensory avoidance   13, 14
Sensory awareness techniques   133
Sensory-enhanced yoga method   146, 183
Sensory-enhanced yoga program   113, 186
Sensory-enhanced yoga vinyasas   259–263
Sensory-enhanced moon salute   259–262
  benefits of sensory-enhanced moon salute   262–263
Sensory homeostasis   16
Sensory hypothesis of PTSD   41–43, 42f
  inverse relationship   43–45, 44f, 47t–51t
Sensory input, therapeutic   36
Sensory modulation   13
Sensory processing. See also Post-traumatic stress disorder (PTSD)
  and PTSD   15–17, 15f, 16f
Sensory processing disorder (SPD)   13
Sensory sensitivity
  definition   14t
  examples of   14
Sensory-enhanced yoga   113–124
  definition   118
  guiding principles   122–124
  kosha model   114–118
  path to self-awareness and integration   113–114
  purpose   118–119
Serotonin   32
Sexual trauma, definition   67–68
Sexual violence, impact of   67
Shushumna   140
Single-photon emission computerized tomography (SPECT)   35–36
Sitkari Breath   150
Social connection   71
Social engagement system   30
Solidarity and community, fostering   94
Somatosensory cortex   26. See also Cortical structures
SPECT. See Single-photon emission computerized tomography
Stimulus discrimination   13
Subcortical structures. See also Post-traumatic stress disorder (PTSD)
  amygdala   22
  hypothalamus   22
  locus ceruleus   21
  periaqueductal gray (PAG)   21–22
  pituitary   22–23
  thalamus   23
Subgenual anterior cingulate cortex   25
Sun Salutation   262
Sympathetic nervous system (SNS)   22, 27
Sympathetic system   30

T

Tension/relaxation exercise   212–213
Thalamus   23, 27, 36, 48t. See also Subcortical structures
The Heart of Yoga   146
Therapeutic sensory input   36
Therapeutic yoga forms
  cat/cow   224–225, 224f
  child   231, 231f
  down dog to up dog flow   230–231, 230f
  downward-facing dog   229–230, 229f
  dynamic sidelying twist   222–223, 222f–223f
  knees to chest   218f, 219
  leg stretches with yoga strap   219–221f, 219f–221f
  modified dynamic vajrasana   227–228, 227f–228f
  modified hare to knee-down up dog   228–229, 228f–229f
  supine half-moon stretch   218, 218f
  supine symmetrical stretch   217, 217f
  supine twist   221, 221f
  thread the needle   226f, 227
  tiger flow to spinal balance   225–226, 225f–226f
  yoga forms from table   223–224, 223f
Top-down executive inhibition   41
Total Force Fitness (TFF)   62
Transdisciplinary model for post-traumatic growth   66, 113, 120, 121f, 195
Transferability, facilitating   96
Trauma Center's yoga program   102
Trauma Informed Mind Body program (TIMBo)   71–74
Trauma-Informed Yoga (TIY)   84
Trauma-Sensitive Yoga (TSY)   69, 70, 102
Triple network model of PTSD   38–41, 40f

U

Ujjayi Breath   149–150
Ultradian rhythm   141
Unmyelinated vagus   30

V

Ventromedial prefrontal cortex (VMPFC)   32, 50t, 182

W

Wellness Survey for Post-Traumatic Growth   198–199, 199t–200t
Window of tolerance   31, 31f
Working memory   26

INDEX continued

Y

Yoga
  on ANS/HPA axis   34
  in mind-body practices   43
  sense of safety for healing   125
Yoga forms using a chair
  dynamic cat to cobra   257–258, 257f
  dynamic knee to chest to extended leg   249, 250f
  head to knee in chair   258, 258f
  leg stretches in chair   250, 251f
  seated cat/cow   251–252, 252f
  seated half-moon stretch   248–249, 250f
  seated mountain   247, 248f
  seated thread the needle   252–253, 254f
  seated warrior   253–256, 253f–256f
  setting sun   252, 253f
  sun breath twists   250–251, 252f
  two-stage forward fold   256–257, 257f

Yoga in prison, recovery/empowerment
  asana, class structure, and language, choices in   85
  case study   80–83
  critical theories and methods in research   85
  curricula development   85
  embodied mindfulness practices in criminal justice system   78–79
  for traumatised people   78
  overview   77–78
  prison setting, impacts of   84–85
  self-awareness and systemic oppression   85
  trauma-informed yoga training   84
Yoga practice, brain studies for
  cortical findings   46–47
  insula findings   46
  limbic findings   45
  thalamic findings   45–46
Yoga session
  body sensing   210
  listening to the body and mind   210
  noticing sensation with body at rest   213
  positioning   210
  sample script for savasana   214
  sensing surroundings   210
  short grounding savasana   215
  tension/relaxation exercise (body sensing)   212–213
Yoga therapy session   206
Yoga with survivors of sexual trauma
  case study   71–74
  choices of asana, pranayama   75
  diverse cultural perspectives and experiences   75
  language and environment   75
  overview   67–68
  review of literature   68–71
  root teaching   75–76
Yogic breath   148